Contents

Illustration Credits

Hockenberry, M.J. (2009). *Wong's essentials of pediatric nursing.* (8th ed.). St. Louis: Mosby: Figure 31-1

Lewis, S.M., et al. (2007). *Medical-surgical nursing: assessment and management of clinical problems.* (7th ed.). St. Louis: Mosby: Figure 22-1

Novak, J.C. & Broom, B.L. (1995). *Ingalls & Salerno's maternal and child health nursing.* (8th ed.). St. Louis: Mosby: Figure 26-1

Potter, P.A. & Castaldo, P. (2003). *Study guide to accompany Potter: Basic nursing.* (5th ed.) St. Louis: Mosby: Figure 4-2

Potter, P.A. & Perry, A.G. (2009). *Fundamentals of nursing: concepts, process, and practice.* (7th ed.). St. Louis: Mosby: Figure 23-1

Thompson, J.M., et al. (1997). *Mosby's clinical nursing.* (4th ed.). St. Louis: Mosby: Figure 31-2

The Evolution of Nursing

chapter

1

Answer Key: Textbook page references are provided as a guide for answering these questions. A complete answer key was provided for your instructor.

HISTORY OF NURSING

Objectives

- Describe the evolution of nursing and nursing education from early civilization to the 20th century.
- Identify the major leaders in the history of the development of nursing in America.

1. Nursing evolves along with changes in: *(1)* _____

_____

_____

2. In early civilization, care of the sick was primarily provided by: *(2)* _____

_____

_____

3. There is evidence that medical treatment existed in ancient Egypt; this treatment included: *(2)*

_____

_____

4. Medicine progressed from the initial belief that illness was caused by: *(2)*_____

_____

_____

5. Discuss the monastic factors that influenced the practice of nursing. *(2-3)*_____

_____

_____

6. What factors influenced the evolution of nursing from occupation to profession? *(4)* _____

   _____

   _____

7. Identify the six ways in which the "Nightingale nurses" improved patient care and advanced the practice of nursing. *(4)*

   _____

   _____

8. Describe the effect that World War I and World War II had on nursing. *(5-6)*_____

   _____

   _____

9. Identify the major events in America in the 19th century that led to the development of the current nursing education programs. *(4)*

   _____

   _____

10. List the four major concepts that are the basis for nursing theories and models. *(17-18)* _____

    _____

    _____

Multiple Choice

11. Hippocrates is credited with development of: *(2)*
    1. a public system of health care.
    2. a public system of safety.
    3. a holistic approach to patient care.
    4. early guidelines for health care.

12. Phoebe, one of the first deaconesses, was known for providing: *(2)*
    1. the first free hospital in Rome.
    2. care to the poor and sick in their homes.
    3. care for prisoners.
    4. care for those who were mentally ill.

13. Florence Nightingale applied the principles of nursing she learned in Germany to care of soldiers during the: *(3)*
    1. Civil War.
    2. Spanish-American War.
    3. Great Plague.
    4. Crimean War.

14. Which of the following individuals is credited with the establishment and development of the Red Cross? *(5)*
    1. Dorothea Dix
    2. Florence Nightingale
    3. Clara Barton
    4. Lavinia Dock

15. Which of the following individuals crusaded for elevation of the standards of care for the mentally ill? *(5)*
    1. Dorothea Dix
    2. Mary Ann Ball
    3. Clara Barton
    4. Florence Nightingale

16. The American Society of Superintendents of Training Schools became a committee of the: *(5)*
    1. Association of Practical Nurse Schools.
    2. National Federation of Licensed Practical Nurses.
    3. National League for Nursing Education.
    4. American Nurses Association.

17. Orem's theory of nursing could be described as: *(17-18)*
    1. nursing care that becomes necessary when a patient is unable to fulfill biological, psychological, developmental, or social needs.
    2. a patient's environment is arranged to facilitate the body's reparative processes.
    3. caring is the central and unifying domain for nursing knowledge and practice.
    4. patients must adapt to circumstances based on physiologic, psychological, sociologic, and dependence-independence adaptive models.

NURSING ORGANIZATIONS

Objectives

- Identify the major organizations in nursing.
- Define the four purposes of NAPNES and NFLPN.

18. Identify the role of the NLN in nursing education. *(9)* _____

   _____

   _____

19. List the purposes of NAPNES and NFLPN. *(9)* _____

   _____

   _____

PRACTICAL NURSING

Objectives

- List the major developments of practical and vocational nursing.
- Define practical and vocational nursing.
- Describe the purpose, role, and responsibilities of the practical or vocational nurse.

20. Identify the major development or event that occurred in the given year and give a brief description of the change that it brought about in practical and vocational nursing. *(8)*

   a. 1892 _____

   b. 1917 _____

   c. 1941 _____

   d. 1949 _____

   e. 1957 _____

   f. 1996 _____

21. The definition that is adapted from NAPNES defines practical and vocational nursing as: *(9)*

_____

_____

22. Discuss the role and responsibilities of the practical or vocational nurse in today's health care system. *(18)*

_____

_____

23. Discuss the benefits of a professional appearance. *(6)* _____

_____

_____

Multiple Choice

24. The duties and responsibilities of the LPN/LVN are determined by the: *(9)*
    1. National League of Nursing.
    2. American Nurses Association.
    3. Vocational Nursing Program.
    4. State Board of Nursing.

25. The content areas for the NCLEX-PN® are determined by the: *(9)*
    1. National League of Nursing.
    2. Council of State Boards of Nursing.
    3. American Nurses Association.
    4. Vocational Nursing Program.

26. Because of demographic changes in the population, increased need for nursing care is necessary in the care of: *(7)*
    1. newborns.
    2. adolescents.
    3. adults.
    4. the elderly.

27. Significant women's health care issues that have most recently guided nursing care include: *(7)*
    1. immunizations, such as the human papillomavirus (HPV) vaccine.
    2. the need for mammography.
    3. the importance of routine pap smears.
    4. the importance of prenatal care

28. Recognizing patients as individuals and making sure that they receive quality care is ensured by nurses providing care according to: *(7)*
    1. nurse practice acts.
    2. Patient's Bill of Rights.
    3. state boards of nursing guidelines.
    4. American Nurses Association recommendations.

29. Nurses are involved in disaster preparedness plans in which of the following ways? (Select all that apply) *(7)*
    1. Triaging of casualties
    2. Vaccination research
    3. Functioning as attendant nurses
    4. Crisis response team members

HEALTH CARE DELIVERY

Objectives

- Identify the components of the health care system.
- Identify the participants in the health care system.
- Describe the complex factors involved in the delivery of patient care.

30. Identify the participants in the health care delivery system and their roles and responsibilities. *(13)*

    _____

    _____

31. Identify three economic factors that influence contemporary health care delivery. *(13)* _____

    _____

    _____

32. Provide a brief description of the following. *(14)*

    a. Malpractice insurance: _____

    _____

    b. Cross-training: _____

    _____

    c. Case management:_____

    _____

33. What is the purpose of the Patient's Bill of Rights? *(15)*_____

    _____

    _____

34. Briefly describe the concepts of health promotion and illness prevention. *(12)* _____

    _____

    _____

Multiple Choice

35. Utilizing Maslow's Hierarchy of Needs, the nurse gives priority to which of the following problems of the patient? *(12)*
    1. Loneliness
    2. Inability to eat
    3. Anxiety
    4. Safety

36. Utilizing Maslow's hierarchy of needs, which of the following needs is basic and should be addressed first? *(12)*
    1. Safety and security
    2. Self-actualization
    3. Physiologic
    4. Love and belonging

37. Social factors that affect health and illness are: *(12)*
    1. smoking and stress.
    2. health care insurance and advanced technology.
    3. excessive body weight and alcoholism.
    4. lifestyle and personal financial hardship.

Legal and Ethical Aspects of Nursing

Answer Key: Textbook page references are provided as a guide for answering these questions. A complete answer key was provided for your instructor.

LEGAL PROCESS

Objective

- Summarize the structure and function of the legal system.

1. The two basic categories of law are: *(23)*_____

_____

_____

2. What is the difference between statutory and common law? *(23)*_____

_____

_____

3. Identify the steps in the legal process for civil litigation. *(23)* _____

_____

_____

4. Why would an appeal be filed in a lawsuit? *(23)*_____

_____

_____

5. What does it mean to be *liable* for an action? *(24)* _____

_____

_____

Multiple Choice

6. The function of criminal law is to: *(23)*
   1. make the aggrieved person whole.
   2. restore the person to where he or she was.
   3. punish and prevent further crime.
   4. establish fault.

7. The function of civil law is to: *(23)*
   1. establish fault.
   2. make the aggrieved person whole.
   3. punish and prevent further crime.
   4. prevent an appeal.

8. The individual who files the complaint in a civil litigation is referred to as the: *(23)*
   1. defendant.
   2. respondent.
   3. plaintiff.
   4. prosecutor.

9. In a criminal case, the conduct or issue in question is considered to be a crime against: *(23)*
   1. the court.
   2. the respondent.
   3. the plaintiff.
   4. society.

LEGAL RELATIONSHIPS

Objective

- Discuss the legal relationship existing between the nurse and the patient.

10. Discuss the concept of accountability and the legal relationship. *(24)* _____

_____

_____

11. Discuss areas in which the nursing staff failed to follow standards of care in the case *Darling v. Charleston Community Memorial Hospital.* *(24)*

_____

_____

Multiple Choice

12. It can be said that a nurse safeguards the nurse-patient relationship when he or she acts: *(24)*
    1. as a clinical nurse specialist with years of experience.
    2. as an experienced nurse in a specialty area.
    3. as other nurses with similar education and experience and in similar situations.
    4. in accordance with the law.

13. The nurse administers the wrong dose of a medication to a patient, and the patient experiences adverse effects as a result of this action. The nurse is considered: (Select all that apply) *(24)*
    1. liable.
    2. accountable.
    3. criminal.
    4. deliberate.

REGULATION OF PRACTICE

Objectives

- Explain the importance of maintaining standards of care.
- Give examples of ways the nursing profession is regulated.

14. What are the purposes of the standards of care? *(24)* _____

_____

_____

15. Evidence that nursing standards are being or have been maintained includes: *(24)* _____

_____

_____

16. How is nursing practice regulated by nurse practice acts and professional organizations? *(25)* _____

_____

_____

17. Explain the interstate compact. *(25)* _____

_____

_____

Multiple Choice

18. Select the action(s) that would be considered a breach in the standards of nursing care. (Select all that apply) *(25)*
    1. Failure to take an accurate and thorough patient history
    2. Failure to notify physician of patient lab values in a timely fashion
    3. Failure to protect patient and prevent patient falls
    4. Failure to introduce self to patient and family members
    5. Failure to give appropriate discharge instructions to the patient

LEGAL ISSUES

Objectives

- Explain nursing malpractice.
- Give examples of ways the licensed practical or vocational nurse can avoid being involved in a lawsuit.
- Give examples of legal issues in health care.
- Discuss federal HIPAA (Health Insurance Portability and Accountability Act of 1996) regulations and the act's impact on the health care system.

19. Briefly define the following elements needed to establish malpractice. *(26)*

    a. Duty: _____

    _____

    b. Breach of duty: _____

    _____

    c. Harm: _____

    _____

    d. Proximate cause: _____

    _____

20. Identify general ways that nurses can avoid involvement in lawsuits. *(29)* _____

    _____

    _____

21. Describe the nurse's role and responsibilities in relation to the following. *(27)*

    a. Confidentiality: _____

    _____

    b. Invasion of privacy:_____

          _____

    c. Reporting of abuse: _____

          _____

    d. Informed consent: _____

          _____

22. Discuss the nurse's primary duties in relation to HIPAA (Health Insurance Portability and Accountability Act of 1996). *(26)*

    _____

    _____

23. Discuss the nurse's responsibilities when obtaining an informed consent from a patient before a procedure. *(27)*

    _____

    _____

Multiple Choice

24. The nurse who uses unnecessary restraints on a patient may be charged with: *(24)*
    1. assault.
    2. battery.
    3. slander.
    4. defamation.

25. When providing first aid in an emergency situation outside a medical facility, it is important for the nurse to have knowledge of the: *(29)*
    1. Nurse Practice Act.
    2. Patient's Bill of Rights.
    3. Good Samaritan Act.
    4. Standards of care.

26. There are staffing issues throughout the medical center, and one of the nurses is "floated" to another unit where this nurse does not want to go. The nurse decides, after receiving the assignment, to leave the unit and go home. The nurse may be found liable specifically for: *(30)*
    1. fraud.
    2. malpractice.
    3. defamation.
    4. abandonment.

27. Select the nursing action that would be considered a breach of patient confidentiality. (Select all that apply) *(27)*
    1. The nurse answers questions asked by the bearer of the patient's health care power of attorney regarding the patient's condition.
    2. The nurse informs the patient's only living relative of the patient's scheduled procedure.
    3. The nurse, who is familiar with the patient's wife, answers her questions over the phone regarding the patient's lab results that have been pending.
    4. Upon being asked to do so by the patient, the nurse waits to explain a scheduled procedure until the patient's husband is present.

ETHICAL PRINCIPLES

Objectives

- Summarize how culture affects an individual's beliefs, morals, and values.
- Identify how values affect decision making.

28. The field of ethics involves the study of: *(31)* _____

   _____

   _____

29. Identify and briefly describe the five fundamental ethical principles. *(32)* _____

   _____

   _____

30. Discuss how values and beliefs are developed and how they affect behavior and decision making. *(31)*

   _____

   _____

31. Gaining insight into your own personal values is a process known as: *(31)* _____

32. List four ways the nurse can meet the needs of the patient while respecting the patient's cultural beliefs and practices. *(31)*

   _____

   _____

ETHICAL PRACTICE

Objectives

- Explain the meaning of a code of ethics.
- Differentiate between a legal duty and an ethical duty.
- Distinguish between ethical and unethical behavior.
- Explain the nurse's role in reporting unethical behavior.

33. A code of ethics serves to: *(32)* _____

_____

_____

34. Indicate whether each of the following involves a legal or an ethical duty. *(31)*

   a. The nurse failed to perform in a reasonable and prudent manner. _____

   _____

   _____

   b. The nurse failed to give the medication to the patient before he was discharged. _____

   _____

   _____

   c. The nurse assigned to care for an AIDS patient requested to change patients with another nurse on the unit.

   _____

   _____

35. Describe the difference between ethical and unethical behavior. *(32)* _____

_____

_____

36. List the priority nursing actions to be implemented in reporting unethical behavior. *(32)*_____

_____

_____

ETHICAL ISSUES

Objective

- Give examples of ethical issues common in health care.

37. Discuss the following ethical issues in health care. *(33)*

    a. Right to refuse treatment: _____

       _____

       _____

    b. "Do not resuscitate" orders: _____

       _____

       _____

    c. Refusal to treat: _____

       _____

       _____

Communication

Answer Key: Textbook page references are provided as a guide for answering these questions. A complete answer key was provided for your instructor.

GOAL OF COMMUNICATION

Objective

- Recognize that communication is inherent in every nurse-patient interaction.

1. What is the goal of communication between the nurse and the patient? *(40)*_____

   _____

   _____

2. Describe the term "two-way communication," and identify when it would be used in a nurse-patient relationship. *(37)*

   _____

   _____

Multiple Choice

3. When giving report during shift change, the night nurse should be aware that a patient may hear the information being exchanged. The patient hearing the information would be referred to as the: *(36)*
   1. receiver.
   2. sender.
   3. unintended receiver.
   4. communicator.

4. In a nurse-patient relationship, when the nurse is communicating with the patient, the type of communication that is least effective is referred to as: *(37)*
   1. two-way communication.
   2. one-way communication.
   3. nonverbal communication.
   4. open-ended communication.

TYPES OF COMMUNICATION

Objectives

- Discuss the concepts of verbal and nonverbal communication.
- Discuss the impact of nonverbal communication.
- Recognize assertive communication as the most appropriate communication style.

5. Identify the types of verbal and nonverbal communication. *(37-38)* _____

_____

_____

6. Explain why consistency between verbal and nonverbal communication is important. *(37)*_____

_____

_____

7. Compare the characteristics of the following styles of communication. *(39)*

Assertive	Aggressive	Unassertive

Multiple Choice

8. An example of nonverbal communication is: *(37-38)*
   1. moaning.
   2. crying.
   3. grimacing.
   4. writing.

9. An example of verbal communication is: *(37-38)*
   1. writing.
   2. grimacing.
   3. smiling.
   4. frowning.

10. Nonverbal communication involves the use of cues. Which of the following is an example of a nonverbal cue? *(38)*
    1. Symbols
    2. Written words
    3. Reading
    4. Physical appearance

11. In the English language, the denotative meaning of the term "hospital" refers to: *(37)*
    1. a facility that generally provides long-term care to patients.
    2. a facility that provides health care treatment to a patient by trained staff.
    3. an organization that depends on volunteers to provide services.
    4. an organization that provides care in the patient's familiar surroundings, such as the patient's home.

12. Choose the term(s) that best describe(s) nonverbal cues. (Select all that apply) *(38)*
    1. Jargon
    2. Tone of voice
    3. Touch
    4. Reading
    5. Rate of voice

THERAPEUTIC COMMUNICATION

Objectives

- Use various therapeutic communication techniques.
- Recognize trust as the foundation for all effective interaction.

13. Discuss tips for building rapport with the patient. *(40)* _____

    _____

    _____

14. Provide examples of the following therapeutic communication techniques. *(43-44)*

    a. Closed questioning: _____

       _____

    b. Stating observations: _____

       _____

    c. Offering information: _____

       _____

    d. Use of humor: _____

       _____

e. Touch: _____

_____

f. Silence:_____

_____

15. When using the communication technique of _____, the nurse acknowledges listening to the patient by nodding or using eye contact. *(43-44)*

Multiple Choice

16. The following is an example of which therapeutic technique? The patient states, "I am worried and don't know what to expect after my biopsy." The nurse replies, "Are you feeling anxious about the results of your biopsy?" *(43-44)*
    1. Reflection
    2. Clarification
    3. Restatement
    4. Paraphrasing

17. An example of activity involving the personal zone is when the nurse: *(46)*
    1. bathes the patient.
    2. sits in a chair and speaks with the patient.
    3. speaks to a small group of expectant parents.
    4. gives a lecture to a large auditorium filled with newly hired staff members.

18. The nurse is aware that providing an opportunity for receiving feedback from the patient is a way of maintaining therapeutic communication. This is an example of which of the following therapeutic communication techniques? *(42)*
    1. Active listening
    2. Therapeutic silence
    3. Minimal exchange
    4. Conveying acceptance

19. The patient will be discharged from the hospital tomorrow. During the discharge teaching, the patient states, "I don't know how I will be able to care for myself after I leave the hospital." The nurse responds, "You don't know how you will take care of yourself when you leave the hospital?" This is an example of which technique? *(43)*
    1. Restating
    2. Reflection
    3. Paraphrasing
    4. Summarizing

20. In completing the patient's history, the nurse asks the patient, "What type of surgeries have you had in the past?" This is an example of which of the following therapeutic communication techniques? *(43-44)*
    1. Clarifying
    2. Paraphrasing
    3. Restating
    4. Open-ended questioning

FACTORS THAT AFFECT COMMUNICATION

Objectives

- Identify various factors that can affect communication.
- Discuss potential barriers to communication.

21. Identify the factors that may affect communication, and provide an example of each. *(46)*_____

_____

_____

22. For each of the following blocks to communication, provide an example of a response that should be avoided by the nurse. *(51)*

    a. Giving advice: _____

    _____

    b. Defensiveness: _____

    _____

    c. Value judgment:_____

    _____

Multiple Choice

23. When communicating with an older adult, the nurse is aware that it is important to: *(48)*
    1. speak loudly.
    2. allow time for processing information.
    3. provide a dark, quiet environment.
    4. avoid hearing the patient's stories.

24. When communicating with a patient of an unfamiliar culture, the nurse knows that: (Select all that apply) *(47-48)*
    1. formal names are preferred in most cultures.
    2. there may be differences in the interpretation of social versus clock time.
    3. the practice and meaning of touch varies among cultures.
    4. the meaning that eye contact conveys may differ among cultures.

COMMUNICATION IN SPECIAL SITUATIONS

Objectives

- Apply the nursing process to patients with impaired verbal communication.
- Apply therapeutic communication techniques to patients with special communication needs.

25. Identify at least five nursing interventions for a patient with impaired communication. *(52)*_____

_____

_____

26. A 58-year-old man was admitted to the medical-surgical unit with a diagnosis of left-sided CVA (stroke). During the admission process, the nurse observed that the patient's speech was unclear and his words were slurred. The nurse also observed that when the patient was asked a question that could be answered with a "yes" or "no" response, he could answer the question by moving his head to imply "yes" or "no." Apply the nursing process to the given situation. *(52)*

    a.   Identify problems observed by the nurse during the admission process. _____

        _____

    b.   Write a nursing diagnosis based on the identified problems._____

        _____

    c.   Write a realistic goal for the nursing diagnosis. _____

        _____

    d.   Identify at least two nursing actions that can be implemented._____

        _____

    e.   Write a statement that reflects the evaluation of the outcome._____

        _____

Multiple Choice

27. The patient tells the nurse, "I'm supposed to check my blood sugar at least three times each day, but I can't always find the test sticks and they're very expensive." The nurse uses which specific therapeutic technique of clarification when responding: *(43)*
    1. "When did you last check your blood sugar?"
    2. "I'll speak with the physician about your situation."
    3. "I see that you know how important it is to check your blood sugar."
    4. "Let me make sure I understand what your concern is with the blood sugar testing."

28. When communicating with a patient who has expressive aphasia, the nurse is aware that it is important to: *(52)*
    1. ask open-ended questions.
    2. ask questions that can be answered with a "yes" or "no."
    3. refer to the family members for information.
    4. allow a short time for the patient to respond.

Vital Signs

Answer Key: Textbook page references are provided as a guide for answering these questions. A complete answer key was provided for your instructor.

PURPOSE AND GUIDELINES

Objectives

- Discuss the importance of accurately assessing vital signs.
- Discuss methods by which the nurse can ensure accurate measurement of vital signs.
- Identify the guidelines for vital signs measurement.
- Discuss frequency of vital signs measurement.
- State the normal limits of each vital sign.
- List the factors that affect vital signs readings.
- Identify the rationale for each step of the vital sign procedures.

1. Accurate assessment of vital signs provides the nurse with: *(56)* _____

   _____

   _____

2. A myocardial contraction that occurs at a regular rhythm but at a rate greater than 100 beats per minute is known as _____. *(70)*

3. The second blood pressure reading that is a result of the decreased pressure in the arteries when the ventricles are resting is known as _____. *(78)*

4. For the following vital signs, identify factors that may influence them and how they are affected.

   a. Temperature: *(62)*_____

      _____

   b. Pulse: *(70)* _____

      _____

   c. Respirations: *(76)* _____

      _____

   d. Blood pressure: *(79)*_____

      _____

5. What are the general guidelines for taking vital signs? *(59)* _____

    _____

    _____

Multiple Choice

6. The nurse is aware that in an acute care facility, the patient's vital signs are measured a minimum of: *(59)*
    1. every 2 hours.
    2. every 4 hours.
    3. every 8 hours.
    4. every 12 hours.

7. The purpose of baseline vital signs includes: (Select all that apply) *(59)*
    1. comparison with vital signs obtained later.
    2. an indication of the patient's normal range of vital signs.
    3. identification of a change in vital signs.
    4. an indication of the patient's past medical history.

TEMPERATURE

Objective

- Accurately assess oral, rectal, axillary, and tympanic temperatures.

8. The _____ site is considered the *least* accurate site for temperature measurement. *(69)*

9. Identify the sites for temperature measurement and the expected temperature reading for each. *(69)*

    _____

    _____

10. Convert the following temperature readings. *(61)*
    a. 37° C   =   _____ ° F
    b. 101.2° F   =   _____ ° C
    c. 39.2° C   =   _____ ° F
    d. 97.8° F   =   _____ ° C

11. Identify signs and symptoms associated with an elevated temperature. *(62)* _____

    _____

    _____

12. What should the nurse do if the patient's temperature is above normal? *(62)* _____

    _____

    _____

Multiple Choice

13. A patient's temperature is 93.2° F. This temperature is referred to as: *(62)*
    1. fever.
    2. hyperthermia.
    3. hypothermia.
    4. pyrexia.

14. Normal body cells are at risk for damage when the temperature exceeds: *(62)*
    1. 100.4° F (38° C).
    2. 104.0° F (40° C).
    3. 105.0° F (40.5° C).
    4. 110.0° F (43.3° C).

15. Normal body temperature can change throughout the day. It is important for the nurse to know that the lowest body temperature can occur between the hours of: *(61)*
    1. 4 PM and 6 PM.
    2. 3 PM and 6 PM.
    3. 2 AM and 9 AM.
    4. 1 AM and 4 AM.

16. It is important for a nurse to know that normal body temperature can range from: *(61)*
    1. 96° F to 98.2° F (35.6° C to 36.8° C).
    2. 98.2° F to 99° F (36.8° C to 37.2° C).
    3. 97° F to 99.6° F (36.1° C to 37.5° C).
    4. 96.2° F to 100.2° F (35.7° C to 37.9° C).

17. When obtaining a rectal temperature from an adult, the nurse inserts the electronic thermometer probe into the rectum approximately: *(66)*
    1. ½ inch.
    2. 1½ inches.
    3. 2 inches.
    4. 3 inches.

PULSE

Objectives

- List the various sites for pulse measurement.
- Accurately assess an apical pulse, a radial pulse, and a pulse deficit.

18. Identify the anatomical site for apical pulse measurement. *(75)* _____

19. On the figure, identify the names and sites for assessment of peripheral pulses. *(74)*

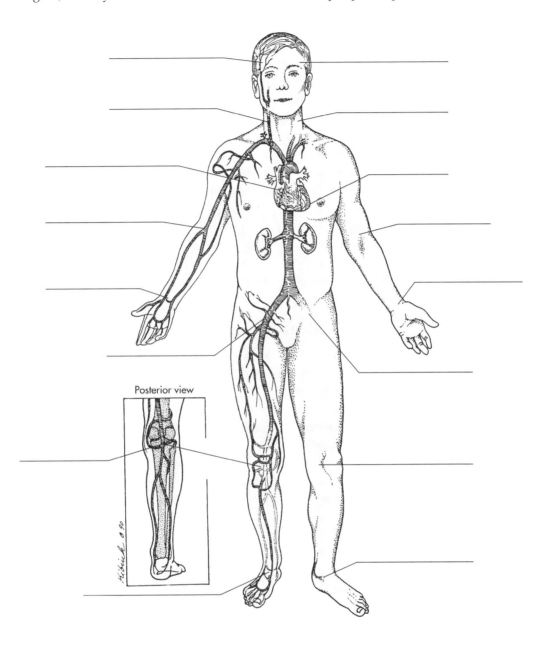

Posterior view

20. Identify nursing actions to implement if the patient's pulse is not within normal limits. *(74)* _____

_____

_____

21. Describe the nursing actions and rationale for apical and radial pulse measurement. *(75)* _____

_____

_____

Multiple Choice

22. Pulse deficit is described as the difference between the radial and: *(73)*
    1. femoral pulse rates.
    2. brachial pulse rates.
    3. apical pulse rates.
    4. carotid pulse rates.

23. The patient's pulse is difficult to assess and disappears with slight pressure. The pulse strength is described as: *(71)*
    1. absent.
    2. weak.
    3. thready.
    4. abnormal.

24. The patient's pulse is easily palpable but disappears when moderate pressure is applied. The pulse strength is described as: *(71)*
    1. thready.
    2. weak.
    3. normal.
    4. abnormal.

25. When assessing the apical pulse, the nurse counts the pulse rate for: *(75)*
    1. 20 seconds and multiplies by 3.
    2. 60 seconds and does not multiply.
    3. 30 seconds and multiplies by 2.
    4. 15 seconds and multiplies by 4.

26. The nurse determines that further teaching is required when the student is observed: (Select all that apply) *(71)*
    1. palpating the carotid pulses bilaterally.
    2. assessing the apical pulse for a full minute.
    3. measuring the popliteal artery at the dorsum of the foot.
    4. using the pads of the index and middle fingers to obtain a radial pulse.

27. The average adult heart rate is: *(70)*
    1. 40 to 80 beats per minute.
    2. 60 to 100 beats per minute.
    3. 80 to 120 beats per minute.
    4. 100 to 140 beats per minute.

RESPIRATION

Objective

- Describe the procedure for determining the respiratory rate.

28. In determining the respiratory rate, the nurse counts for _____ seconds. *(78)*

29. A rapid respiratory rate is described as _____. *(76)*

30. The respiratory rate may be increased by: *(76)*_____

_____

_____

31. Describe the nursing actions and the rationale for measurement of respirations. *(78)* _____

_____

_____

32. What should the nurse do if the patient's respirations are rapid and labored? *(77)* _____

_____

_____

Multiple Choice

33. Respiratory rate is controlled by the: *(76)*
    1. cerebellum.
    2. spinal cord.
    3. medulla oblongata.
    4. cerebrum.

34. The nurse is aware that a patient's respiratory rate may be increased by: *(76)*
    1. narcotics.
    2. acute pain.
    3. hypothermia.
    4. brainstem injury.

35. The best time for the nurse to count respirations is: *(77)*
    1. immediately after the patient wakes up.
    2. following any strenuous activity.
    3. before and after each meal, and before administering medications to the patient.
    4. immediately following measurement of the radial pulse while the fingers are still in place over the artery.

BLOOD PRESSURE

Objectives

- Accurately assess the blood pressure.
- Describe the benefits of and precautions to follow for self-measurement of blood pressure.

36. When obtaining the patient's blood pressure, the cuff is deflated at a rate of
    _____. *(83)*

37. The pulsating sounds that are heard when assessing the patient's blood pressure are known as
    _____ sounds. *(80)*

38. When should the blood pressure be assessed in the lower extremities? *(82, 84)* _____

_____

_____

39. Describe the nursing actions and the rationale for measurement of blood pressure. *(82-83)* _____

_____

_____

40. What nursing actions should be implemented if the patient's blood pressure is below normal? *(79-80)*

_____

_____

41. Identify on the aneroid gauge where the Korotkoff sounds were heard for a blood pressure of 136/78 mm Hg. *(81)*

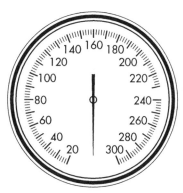

Multiple Choice

42. A high blood pressure reading may result if the blood pressure cuff is: *(82)*
    1. too large.
    2. too small.
    3. placed low on the arm.
    4. placed high on the arm.

HEIGHT AND WEIGHT

Objective

- Accurately assess the height and weight measurements.

43. To obtain an accurate weight measurement, the nurse should: *(87)*_____

_____

_____

44. Describe the nursing actions and rationale for measurement of height and weight. *(87)* _____

_____

_____

45. It is important for the nurse to know how to convert a weight in pounds to the equivalent in kilograms. *(87)*
    a. A patient who weighs 44 lbs weighs _____ kg.
    b. A patient who weighs 210 lbs weighs _____ kg.

46. Fluid balance may be assessed by weighing the patient. If the patient weighs 1 kg less today than yesterday, how much fluid was lost? *(87)*

_____

_____

DOCUMENTATION AND REPORTING

Objectives

- Accurately record and report vital signs measurements.
- State the normal limits of each vital sign.

47. Identify the expected vital signs for the following age groups. *(60)*

	Pulse	**Respirations**	**Blood Pressure**
a. Neonate			
b. Toddler			
c. Adolescent			
d. Adult			

48. In most health care facilities, vital signs are documented on a _____. *(61, 63)*

49. What vital signs measurements should be reported immediately? *(59)* _____

_____

_____

Multiple Choice

50. The nurse receives the end-of-shift report from another staff member. Based on the following assessment information for the adult patients on the unit, it is a priority for the nurse to visit which patient first? *(60)*
    1. BP–120/80, P–68, R–16
    2. BP–110/74, P–72, R–14
    3. BP–130/90, P–80, R–18
    4. BP–120/90, P–62, R–10

51. The nurse documents a pulse that feels full and springlike, even with pressure, as: *(71)*
    1. 1+.
    2. 2+.
    3. 3+.
    4. 4+.

Physical Assessment

Answer Key: Textbook page references are provided as a guide for answering these questions. A complete answer key was provided for your instructor.

DISEASE AND DIAGNOSIS

Objectives

- Discuss the difference between a sign and a symptom.
- Compare and contrast the origins of disease.
- List the four major risk categories for development of disease.
- Discuss frequently noted signs and symptoms of disease conditions.
- List the cardinal signs of inflammation and infection.

1. Identify the difference between a sign and a symptom. *(93-94)* _____

_____

_____

2. Identify whether each of the following is a sign or a symptom. *(93-94)*

    a. Headache: _____

    b. Nausea: _____

    c. Anxiety: _____

    d. Vomiting: _____

    e. Drainage: _____

3. Identify at least five possible etiologies of disease. *(93)* _____

_____

_____

4. The four major risk categories for the development of disease are: *(95)* _____

_____

_____

5. The cardinal signs of infection and inflammation are: *(95)* _____

_____

_____

6. _____ is a sign comprising an abnormal "swishing" sound heard over an artery. *(110)*

Multiple Choice

7. The nurse recognizes that an example of a hereditary disease is: *(95)*
   1. mitral valve prolapse.
   2. tuberculosis.
   3. cystic fibrosis.
   4. congestive heart failure.

8. Congenital diseases: *(94)*
   1. appear at birth.
   2. are transmitted from parent to child.
   3. have unknown etiology.
   4. are a result of infection.

9. Deficiency diseases are a result of: *(94)*
   1. lack of nutrients.
   2. abnormal growth of tissue.
   3. exposure to microorganisms.
   4. harmful substances.

10. The risk factor that can lead to the development of coronary artery disease is: *(95)*
    1. osteoporosis.
    2. cancer.
    3. trauma.
    4. diabetes.

11. A lifestyle risk that can lead to the development of lung disease is: *(95)*
    1. air pollution.
    2. asbestos.
    3. smoking.
    4. malnutrition.

12. While obtaining the vital signs, the nurse observed that the patient was sweating profusely. The term used to describe this sign is: *(96)*
    1. diaphoresis.
    2. cyanosis.
    3. ecchymosis.
    4. pruritus.

13. When assessing the patient's skin color, the nurse noted that the skin and the mucous membranes had a bluish discoloration. The term used to describe this sign is: *(96)*
    1. jaundice.
    2. pallor.
    3. cyanosis.
    4. ecchymosis.

14. While transferring the patient from the stretcher to the bed, the nurse observed that the patient was experiencing difficulty breathing. The term used to describe this sign is: *(96)*
    1. orthopnea.
    2. dyspnea.
    3. tachypnea.
    4. asthenia.

15. The patient's oral temperature is 101.2° F. The term used to describe this sign is: *(96)*
    1. edema.
    2. fever.
    3. pruritus.
    4. jaundice.

16. The patient informed the nurse that she was not hungry and had been experiencing loss of appetite for several days. The term used to describe this symptom is: *(96)*
    1. lethargy.
    2. dyspnea.
    3. anorexia.
    4. erythema.

17. When assessing the older adult, the nurse is aware that slumping, irritability, or sighing can indicate that the patient is exhibiting signs related to the symptom of: *(106)*
    1. dyspnea.
    2. fatigue.
    3. orthopnea.
    4. erythema.

18. Choose the data that are considered objective data. (Select all that apply) *(93)*
    1. Pulse
    2. Nausea
    3. Pain
    4. Fear
    5. Cyanosis

19. Choose the data that are considered subjective data. (Select all that apply) *(93-94)*
    1. Blood pressure
    2. Edema
    3. Pain
    4. Erythema
    5. Pruritus

MEDICAL EXAMINATION

Objectives

- Describe the nursing responsibilities when assisting a physician with the physical examination.
- List equipment and supplies necessary for the physical examination and assessment.

20. When assisting the physician with the physical examination, the nurse is responsible for: *(97)* _____

    _____

    _____

21. For the following parts of the examination, identify the position(s) of the patient. *(99)*

    a.   Head and neck: _____

    b.   Thorax:_____

    c.   Abdomen: _____

    d.   Female genitalia: _____

    e.   Musculoskeletal system:_____

22. Identify the equipment needed to assess or examine the following. *(98)*

    a.   Vital signs:_____

    b.   Lung sounds: _____

    c.   Reflexes:_____

23. Discuss the nursing responsibilities related to the psychological preparation of the patient for a physical examination. *(97)*

    _____

    _____

NURSING ASSESSMENT

Objectives

- Explain the necessary skills for the physical examination and nursing assessment.
- Discuss the nurse-patient interview.
- List the essentials to obtaining a patient's health history.
- Discuss the sequence of steps when performing a nursing assessment.
- Explain ways to develop cultural sensitivity.

24. Provide examples of questions that may be asked by the nurse to obtain information during a review of systems. *(103)*

    a.   Respiratory: _____

    _____

    b.   Endocrine:_____

    _____

c. Gastrointestinal: _____

_____

25. When preparing to check the patient's pupillary reflexes, the nurse must first _____. *(109)*

26. Identify the skills used in the physical examination and nursing assessment and the purpose of each one. *(106-107)*

_____

_____

_____

_____

27. Identify two elements that can enhance the nurse-patient interview. *(101)*_____

_____

_____

28. The objectives of obtaining the nursing health history are: *(101-102)* _____

_____

_____

29. List the essential information obtained in a health history that will assist the nurse in developing the patient's plan of care. *(102-106)*

_____

_____

30. Identify ways that the nurse may develop cultural sensitivity in relation to the physical examination. *(104)*

_____

_____

31. What does each letter or word represent in the mnemonic device for assessing patients? *(108)*

a. A: _____

b. B: _____

c. C: _____

d. In: _____

e. Out: _____

f. P:_____

g. S:_____

32. Identify areas included in a cardiovascular assessment. *(113-115)* _____

_____

_____

Multiple Choice

33. The nurse uses the OPQRST method for obtaining the most information about the patient's present health concerns. The P in the OPQRST method refers to the: *(102)*
    1. quality of the concern.
    2. cause of the concern.
    3. severity of the concern.
    4. beginning of the concern.

34. The most frequently used skill in the physical nursing assessment is: *(107-108)*
    1. inspection.
    2. palpation.
    3. percussion.
    4. auscultation.

ASSESSMENT FINDINGS

Objective

- Discuss normal assessment findings in the head-to-toe assessment.

35. Identify whether the following findings are expected or unexpected. *(107-118)*

    a. Decreased skin turgor: _____

    b. Fruity breath: _____

    c. Pupils round and reactive to light: _____

    d. Barrel chest:_____

    f. Two-second capillary refill: _____

    g. Adventitious breath sounds: _____

    h. No abdominal sounds: _____

    i. Bilateral, palpable pedal pulses: _____

DOCUMENTATION

Objective

- Describe documentation of the physical examination and nursing assessment.

36. How are physical assessment results usually documented? *(117-118)* _____

_____

_____

37. What is important for the nurse to do when documenting findings? *(117-118)* _____

_____

_____

Multiple Choice

38. The nurse documents that the patient has crackles. This is determined by the nurse as a result of auscultating: *(111-112)*
    1. short, discrete, bubbling sounds on inspiration.
    2. high-pitched musical sounds on inspiration.
    3. grating sounds on expiration.
    4. coarse gurgling on expiration.

Nursing Process and Critical Thinking

Answer Key: Textbook page references are provided as a guide for answering these questions. A complete answer key was provided for your instructor.

PHASES OF THE NURSING PROCESS

Objectives

- Explain the use of each of the six phases of the nursing process.
- List the elements of each of the six phases of the nursing process.

1. The six phases of the nursing process are: *(122)*_____

_____

_____

2. "Readiness for enhanced nutrition" is an example of a _____ nursing diagnosis. *(126)*

Multiple Choice

3. The nursing process: *(121)*
   1. provides the patient with quality care.
   2. focuses on a specific patient-related problem.
   3. provides a framework for the practice of nursing.
   4. ensures positive outcomes.

4. The patient's information and data are collected during the: *(122)*
   1. assessment phase.
   2. planning phase.
   3. implementation phase.
   4. evaluation phase.

5. During which phase of the nursing process does the nurse identify the health problems? *(123-124)*
   1. Assessment
   2. Diagnosis
   3. Planning
   4. Implementation

6. The nurse sets priorities for nursing intervention in the: *(128)*
   1. assessment phase.
   2. diagnosis phase.
   3. planning phase.
   4. implementation phase.

7. The nurse instructs the patient on the use of her inhaler. During which phase of the nursing process does this take place? *(131)*
   1. Diagnosis
   2. Planning
   3. Implementation
   4. Evaluation

ASSESSMENT

Objective

- Describe the establishing of the database.

8. What sources are used to obtain information for the patient database? *(122-123)* _____

   _____

   _____

9. Explain the difference between objective and subjective data. *(122)* _____

   _____

   _____

Multiple Choice

10. After collecting and validating the data, the nurse organizes and clusters the data. Data clustering refers to: *(123)*
    1. the evaluation of the patient data.
    2. focusing on the patient's problems.
    3. the grouping of related cues.
    4. the analysis of related outcomes.

11. It is best to perform a focused assessment when a patient is: (Select all that apply) *(122)*
    1. admitted to a long-term care facility.
    2. critically ill.
    3. disoriented.
    4. unable to respond to the nurse.

12. During a patient assessment, biographical data would include: *(123)*
    1. the patient's medications taken at home.
    2. the reason for the patient's admission to the facility.
    3. age, obtained weight, and place of employment.
    4. a history of any medical conditions.

DIAGNOSIS

Objectives

- Discuss the steps used to formulate a nursing diagnosis.
- Differentiate among types of health problems.

13. Identify the four components of a nursing diagnosis. *(124-126)* _____

_____

_____

14. Write a possible nursing diagnosis based upon the following situations. *(126)*

   a. A 52-year-old patient is admitted after episodes of severe vomiting. _____

   _____

   _____

   b. A 75-year-old patient with right hemiparesis arrives seeking care following a cerebral vascular accident (stroke).

   _____

   _____

15. What are the four types of nursing diagnosis statements? *(126)* _____

_____

_____

Multiple Choice

16. The nursing diagnosis is defined as: *(124)*
    1. the identification of a disease or condition that involves problems with structures.
    2. problems that nurses cannot prescribe a treatment for.
    3. a clinical judgment about individual, group, or community responses to actual or potential health problems.
    4. problems that are identified as a result of the planning phase.

17. At the completion of the nursing assessment phase, the nursing diagnosis statement is formulated and a possible diagnosis statement may be written by the nurse. The possible or "risk diagnosis" statement is written when the: *(126)*
    1. actual factors are present in a circumstance.
    2. factors are predicted to occur in a circumstance.
    3. medical aspects of a circumstance are unsafe.
    4. cues obtained from the patient indicate no problems exist.

18. Based on the definition of a collaborative problem, which of the following problems would be an example of one? *(126)*
    1. Pain
    2. Anxiety
    3. Coping
    4. Edema

OUTCOMES IDENTIFICATION, PLANNING, AND IMPLEMENTATION

Objectives

- Describe the development of patient-centered outcomes.
- Discuss the creation of nursing orders.

19. Identify Maslow's hierarchy of needs beginning with the ones that are given highest priority in patient care situations. *(128)*

    _____

    _____

20. Patient-centered outcomes should be statements that are: *(127-128)* _____

    _____

    _____

21. Write possible patient-centered outcomes using the following terms. *(127-128)*

    a. Describe: _____

       _____

    b. Verbalize:_____

       _____

    c. List:_____

       _____

    d. Demonstrate: _____

       _____

22. What is included in a nursing order? *(129-130)* _____

    _____

    _____

23. Write an example of a nursing order. *(129-130)* _____

_____

_____

24. Provide examples of possible nursing actions that may be implemented for a patient with a nursing diagnosis of "Risk for impaired skin integrity, due to loss of mobility on right side." *(129-130)*

_____

_____

Multiple Choice

25. A nursing order is created to provide: *(129-130)*
    1. specific written instructions for all caregivers.
    2. a general statement that conveys information.
    3. a statement providing general information for nursing interventions.
    4. information for the formulation of a care plan.

26. Which of the following are nursing interventions? (Select all that apply) *(129)*
    1. Monitoring the patient for problems or complications
    2. Performing an activity for a patient
    3. Teaching the patient or family about health maintenance
    4. Advising a patient on the type of medication necessary for the patient's condition

EVALUATION

Objective

- Explain the evaluation of a nursing care plan.

27. Describe the steps in the evaluation of the nursing care plan. *(131-132)* _____

_____

_____

28. What are the possible evaluation outcomes? *(131-132)*_____

_____

_____

CARE PLANS AND CLINICAL PATHWAYS

Objectives

- Demonstrate the nursing process by writing a nursing care plan.
- Describe the use of clinical pathways in managed care.

29. Identify the purpose and advantages of clinical pathways. *(133)* _____

_____

_____

30. Write a nursing care plan for the following patient situation. *(133)*

Ms. M., 48 years of age, is admitted to the medical-surgical unit after an abdominal hysterectomy. Her vital signs are stable. The IV in her left forearm is patent, without swelling or tenderness. The dressings are dry and intact. Ms. M. has a Foley catheter in place that is draining clear, yellow urine. Ms. M. was just transferred from the surgical recovery unit. Ms. M. is expressing severe pain.

_____

_____

_____

_____

_____

_____

GROUPS

Objective

- Explain the activities of NANDA, NIC, and NOC.

31. Describe the general activities of NANDA, NIC, and NOC. *(124-125)* _____

_____

_____

32. Identify at least two benefits of using the standardized language of NANDA, NIC, and NOC. *(124-125)*

_____

_____

CRITICAL THINKING

Objective

- Discuss critical thinking.

33. Provide specific examples of how critical thinking is applied in clinical nursing situations. *(134-135)*

_____

_____

34. Describe the term "evidence-based practice." *(131)* _____

_____

_____

Documentation

chapter

7

Answer Key: Textbook page references are provided as a guide for answering these questions. A complete answer key was provided for your instructor.

PURPOSES

Objectives

- List the five purposes for written patient records.
- Explain the relationship of the nursing care plan to care documentation and patient care reimbursement.

1. The person who is appointed to examine patients' charts and health records to assess quality of care is known as _____. *(139-140)*

2. The _____ is a system used to consolidate patient orders and care needs in a centralized, concise way. *(145)*

3. The five basic purposes of written patient records are: *(138-139)* _____

   _____

   _____

4. Explain how home health care documentation relates to reimbursement. *(151)* _____

   _____

   _____

Multiple Choice

5. A system that is used by Medicare for reimbursement of patient care services is: *(139)*
   1. focused medical factor–related grouping.
   2. diagnosis-related group.
   3. quality assurance or improvement.
   4. problem-oriented diagnosis-related group.

6. The most accurate definition of *the patient's chart* is: *(138)*
   1. a system used to consolidate patient orders and care needs in a centralized, concise way.
   2. a legal record used to meet the many demands of the health system.
   3. written information contained in the patient records.
   4. subjective and objective assessment, plan, evaluation; in this more compact form, the care given or action taken is included in the plan notations.

METHODS AND FORMS

Objectives

- Describe the differences between traditional and problem-oriented medical records.
- Describe the purpose of and the relationship between the Kardex and the nursing care plan.
- Describe the differences in documenting care using activities of daily living and physical assessment forms, and narrative, SOAPE, and focus formats.
- Discuss issues related to computerization in documentation.
- Discuss documentation and clinical pathways.

7. Explain the major differences between a traditional patient record and a problem-oriented (POMR) record. *(142-143)*

_____

_____

8. a. What is the purpose of an incident report? *(145)* _____

_____

_____

b. Is the incident report included in the patient's record? *(148)* _____

_____

_____

9. Describe the relationship between the Kardex and the patient chart. *(145)*_____

_____

_____

10. What are the advantages and disadvantages of computer documentation? *(152-153)* _____

_____

_____

11. Identify the primary benefit of documenting with clinical pathways. *(149, 151)* _____

_____

_____

Multiple Choice

12. Focus charting contains: *(144)*
    1. nursing action and patient response.
    2. a description of the patient's present condition.
    3. objective and subjective assessment data.
    4. nursing diagnosis, action, and patient's response.

13. Charting by exception: *(145)*
    1. provides comprehensive nurse's notes.
    2. provides a more organized flow in the nurse's notes.
    3. decreases the time needed to complete the nurse's notes.
    4. summarizes the information in the nurse's notes.

14. What type of charting format usually requires the most time to complete? *(142)*
    1. SOAP
    2. Focus
    3. PIE
    4. Narrative

15. What type of charting format most reflects the nursing process? *(144)*
    1. Narrative
    2. Traditional
    3. Focus
    4. PIE

16. What documentation is included in the "P" when using the PIE method of charting? *(145)*
    1. Patient response
    2. Problem list
    3. Assessment
    4. Plan

17. The POMR is divided into which four major sections? *(142)*
    1. History and physical examination, physician's orders, nurse's notes, and progress notes
    2. Database, problem list, plan, and progress notes
    3. Subjective data, objective data, diagnostic tests, and progress notes
    4. Physician's orders, nurse's notes, lab reports, and progress notes

18. The problem-oriented medical record: *(142)*
    1. uses a patient problem list as index for chart documenting.
    2. uses a narrative format for documenting in the nurse's notes.
    3. uses care plans for documenting in the nurse's notes.
    4. emphasizes the use of specific forms for charting.

19. The charting format most commonly used for documentation of clinical pathways is: *(149, 151)*
    1. focus charting.
    2. traditional charting.
    3. charting by exception.
    4. narrative charting.

GUIDELINES

Objectives

- Describe the basic guidelines for and mechanics of charting.
- State important legal aspects of chart ownership, access, confidentiality, and patient care documentation.

20. The essential elements of documentation are: *(138)* _____

_____

_____

21. What are the basic guidelines for charting? *(140-141)*_____

_____

_____

22. Confidentiality of the patient's medical record is guaranteed by: *(152)*_____

_____

_____

23. Identify the important legal aspects for the following. *(152)*

    a.   Record ownership:_____

_____

    b.   Access: _____

_____

    c.   Confidentiality: _____

_____

24. Military time is used in most hospitals to document the time care is given. Convert the following civilian times to military time. *(151)*
    a.   3:00 PM   =   _____
    b.   7:30 PM   =   _____
    c.   6:00 PM   =   _____
    d.   Midnight =   _____

Multiple Choice

25. When an error is made by the nurse in charting: *(140)*
    1. it is reported to the charge nurse, and the nurse continues with the charting.
    2. Wite-out (correction fluid) is used to correct the error, and the nurse continues with the charting.
    3. the charting is started over on a new sheet.
    4. a line is drawn through the error and initialed, and then the nurse continues with the charting.

26. Confidentiality is most often maintained with use of computer charting through the: *(155)*
    1. assignment of individual passwords.
    2. legal signature of the nurse.
    3. use of patient code names.
    4. use of assigned individual patient unit numbers.

27. The patient can gain access to his or her records or chart: *(152)*
    1. in all states.
    2. immediately upon request of the information.
    3. through a formal written request.
    4. by following established procedures of the facility or institution.

28. Inadequate documentation that is commonly involved in cases of malpractice include: (Select all that apply) *(140-141)*
    1. documenting incorrect data.
    2. charting nursing actions in advance.
    3. charting incorrect times at which events occurred.
    4. failing to record verbal orders or failing to have them signed.

HEALTH CARE SITES

Objectives

- Discuss long-term health care documentation.
- Discuss home health care documentation.

29. In relation to documentation, the Omnibus Budget Reconciliation Act (OBRA) of 1987 requires: *(152)*

_____

_____

30. Briefly identify how long-term care and home health care documentation are different from acute care (hospital) documentation. *(151-152)*

_____

_____

Cultural and Ethnic Considerations

Answer Key: Textbook page references are provided as a guide for answering these questions. A complete answer key was provided for your instructor.

CULTURE AND ETHNICITY

Objective

- Describe ways that culture affects the individual.

1. The term that describes learned beliefs, customs, and practices shared by a group and passed to another generation is _____. *(158)*

2. A group of people who share common social and cultural heritage based on traditions and national origin is referred to as _____. *(161)*

Multiple Choice

3. The nurse anticipates that the older adult patient will be: *(160)*
   1. more tolerant of other cultures.
   2. moving away from traditions and rituals.
   3. farther removed from their religious beliefs and practices.
   4. resistant to attempts to change trusted home remedies and practices.

4. A group that shares primary characteristics with another but has some different behaviors and ideas describes a(n): *(158)*
   1. ethnic group.
   2. dominant group.
   3. subculture.
   4. race.

CULTURALLY RELATED ASSESSMENTS

Objectives

- Explain how personal cultural beliefs and practices can affect nurse-patient and nurse-nurse relationships.
- Identify and discuss cultural variables that may influence health behaviors.

5. Describe how the following cultural variables influence health behaviors. *(159-160)*

   a. Family structure and roles:_____

   _____

   b. Religious beliefs: _____

   _____

   c. Health-practice traditions: _____

   _____

6. Compare and contrast two different cultural groups in relation to the following. *(163-164)*

   a. Time orientation: _____

   _____

   b. Dietary preferences:_____

   _____

   c. Birth rites: _____

   _____

Multiple Choice

7. Which of the following statements reveals the influence of culture on health beliefs? (Select all that apply) *(170-171)*
   1. Western cultures have traditionally used the biomedical method of treating illness.
   2. All cultures value traditional medicine.
   3. The response to health and illness varies among different cultures.
   4. Based on cultural data, the nurse makes certain assumptions about the patient.

8. Which of the following religious groups believes that blood transfusions violate God's laws? *(165-169)*
   1. Quakers
   2. Mennonites
   3. Jehovah's Witnesses
   4. Roman Catholics

9. The nurse caring for a diverse group of patients anticipates that special intervention at the time of death will be provided for the patient who is: *(165-169)*
   1. Eastern Orthodox.
   2. Pentecostal.
   3. a Disciple of God.
   4. Seventh Day Adventist.

NURSING PROCESS

Objectives

- Identify the importance of transcultural nursing.
- Explain how the nurse can use cultural data to help develop therapeutic relationships with the patient.
- Discuss the use of the nursing process when caring for culturally diverse patients.

10. How does the nurse integrate transcultural nursing into practice? *(159-160)*_____

_____

_____

11. List considerations related to cultural differences that nurses need to be aware of when caring for an older adult. *(160)*

_____

_____

12. Identify nursing interventions that may be used to communicate with a non–English-speaking patient. *(162)*

_____

_____

13. In order to assist the patient to meet his or her needs, the nurse wants to complete an accurate assessment. How should the nurse ask the patient about the following? *(162-163)*

a. Language: _____

_____

b. Illness: _____

_____

c. Family structure: _____

_____

d. Dietary practices: _____

_____

e. Use of folk medicine:_____

_____

14. Write a nursing diagnosis that can be modified to reflect the problems of a culturally diverse patient. *(171-172)*

Multiple Choice

15. Transcultural nursing is: *(159-160)*
    1. nursing care that is given to a group of patients who share specific beliefs.
    2. nursing care based on a specific group's behavior and needs.
    3. the implementation of culturally appropriate nursing care.
    4. the implementation of generalized standards of care to meet needs of all patients.

16. When communicating with a patient who has a limited grasp of English, the nurse should: *(162-163)*
    1. speak loudly.
    2. keep questions brief and simple.
    3. use sign language and get an interpreter.
    4. provide detailed directions.

17. In assisting a female patient who is Muslim American, the nurse anticipates her cultural needs during a physical examination by: *(168)*
    1. covering body parts as much as possible.
    2. examining her in the presence of her husband.
    3. maintaining close eye contact throughout the examination.
    4. requesting that a male physician perform the entire examination.

18. In reviewing the dietary needs of a group of patients, the nurse notices that there is a shared restriction for patients who are of the Pentecostal, Church of the Nazarene, and Mormon faiths. This dietary restriction includes: *(168-169)*
    1. mixing of dairy and meat products.
    2. ingestion of pork and corn-based flour products.
    3. use of alcohol and tobacco.
    4. ingestion of caffeinated beverages.

19. When communicating with a patient, the nurse knows that eye contact may have to be avoided with which cultures? (Select all that apply) *(175)*
    1. Italian American
    2. elderly Native American
    3. Hispanic
    4. Middle Eastern

Life Span Development

Answer Key: Textbook page references are provided as a guide for answering these questions. A complete answer key was provided for your instructor.

FAMILY

Objectives

- Differentiate among the types of family patterns and their functions in society.
- Describe different types of stresses that commonly affect today's families.

1. Conception (fertilization) can be described as the union between _____ and _____.
   (181)

2. Families are composed of two or more people who are united by _____. *(182-183)*

3. List the four family patterns and describe how each one functions. *(183-184)* _____

   _____

   _____

4. Identify factors that have contributed to the changes that families of today have undergone and are still undergoing. *(183)*

   _____

   _____

5. Discuss the qualities of functional families. *(184)* _____

   _____

   _____

6. Three common causes of family stress are: *(186-187)* _____

   _____

   _____

Multiple Choice

7. The nuclear family is: *(183)*
   1. biological parents, offspring, and grandparents.
   2. biological parents, offspring, grandparents, aunts, and uncles.
   3. biological parents and their offspring.
   4. traditional family and some additional family members.

8. A social contract family consists of: *(184)*
   1. remarried adults and children.
   2. same-sex couple with foster or adoptive children.
   3. the family unit with adopted children.
   4. an unmarried couple living together and sharing roles and responsibilities.

9. The nurse is assessing how the patient's family functions. The nurse determines that the family is primarily autocratic based upon the observation of the: *(184)*
   1. mother assuming primary dominance in decision making.
   2. parents implementing strict rules and expectations.
   3. uncle controlling the finances.
   4. children participating in negotiations.

10. The disengagement phase of parenthood can be best described as: *(186)*
    1. beginning at the birth or adoption of the first child.
    2. extending from the wedding up until the birth of the first child.
    3. the period of family life when the grown children depart from the home.
    4. the last stage of the life cycle, which requires the individual to cope with a large range of changes.

GROWTH AND DEVELOPMENT

Objectives

- Describe the physical characteristics at each stage of the life cycle.
- List the psychosocial changes at the different stages of development.
- Discuss Erikson's stages of psychosocial development.
- Describe Piaget's four stages of cognitive development.

INFANCY, TODDLERHOOD, PRESCHOOL AGE, SCHOOL AGE

Objective

- Describe the cognitive changes occurring in the early childhood period.

11. _____ is a function or gradual process of change from simple to complex. *(188-189)*

12. Children may be affected by stress. Identify at least five common signs of stress in children. *(186)*

_____

_____

13. Identify the major physical and psychosocial changes that occur from infancy through school age. *(189-198)*

	Physical Changes	**Psychosocial Changes**
a. Infant		
b. Toddler		
c. Preschooler		

Multiple Choice

14. Height increases approximately _____ a month for the first 6 months of life. *(189)*
    1. ½ inch
    2. 1 inch
    3. 2 inches
    4. 3 inches

15. By the time an infant is 1 year of age, the child will have: *(189)*
    1. doubled his or her birth weight.
    2. gained 1 lb per month.
    3. tripled his or her birth weight.
    4. gained 3 lbs per month.

16. Weight gain after 8 months is attributed to gains in: *(189)*
    1. fat and muscle.
    2. fat and bone.
    3. fat and increased fluid volume.
    4. muscle and bone.

17. Obvious growth in the long bones and increase in height of approximately 2 inches per year for both boys and girls are physical characteristics of: *(198)*
    1. preschoolers.
    2. toddlers.
    3. school-age children.
    4. adolescents.

18. By the age of 2½ years, the toddler has: *(189)*
    1. complete primary dentition, 20 teeth.
    2. approximately 16 teeth.
    3. approximately 12 teeth.
    4. approximately 30 teeth.

19. The infant uses the senses to learn about self and environment in the: *(190)*
    1. formal operational stage.
    2. preoperational stage.
    3. sensorimotor stage.
    4. concrete operational stage.

20. The toddler gradually begins to "de-center" (becomes less egocentric and understands other points of view) in the: *(194)*
    1. formal operational stage.
    2. preoperational stage.
    3. sensorimotor stage.
    4. concrete operational stage.

21. The school-age child is able to think about abstractions and hypothetical concepts and is able to move in thought "from the real to the possible" in the: *(200)*
    1. formal operational stage.
    2. preoperational stage.
    3. sensorimotor stage.
    4. concrete operational stage.

22. The preoperational thought stage of early childhood extends from: *(194)*
    1. 1 to 3 years of age.
    2. 2 to 7 years of age.
    3. 5 to 9 years of age.
    4. 9 to 12 years of age.

23. The parent tries to hand the child over to a caregiver at the day care center, but the child reacts by crying and clinging. The nurse anticipates this behavior will begin in children at the age of: *(190)*
    1. 3 months.
    2. 8 months.
    3. 1 year.
    4. 2 years.

24. The nurse is teaching the parents of an infant what the principles are for introduction of foods. The nurse provides accurate information when informing the parents that: (Select all that apply) *(191)*
    1. citrus fruits may be given before the infant is 6 months of age.
    2. foods should be mixed together for improved taste.
    3. cereals should be started before vegetables and meats.
    4. it is best to introduce only one new food at a time, allowing several days between new foods.

ADOLESCENCE

Objective

- Discuss the developmental tasks of the adolescent period.

25. Identify at least five developmental tasks of the adolescent. *(204)* _____

_____

_____

Multiple Choice

26. The second major period of rapid physical growth is observed in the: *(201)*
    1. school-age child.
    2. adolescent.
    3. young adult.
    4. middle adult.

27. The most critical indicator of severe depression is: *(204)*
    1. a change in appetite.
    2. an inability to concentrate.
    3. a preoccupation with death.
    4. a verbalization of thoughts of harming oneself.

28. The nurse is working with a group of parents of high school students. During the discussion, the following statements are made by the parents. Based on an understanding of the needs of adolescents, which statement requires follow-up by the nurse? *(202)*
    1. "We try to set reasonable limits on dating."
    2. "The car has to be back home by 9:00 PM on school nights."
    3. "We think that there should be as much experimentation and freedom as possible."
    4. "The number of after-school activities are tremendous, so we discuss how many things are realistic."

YOUNG AND MIDDLE ADULTHOOD

Objectives

- List the developmental tasks for early adulthood.
- Describe the developmental tasks for middle adulthood.

29. Provide examples of the developmental tasks for the early and the middle adult. *(204, 206)* _____

_____

_____

30. A leading cause of death for the young adult is _____. *(206)*

Multiple Choice

31. Generativity can best be defined as: *(208)*
    1. the ability to relate one's deepest hopes and concerns to another person.
    2. the task of reorganization, reevaluation, and acceptance.
    3. accepting responsibility for and offering guidance to the next generation and adapting to physical and role changes.
    4. a time of satisfaction and pleasure.

32. Developmental tasks of early adulthood include: (Select all that apply) *(204)*
    1. development of career and job satisfaction.
    2. acceptance of self and others.
    3. maximizing personal worth and identity.
    4. making decisions regarding careers, marriage, and children.

LATE ADULTHOOD

Objectives

- Define aging.
- Discuss theories of aging.
- Describe the normal age-related changes affecting the major body systems.
- Discuss the effect of the aging process on personality, intelligence, learning, and memory.

33. A form of discrimination and prejudice against older adults is referred to as _____. *(209)*

34. Define the aging theory of biological programming: *(210)*_____

_____

_____

35. Describe the physical changes that occur in each of the following systems as a result of the aging process. *(212-213)*

    a. Sensory: _____

    _____

    b. Integumentary:_____

    _____

   c. Cardiovascular: _____

      _____

   d. Respiratory: _____

      _____

   e. Gastrointestinal: _____

      _____

   f. Genitourinary: _____

      _____

   g. Musculoskeletal: _____

      _____

   h. Neurologic: _____

      _____

36. What influence does the aging process have on the following? *(213-215)*

   a. Personality: _____

      _____

   b. Intelligence and learning: _____

      _____

   c. Memory: _____

      _____

Multiple Choice

37. Aging is best defined as a: *(209-210)*
   1. period of decline in social activities.
   2. period in which senility increases.
   3. normal condition of human existence that can be affected by health habits and family.
   4. normal state in which changes in physiological conditions are universal and inevitable.

38. The nurse is assessing an older adult patient and recognizes that the following is an unexpected finding associated with the aging process: *(212)*
   1. Presbyopia
   2. Opacity of the lens
   3. Decreased depth perception
   4. Slowed accommodation

Loss, Grief, Dying, and Death

Answer Key: Textbook page references are provided as a guide for answering these questions. A complete answer key was provided for your instructor.

GRIEF AND LOSS

Objectives

- Explain how the concept of loss affects the grief reaction.
- Recognize the five aspects of human functioning and how each interacts with the others during the grieving and dying process.

1. The condition of being subject to death is known as _____. *(219)*

2. Grief is a pattern of physical and emotional responses to bereavement, separation, or _____. *(218)*

3. Briefly describe the concepts of loss and grief. *(218)* _____

   _____

   _____

4. Identify at least seven factors that influence the experience of loss. *(220)* _____

   _____

   _____

5. Discuss how physical and social aspects of human functioning influence the grieving process. *(220-223)*

   _____

   _____

6. Describe grief therapy. When was it introduced? *(219)* _____

   _____

   _____

Multiple Choice

7. Maturational loss is best defined as: *(219)*
   1. a loss occurring suddenly in response to a specific external event.
   2. any significant loss that requires adaptation through the grieving process.
   3. a loss resulting from normal life transitions.
   4. events such as the death of a loved one, divorce, the breakup of a relationship, or the loss of a job.

8. Situational loss can best be defined as: *(219)*
   1. a loss occurring suddenly in response to a specific external event.
   2. any significant loss that requires adaptation through the grieving process.
   3. a loss resulting from normal life transitions.
   4. events such as the death of a loved one, divorce, the breakup of a relationship, or the loss of a job.

STAGES OF GRIEF AND DYING

Objectives

- Describe the stages of dying.
- Identify needs of the grieving patient and family.
- Discuss support for the grieving family.
- Discuss approaches to facilitate the grieving process.

9. Identify Kübler-Ross's stage of dying in each of the following examples of patient responses. *(223)*

   a. "No, not me." _____

   b. "I just want to live until my daughter gets married." _____

   c. "It's not fair. I can't stand this!" _____

10. Identify the nursing assessments and interventions for the patient and/or family experiencing death and grieving. *(224-228)*

	Assessment	Interventions
a. Physical needs		
b. Emotional needs		
c. Spiritual needs		

11. A sign, symptom, or behavior associated with dysfunctional grieving (unresolved grief) is
_____. *(222-224)*

12. It is important that the nurse have knowledge and an understanding of survivors' reactions to be able to identify and meet the needs of the grieving family. List and describe Martocchio's manifestations of grief or survivors' reactions. *(244)*

_____

_____

Multiple Choice

13. Following the loss of a loved one, an individual may experience a sense of presence. These perceptions typically manifest by which of the following experiences? (Select all that apply) *(221)*
    1. Dreams
    2. Hallucinations
    3. Perceptions of smell
    4. General feelings of the deceased's presence

NURSING PROCESS

Objectives

- Identify unique physical signs and symptoms of the near-death patient.
- Discuss nursing interventions for the dying patient.
- Describe techniques in assisting the dying patient to say good-bye.
- Identify how the changes in the health care system affect nursing interventions for the dying patient.
- Describe nursing responsibilities in the care of the body after death.

14. Write a nursing diagnosis, patient outcome, and nursing interventions based on the following situation. *(224-225, 229)*

   The patient lost her husband in an automobile accident a year ago. She is still experiencing insomnia and feelings of worthlessness and anger, and she continues to avoid family and social functions.

   _____

   _____

   _____

   _____

15. Provide examples of how nurses cope with grief when they deal with their dying patients. *(221-222)*

   _____

   _____

16. What are the priority needs of the dying patient? *(240)* _____

    _____

    _____

17. What are some techniques that nurses may use to assist patients to say good-bye? *(237-238)* _____

    _____

    _____

18. Number the following nursing actions in the order that they should be done for postmortem care, from first to last. *(241-243)*

    _____ Remove all tubing and other devices.
    _____ Wash hands and don gloves.
    _____ Place patient in supine position.
    _____ Bathe patient as necessary.
    _____ Close patient's eyes and mouth if needed.
    _____ Allow family to view body and remain in the room.

Multiple Choice

19. Signs and symptoms that the nurse would expect to assess in the patient nearing death include: (Select all that apply) *(239-240)*
    1. lowered blood pressure.
    2. rapid, bounding pulse.
    3. irregular respiratory pattern.
    4. constricted and fixed pupils.

SPECIAL SUPPORTIVE CARE

Objective

- List nursing interventions that may facilitate grieving in special circumstances.

20. Identify nursing interventions in the following special circumstances. *(231-233)*

    a. Perinatal death: _____

    _____

    b. Pediatric death: _____

    _____

    c. Gerontologic death: _____

    _____

d. Suicide: _____

_____

ISSUES RELATED TO DEATH AND DYING

Objectives

- Explain advance directives, which include the living will and the durable power of attorney.
- Explain concepts of euthanasia, do-not-resuscitate (DNR) orders, organ donations, fraudulent methods of treatment, and the Dying Person's Bill of Rights.

21. Provide examples of fraudulent methods of treatment that may be offered to the dying patient or family. *(237)*

_____

_____

Multiple Choice

22. The terminally ill patient has been experiencing severe pain and has requested that the doctor assist her to end her suffering. The appropriate term used when referring to the action of ending this patient's life is: *(233)*
    1. euthanasia.
    2. passive suicide.
    3. brain death.
    4. mercy killing.

23. The patient in Room 318 has a DNR order. The licensed vocational nurse knows that a DNR order means: *(234)*
    1. withholding of nutrition.
    2. administering pain medication.
    3. not administering CPR if the patient stops breathing.
    4. discontinuing all intravenous lines (IVs).

24. The Uniform Anatomical Gift Act: *(235-236)*
    1. stipulates that physicians who certify death shall not be involved in removal or transplant of organs.
    2. prohibits selling or purchasing organs.
    3. facilitates this area of medical and nursing research.
    4. stipulates that at the time of death a qualified health care provider must ask family members to donate organs.

25. The goal of the Dying Person's Bill of Rights is to: *(236)*
    1. assist the nurses in providing appropriate care.
    2. list the treatment options of the patient.
    3. provide guidelines for the health care agencies.
    4. ensure death with dignity for the patient.

26. An advance directive: *(235)*
    1. appoints a health care surrogate to make decisions in the event the patient or individual is incompetent.
    2. provides for decisions related to the patient's financial needs.
    3. describes the patient's wishes about his or her estate when death is near.
    4. describes the patient's wishes about his or her care when death is near.

27. The nurse is working in a pediatric outpatient clinic. There is an 8-year-old child whose grandfather has just died. The nurse anticipates, based on the developmental level, that the child will respond by saying the following: *(223, 232)*
    1. "Grandpa will come back soon."
    2. "Grandpa was old and supposed to die."
    3. "I was bad at school and talked back to Mom. That's why Grandpa died."
    4. "It was better that Grandpa died quickly and didn't have to suffer a long time."

28. Durable power of attorney: *(234)*
    1. appoints a health care surrogate to make decisions in the event the patient or individual is incompetent.
    2. provides for decisions related to the patient's financial needs.
    3. describes the patient's wishes about his or her estate when death is near.
    4. describes the patient's wishes about his or her care when death is near.

Admission, Transfer, and Discharge

chapter

11

Answer Key: Textbook page references are provided as a guide for answering these questions. A complete answer key was provided for your instructor.

PATIENT RESPONSE TO HOSPITALIZATION

Objectives

- Describe common patient reactions to hospitalization.
- Identify nursing interventions for common patient reactions to hospitalization.

1. Provide examples of nursing interventions for the following reactions to hospitalization. *(248-249)*

   a. Fear of the unknown: _____

   _____

   b. Loss of identity: _____

   _____

   c. Disorientation: _____

   _____

   d. Separation anxiety and/or loneliness: _____

   _____

Multiple Choice

2. The practical or vocational nurse is aware that separation anxiety can be expressed in older adults by: *(249)*
   1. quietness.
   2. crying.
   3. calling for the nurse.
   4. fear.

3. The nurse is aware that separation anxiety can be expressed in children by: *(248-249)*
   1. quietness.
   2. crying.
   3. calling for the nurse.
   4. fear.

4. Fear of the unknown can be related to Maslow's need for: *(248)*
    1. self-esteem.
    2. self-actualization.
    3. safety.
    4. belonging.

5. Loss of identity can be related to Maslow's need for: *(249)*
    1. self-esteem.
    2. self-actualization.
    3. safety.
    4. belonging.

ADMISSION

Objective

*   Discuss the nurse's responsibilities in performing an admission.

6. Provide the rationale for each of the following nursing actions related to the admission of the patient to the care unit. *(249-250)*

    a. Checking and verifying of ID band: _____

    _____

    b. Assessing immediate needs: _____

    _____

    c. Explaining hospital routines, such as visiting hours, mealtime, and morning wake-up: _____

    _____

7. List the information that should be included when orienting the patient to the room. *(251)*_____

    _____

    _____

TRANSFER

Objective

*   Describe how the nurse prepares a patient for transfer to another unit or facility.

8. When transferring a patient to another unit or facility, the nurse should _____. *(257)*

DISCHARGE

Objectives

- Discuss discharge planning.
- Explain how the nurse prepares a patient for discharge.
- Identify the nurse's role when a patient chooses to leave the hospital against medical advice.

9. Ideally, discharge planning begins _____. *(259)*

10. Identify two examples of health care disciplines other than nursing that are involved in referrals, and explain their role in the discharge process. *(260-262)*

   _____

   _____

11. Provide the rationale for each of the following nursing actions in the discharge of a patient. *(262-263)*

   a. Makes certain there is a written discharge order: _____

   _____

   b. Arranges for patient and family to visit the business office and check to see that a release has been given:

   _____

   c. Notifies the family or person who will be transporting the patient to home: _____

   _____

   d. Gathers equipment, supplies, and prescriptions that the patient is to take home: _____

   _____

   e. Assists the patient in dressing and packing items to go home: _____

   _____

Multiple Choice

12. When a patient wishes to leave the hospital against medical advice (AMA), the nurse's first responsibility is to: *(263)*
   1. notify the physician.
   2. document the incident thoroughly in the nurse's notes.
   3. detain the patient.
   4. request that the patient sign the special release form (AMA form).

13. After the patient has been discharged AMA, the nurse: *(263)*
   1. notifies the accounting department.
   2. notifies the supervisor.
   3. documents the incident thoroughly in the nurse's notes.
   4. reports the AMA to the risk manager.

NURSING PROCESS

Objectives

- Identify guidelines for admission, transfer, and discharge of a patient.
- Discuss the nursing process and how it pertains to admitting, discharging, and transferring the patient.

14. Discuss factors that the nurse should consider when admitting, transferring, or discharging an older adult patient. *(249)*

_____

_____

15. Identify at least two guidelines that can be used when communicating with patients from various cultural backgrounds during the admission, transfer, or discharge process. *(250)*

_____

_____

16. Provide an example of a general nursing diagnosis that may be appropriate for a patient during the admission, transfer, or discharge process. *(256-257)*

_____

_____

17. The nurse is aware that admission to a health care facility evokes anxiety and fear in many patients; therefore, the nurse should convey _____ towards the patient, as evidenced by the nurse recognizing, understanding, and to some extent sharing the emotions that the patient is experiencing. *(249)*

Multiple Choice

18. Planning the discharge of a patient should begin: *(259)*
    1. the day of discharge.
    2. the day before discharge.
    3. as soon as possible after admission.
    4. two to three days after admission.

19. During the admission of a patient to a health care facility, the responsibilities of the admitting clerk or secretary include: (Select all that apply) *(249-250)*
    1. obtaining identifying information from the patient.
    2. giving the patient information on Health Information Portability and Accountability Act (HIPAA) guidelines.
    3. placing the correct ID band on the patient's wrist.
    4. obtaining the list of current medications from the patient.

20. An elderly Chinese-American male patient is admitted to Room 412, which is a semiprivate room, at 1:00 PM. The patient demonstrates signs of being very anxious, most likely in relation to: *(250)*
    1. separation from his children.
    2. sharing the room with a roommate.
    3. being admitted to a room containing the number "4."
    4. being admitted during a busy part of the hospital day.

Medical-Surgical Asepsis and Infection Prevention and Control

chapter

12

Answer Key: Textbook page references are provided as a guide for answering these questions. A complete answer key was provided for your instructor.

TERMS

Objective

- Define the key terms listed.

1. Define the following terms.

   a. Carrier: *(271)*_____

   _____

   b. Endogenous: *(275)* _____

   _____

   c. Exogenous: *(275)* _____

   _____

   d. Fomite: *(272)* _____

   _____

   e. Vector: *(272)* _____

   _____

ASEPSIS

Objectives

- Explain the difference between medical and surgical asepsis.
- Identify principles of surgical asepsis.

2. Describe the difference between medical and surgical asepsis. *(267)*_____

_____

_____

3. Identify the seven major principles of sterile technique, and for each principle provide at least one example of how the nurse implements it. *(292)*

_____

_____

INFECTION AND INFLAMMATION

Objectives

- Discuss the events in the inflammatory response.
- Describe the signs and symptoms of a localized infection and those of a systemic infection.

4. Describe an inflammatory response and the stages of the infectious process. *(273-274)*_____

_____

_____

5. Identify the differences between localized and systemic responses to infection. *(273)*_____

_____

_____

CHAIN OF INFECTION

Objectives

- Explain how each element of the chain of infection contributes to infection.
- List five major classifications of pathogens.
- Differentiate between *Staphylococcus aureus* and *Staphylococcus epidermidis* in terms of virulence.
- Discuss nursing interventions used to interrupt the sequence in the infection process.
- Discuss examples of how to prevent infection for each component in the chain of infection.

6. For the chain of infection, identify how each component contributes to infection and nursing interventions to prevent or control the spread of infection. *(267-273)*

	Contribution to Infectious Process	Nursing Actions
a. Infectious agent		
b. Reservoir		
c. Exit route		
d. Method of transmission		
e. Entrance		
f. Host		

7. Identify the five major classifications of pathogens and one example of a microorganism for each. *(268-271)*

_____

_____

8. How do *S. aureus* and *S. epidermidis* differ from each other in terms of virulence? *(269-270)* _____

_____

_____

9. Identify the normal body defense mechanisms and factors that may alter each. *(274)*

   a. Skin: _____

   _____

   b. Respiratory tract: _____

   _____

   c. Gastrointestinal tract: _____

   _____

10. The nurse recognizes that the best way to interfere with the transmission of microorganisms is
    _____. *(277-278)*

Multiple Choice

11. The patient has a large midline abdominal incision. With the specific purpose of reducing a possible reservoir of infection, the nurse: *(271)*
    1. wears gloves and mask at all times.
    2. isolates the patient's personal articles.
    3. has the patient cover the mouth and nose when coughing.
    4. changes the dressing when it becomes soiled.

HEALTH CARE–ASSOCIATED INFECTION

Objective

- Explain conditions that promote the onset of health care–associated infections.

12. Describe a health care–associated infection, and identify conditions that may lead to its development.
    (274-275)

    _____

    _____

INFECTION CONTROL

Objectives

- Demonstrate the appropriate procedure for 2-minute hand hygiene.
- Discuss the recommended guidelines of isolation precautions for the health care facility, referred to as standard precautions.
- Demonstrate technique for gowning and gloving.
- Demonstrate the procedure for double-bagging contaminated articles.
- Correctly don and remove sterile gloves using the open technique.
- Describe the accepted techniques of preparation for disinfection and sterilization.
- Discuss health promotion in patient teaching for infection control.

13. Identify at least five miscellaneous guidelines for standard precautions. *(276-277)* _____

_____

_____

14. Discuss at least four areas for patient teaching to prevent the spread of infection in the home environment. *(304)*

_____

_____

15. You discover that your nursing colleague has an allergy to latex. What should you suggest? *(291)*

_____

_____

16. You are observing the nursing assistant performing routine hand hygiene. Identify whether the following actions are appropriate or require more instruction. *(278-279)*

a.   Hands are kept higher than the elbows._____

b.   Faucets are turned off with a dry paper towel. _____

c.   Care is taken to wash around jewelry. _____

17. What is the proper method for disposal of sharps? *(272)*_____

_____

_____

18. For the following patients on isolation precautions, identify the type of room that should be selected. *(286)*

a.   A patient with an active infectious disease:_____

b.   A patient with an immunosuppressive problem: _____

19. Identify the basic principles of isolation. *(290)*_____

_____

_____

20. Identify the proper steps for donning and removing sterile gloves. *(298-301)*_____

_____

_____

21. Describe the procedure for gowning for contact isolation. *(283-284)* _____

_____

_____

22. Articles from the patient's isolation room require double-bagging. Identify if the following actions by the nurse are appropriate or inappropriate. *(284-285)*

    a.   Bag is removed completely from the patient's room._____

    b.   Contaminated bag is dropped into a second bag without touching the edges of the second bag.

    _____

    c.   Gown, gloves, and mask are removed before double-bagging. _____

23. Describe the steps for opening a wrapped sterile package. *(295-296)* _____

_____

_____

24. Explain how sterile solutions should be poured onto a sterile field. *(295, 297)* _____

_____

_____

25. Provide an example of a patient who would require the following precautions. *(286)*

    a.   Airborne precautions: _____

    b.   Droplet precautions: _____

    c.   Contact precautions: _____

26. Identify the major differences between routine hand hygiene and surgical handwashing. *(280)*

_____

_____

27. Identify at least two specific considerations for the older adult patient regarding the infectious process. *(273)*

_____

_____

28. Specify two possible nursing diagnoses for a patient who is susceptible to or affected by an infectious process. *(305)*

_____

_____

Multiple Choice

29. The nurse is preparing a room for a patient with herpes simplex virus. In particular, this type of precaution means that the care should include: *(286)*
    1. a private room with negative air flow.
    2. hand hygiene after filtration masks are removed.
    3. use of gloves and gown upon entering the room.
    4. use of a surgical mask on the patient during transfers.

30. The nurse is preparing a teaching plan for patients about rubella. The nurse informs them that this virus may be transmitted by: *(286)*
    1. mosquitoes.
    2. droplet nuclei.
    3. blood products.
    4. improperly handled food.

31. The nurse is working on a unit with a number of patients who have infectious diseases. One of the most important methods for reducing the spread of microorganisms is: *(277)*
    1. sterilization of equipment.
    2. the use of gloves and gowns.
    3. maintenance of isolation precautions.
    4. hand hygiene before and after patient care.

32. The assignment today for the nurse includes a patient with tuberculosis. In caring for a patient on airborne precautions, the nurse should routinely use: *(287)*
    1. regular masks and eyewear.
    2. gowns and gloves.
    3. surgical handwashing and gloves.
    4. particulate respirator masks and gowns.

33. The nurse is observing the new staff member who is preparing to do a sterile dressing. The nurse determines that the staff member requires correction and additional instruction if observed: *(293, 295-297)*
    1. opening the closest flap of the sterile wrapped package first.
    2. placing the cap of the sterile solution inside up on a clean surface.
    3. opening sterile items and dropping them directly onto the sterile field.
    4. maintaining a 1-inch border around the sterile drape.

34. The nurse is aware that the body has normal defenses against infection. An acidic environment is one defense mechanism that is characteristic of which of the body systems? (Select all that apply) *(274)*
    1. Respiratory system
    2. Gastrointestinal system
    3. Reproductive system
    4. Urinary system

Surgical Wound Care

Answer Key: Textbook page references are provided as a guide for answering these questions. A complete answer key was provided for your instructor.

ASSESSMENT

Objectives

- Discuss the body's response during each stage of wound healing.
- Discuss common complications of wound healing.
- Differentiate between healing by primary and secondary intention.

1. Provide an example for each of the following wound classifications. *(311)*

   a. Clean:_____

   b. Clean-contaminated: _____

   c. Contaminated: _____

2. Describe the following aspects of the stages of wound healing. *(311)*

	Time Frame	Cellular/Tissue Activity
a. Inflammatory phase		
b. Reconstruction phase		
c. Maturation phase		

3. Describe the following types of wound healing. *(311-312)*

    a. Primary:_____

        _____

    b. Secondary:_____

        _____

    c. Tertiary: _____

        _____

4. Identify factors that may impair wound healing. *(313)* _____

    _____

    _____

5. Describe the complications that may occur with wound healing and the nursing assessment and intervention for each. *(313)*

    _____

    _____

6. The trend for care of a postoperative sutured clean wound is to: *(314)* _____

    _____

    _____

WOUND CARE, SUPPORT, AND COMFORT MEASURES

Objectives

- Explain the procedure for applying sterile dry dressing and wet-to-dry dressings.
- Identify the procedure for removing sutures and staples.
- Discuss care of the patient with a wound drainage system such as Hemovac or Davol suction or T-tube drainage.
- Identify the procedure for performing sterile wound irrigation.
- Describe the purposes of and precautions taken when applying bandages and binders.
- List nursing diagnoses associated with impaired skin integrity.

7. What is the purpose of each of the following types of dressings? *(315-316)*

    a. Gauze: _____

    b. Semiocclusive: _____

    c. Occlusive: _____

8. For the following dressings, identify the type of wound that it can be used on. *(316-321)*

   a. Dry dressing: _____

   b. Wet-to-dry: _____

   c. Transparent: _____

9. You are observing a new staff member perform a sterile dry dressing change. How would you correct the following actions, if you observe them? *(317-318)*

   a. The tape is loosened in a direction away from the incision. _____

   _____

   _____

   b. Clean gloves are used to remove the old dressing. _____

   _____

   _____

   c. The area surrounding the incision is cleansed, and then the incision is cleansed using a back-and-forth stroking motion.

   _____

   _____

   d. Montgomery straps are used. _____

   _____

   _____

10. The new staff member proceeds to do a wet-to-dry dressing change. How would you correct the following actions, if you observe them? *(319-320)*

   a. The old dressing is moistened for easy removal. _____

   _____

   _____

   b. The new dressing is left dripping wet. _____

   _____

   _____

    c. The deep wound is packed using forceps. _____

_____

_____

    d. A dry dressing is applied over the wet gauze. _____

_____

_____

11. The nurse is preparing to implement wound irrigations. *(321-323)*

    a. The purpose of wound irrigation is: _____

_____

    b. The equipment needed for irrigation includes: _____

_____

    c. The position of a syringe for irrigation is: _____

_____

    d. The direction of cleansing is: _____

_____

    e. A hand-held shower is positioned: _____

_____

12. The nurse is assessing the amount of drainage that the patient has from a surgical wound and finds that 650 mL has drained from 9:00 AM until now, 11:40 PM. What should the nurse do? *(327)*

_____

_____

13. The patient has a T-tube in place following an abdominal cholecystectomy. The nurse anticipates that the expected output of bile will be _____. *(329-330)*

14. Discuss the specific interventions for irrigating a deep wound. *(322-323)* _____

_____

_____

15. For staple or suture removal, indicate the correct options. *(324-325)*
    a. Sterile or clean procedure? _____
    b. All of the staples are removed at once? _____
    c. Steri-Strips are applied to the site? _____
    d. Intermittent sutures are snipped at skin level away from the knots? _____

16. Identify two nursing diagnoses and patient outcomes associated with wound healing. *(338-340)*_____

    _____

    _____

17. What is the difference between a Penrose drain and a Hemovac or Jackson-Pratt drainage system? *(328-329)*

    _____

    _____

18. What nursing assessment and patient teaching are necessary for a patient with a wound drainage system? *(328-329)*

    _____

    _____

19. Identify at least three home care considerations for wound care. *(339)* _____

    _____

    _____

20. The patient has a wound vacuum-assisted closure. Describe the correct options for the following aspects of this system. *(330-333)*

    a. Type of foam used: _____

    b. Periwound skin care:_____

    c. Maintenance of occlusive seal:_____

    d. Pressure range or average pressure: _____

    e. The alarm sounds when:_____

    f. A leak is present if the nurse: _____

21. Before a bandage or binder is applied, what should the nurse assess? *(334)* _____

    _____

    _____

22. Identify at least five guidelines for bandage and binder application. *(337)*_____

_____

_____

23. Identify the type of bandage turns that should be used for the following body areas. *(336)*

    a. Finger or wrist:_____

    b. Calf or thigh:_____

    c. Joints: _____

    d. Scalp: _____

24. The patient is to have an abdominal binder applied. What is an important consideration for the nurse when implementing this application? *(335)*

_____

_____

Multiple Choice

25. A binder is used for a patient to: *(334)*
    1. reduce ventilatory capacity.
    2. assist in ambulation.
    3. increase circulatory stasis.
    4. provide support.

26. The nurse is preparing to remove the patient's staples. Upon assessment, the nurse determines that the staples should not be removed because: *(325)*
    1. the wound edges are separated.
    2. there is no drainage from the incision.
    3. the patient is anxious about their removal.
    4. a negative cosmetic result could occur.

27. The nurse is preparing to change the patient's dry sterile dressing. Upon attempting the removal of the old dressing, it is found to be adhered to the site. The nurse should: *(316)*
    1. notify the physician.
    2. leave the dressing in place.
    3. pull the dressing off quickly.
    4. moisten the dressing with saline.

28. The nurse notes that the patient's abdominal surgery dressing is saturated with red, watery drainage. The best description of this exudate is: *(314)*
    1. serous.
    2. purulent.
    3. serosanguineous.
    4. sanguineous.

29. A postoperative patient after total abdominal hysterectomy develops a wound evisceration. The nurse's first response is: *(324)*
    1. notify the physician.
    2. make the patient NPO (nothing-by-mouth status).
    3. place the patient in a low Fowler's position with the knees flexed.
    4. cover the wound with a dressing moistened with saline.

30. If, during the postoperative period, a patient develops internal abdominal bleeding that progresses to hypovolemic shock, the signs and symptoms the nurse would expect to see include: (Select all that apply) *(324)*
    1. a drop in blood pressure.
    2. an increased pulse rate.
    3. an increase in urinary output.
    4. the abdomen becoming rigid and distended.

Safety

Answer Key: Textbook page references are provided as a guide for answering these questions. A complete answer key was provided for your instructor.

TERMS

Objective

- Define the key terms as listed.

1. Define or describe the following.

   a. Disaster situation: *(346)* _____

   _____

   b. Hazard Communication Act: *(357)* _____

   _____

   c. RACE: *(359)* _____

   _____

   d. Safety reminder device (SRD): *(361)* _____

   _____

   e. Bioterrorism: *(363)* _____

   _____

ENVIRONMENT

Objective

- Discuss necessary modifications of the hospital environment for the left-handed patient.

2. The patient who has just been admitted to the unit is left-handed. What special instructions will you provide to the nursing assistant for modification of the patient's environment? *(354)*

PROMOTION OF SAFETY

Objectives

- Relate the Occupational Safety Health Administration's (OSHA's) guidelines for violence protection programs to the workplace.
- Summarize safety precautions that can be implemented to prevent falls.

3. Identify at least five risk factors for work-related violence in the health care agency and three ways in which the nurse can be involved in violence prevention. *(356)*

---

4. A patient in the long-term care facility has a history of falls in the home. Identify nursing interventions that may be implemented to prevent falls while the patient resides in the facility. *(344-345)*

---

5. The patient is using an older thermometer at home that contains mercury. The thermometer is dropped and breaks, releasing mercury onto the floor. A priority nursing action with a mercury spill is to: *(355)*

---

6. For the nursing diagnosis *risk for injury/falls*, identify a patient outcome and three nursing interventions. *(365-366)*

Multiple Choice

7. An older adult patient in the extended care facility has been wandering around outside of the room during the late evening hours. The patient has a history of falls. The nurse intervenes by: *(344-345)*
    1. obtaining an order for a bed and chair alarm.
    2. keeping the light on and the television playing all night.
    3. reassigning the patient to a room close to the nurse's station.
    4. having the family members come and check on the patient during the night.

SPECIFIC SAFETY CONCERNS

Objectives

- Relate specific safety considerations to the developmental age and the needs of individuals across the life span.
- Identify nursing interventions that are appropriate for individuals across the life span to ensure a safe environment.
- Identify safety concerns specific to the health care environment.

8. For the following age groups, identify a specific safety concern and a nursing intervention to prevent injury. *(345-346)*

	Safety Concern	Nursing Intervention
a. Infant		
b. Toddler		
c. Older adult		

9. Identify basic precautions that may be implemented by the nurse to promote overall safety in the health care environment. *(344)*

_____

_____

10. Describe how the nurse can promote safe ambulation for the patient in a health care facility. *(344-345)*

_____

_____

11. Identify three additional factors that influence the safety of the older adult in the home or health care environment. *(346)*

_____

_____

12. What are some of the safety risks to the nurse working within the health care environment? *(355-357)*

_____

_____

Multiple Choice

13. A male patient of average body build resides in the extended care facility and requires assistance to ambulate down the hall. The nurse has noticed that the patient has some weakness on the left side. The nurse assists this patient to ambulate by standing at his: *(344-345)*
    1. left side and holding his arm.
    2. right side and holding his arm.
    3. left side and holding one arm around his waist.
    4. right side and holding one arm around his waist.

SAFETY REMINDER DEVICES

Objectives

- Describe safe and appropriate methods for the application of safety reminder devices.
- Discuss nursing interventions that are specific to the patient requiring a safety reminder device.
- Detail measures to create a restraint-free environment.

14. Identify the related principles for the application and the maintenance of safety reminder devices. *(346-353)*

    a. Medical orders:_____

    _____

    b. Patient assessment: _____

    _____

    c. Maintenance of skin integrity and circulation: _____

    _____

    d. Documentation: _____

    _____

15. Describe how the nurse may implement a restraint-free environment for a patient. *(347)*_____

_____

_____

Multiple Choice

16. The patient is newly admitted to the extended care facility and appears to be disoriented. There is a concern for the patient's immediate safety. The nurse is considering the use of a safety reminder device to prevent an injury. When using an SRD the nurse should: (Select all that apply) *(346-353)*
    1. obtain a physician's order.
    2. explain purpose of the SRD to the patient.
    3. explain the purpose of the SRD to the family.
    4. be sure that all of the nursing staff agree that the SRD is necessary.

FIRE SAFETY

Objective

- Cite the steps to be followed in the event of a fire.

17. In the event of a fire in a health care agency, the nurse's top priority is: _____
    (358)

18. The nurse is planning to teach a community group about fire safety in the home. What information should be included in the presentation? *(360)*

_____

_____

19. There is a fire in the health care agency. Identify the nursing interventions for the following individuals. *(357-358)*

    a. A patient who is close to the area of the fire but is unable to ambulate: _____

    _____

    b. Visitors who have gone over to use the elevators: _____

    _____

    c. A patient who has oxygen in use: _____

    _____

20. For the following fires, identify the extinguisher that should be used. *(359)*

    a.   Paper in a wastebasket:_____

    b.   A liquid anesthetic: _____

    c.   An electric intravenous (IV) infusion pump:_____

Multiple Choice

21. While walking through the hallway in the hospital, the nurse notices smoke coming from the wastebasket in the patient's room. Upon entering the room, the nurse finds that there is a fire that is starting to flare up. The nurse should first: *(358)*
    1.   extinguish the fire.
    2.   remove the patient from the room.
    3.   contain the fire by closing the door to the room.
    4.   turn off all of the surrounding electrical equipment.

DISASTER PLANNING

Objective

- Discuss the role of the nurse in disaster planning.
- Discuss high-risk syndromes of bioterrorism.

22. Explain the difference in focus between an internal and an external disaster. *(361)* _____

    _____

    _____

23. What is the role of the nurse in disaster planning? *(361-362)* _____

    _____

    _____

24. Indications that alert the nurse to a possible bioterrorism-related outbreak include: *(363)* _____

    _____

    _____

25. A role of the nurse during a bioterrorist attack is to: *(363-364)* _____

    _____

    _____

26. Identify the signs and symptoms associated with acute radiation syndrome. *(355)*

    a. Hematopoietic:_____

    _____

    b. Gastrointestinal:_____

    _____

    c. Cerebrovascular and/or central nervous system: _____

    _____

Multiple Choice

27. It is suspected that a patient has been exposed to cyanide gas. The nurse is alert to the presence of which one of the following indications? *(364-365)*
    1. Erratic behavior
    2. Nausea and vomiting
    3. Respiratory distress
    4. Vesicle formation

ACCIDENTAL POISONING

Objective

- Describe nursing interventions in the event of accidental poisoning.

28. Identify the specific risks for and prevention of accidental poisoning for each group. *(360-361)*

	Risks	**Preventive Measures**
a. Children		
b. Older adults		

29. A patient is suspected of having ingested a poisonous substance. The nurse should: _____
_____ *(360-361)*

Multiple Choice

30. A mother calls the poison control center after a child has ingested a bottle of baby aspirin. The mother should be instructed to: *(360-361)*
    1. identify the amount of substance ingested.
    2. give the age-appropriate amount of syrup of ipecac.
    3. position the child, lying down, with the head tilted back.
    4. drive the child herself to the nearest emergency department.

31. During a type IV hypersensitivity allergic reaction to latex, the signs and symptoms that nurse would expect the patient to exhibit include: (Select all that apply) *(354)*
    1. hives.
    2. generalized edema.
    3. difficulty breathing.
    4. skin redness and itching.

Body Mechanics and Patient Mobility

Answer Key: Textbook page references are provided as a guide for answering these questions. A complete answer key was provided for your instructor.

BODY MECHANICS

Objectives

- State the principles of body mechanics.
- Explain the rationale for using appropriate body mechanics.

1. Identify four principles of body mechanics for health care workers and the rationale for each one. *(370-371)*

   _____

   _____

2. The nurse is observing a colleague performing patient care. Identify whether the following techniques are appropriate or inappropriate body mechanics. *(370-372)*

   a. Facing away from the work: _____

   b. Positioning the feet 6 to 8 inches apart: _____

   c. Keeping the knees straight: _____

   d. Keeping the head down:_____

   e. Sliding heavy objects: _____

   f. Relaxing the abdominal muscles: _____

POSITIONING

Objective

- Demonstrate execution of Fowler's, supine (dorsal), Sims', side-lying, prone, dorsal recumbent, and lithotomy positions.

3. For the following patient positions, identify the position of the bed and the equipment needed and its placement for patient alignment. *(372-375)*

	Bed Position	**Equipment and Placement for Patient Support**
a. Fowler's		
b. Supine		
c. Sims'		
d. Side-lying		
e. Prone		
f. Dorsal recumbent		
g. Lithotomy		

4. What is the rationale for the use of the following devices? *(377)*

    a. Hand rolls: _____

    _____

    b. Foot boots:_____

    _____

    c. Side rails:_____

    _____

    d. Wedge pillows:_____

    _____

RANGE OF MOTION

Objective

- Explain range-of-motion (ROM) exercises.

5. Identify the purpose, as well as the principles related to performance, of range-of-motion exercises. *(378-379)*

    _____

    _____

6. Describe the range-of-motion exercises that are performed with the following body areas. *(380-381)*

    a. Knee: _____

    _____

    b. Hip: _____

    _____

    c. Wrist: _____

    _____

MOVING PATIENTS

Objective

- Relate appropriate body mechanics to the techniques for turning, moving, lifting, and carrying the patient.

7. Before turning or transferring patients, what patient assessment and preparations should be made? *(387)*

    _____

    _____

8. For the following situations, identify the appropriate nursing intervention. *(382-387)*

    a. A patient who is going to ambulate after not being out of bed for a while: _____

    _____

    b. A patient who is in bed and has a serious head and neck condition needs to be turned: _____

    _____

    c. A patient with left-sided weakness is to move from the bed to a chair: _____

    _____

Multiple Choice

9. The nurse is working with a patient who is only able to minimally assist the nurse in moving from the bed to the chair. The nurse needs to help the patient up. The correct technique for lifting the patient to stand and pivot to the chair is to: *(384-386)*
    1. keep the legs slightly bent.
    2. maintain a narrow base with the feet.
    3. keep the stomach muscles loose.
    4. support the patient away from the body.

10. The patient has had a surgical procedure and is getting up to ambulate for the first time. While ambulating down the hallway, the patient complains of severe dizziness. The nurse should first: *(376)*
    1. call for help.
    2. lower the patient gently to the floor.
    3. lean the patient against the wall until the episode passes.
    4. support the patient and move quickly back to the room.

IMMOBILITY

Objectives

- Discuss the complications of immobility.
- State the nursing interventions to prevent complications of immobility.
- Identify complications caused by inactivity.

11. Identify the complications of immobility and nursing interventions that may be implemented to prevent their occurrence. *(376)*

_____

_____

12. For the following situations, identify the nursing intervention. *(376-377)*

   a. The patient develops a reddened area on the sacrum._____

   _____

   b. While transferring the patient from the bed to a chair, the patient starts to fall. _____

   _____

   c. The patient with right-sided weakness following a cerebrovascular accident (CVA or stroke) is unable to perform range of motion of the right extremities.

   _____

13. The patient has a cast on the lower left leg. Upon completion of a neurovascular assessment, the nurse believes that the patient may be experiencing compartment syndrome as a result of finding _____. *(377-378)*

14. Identify a nursing diagnosis for a patient who has had a CVA with resulting right-sided paresis. *(389-390)*

_____

_____

Multiple Choice

15. It is known that the patient will be immobilized for an extended period. The nurse recognizes that there is a need to prevent respiratory complications and intervenes by: *(376)*
   1. suctioning the airway every hour.
   2. changing the patient's position every 4 to 8 hours.
   3. using oxygen and nebulizer treatments regularly.
   4. encouraging deep breathing and coughing every hour.

16. Patients who are immobilized in health care facilities require that their psychosocial needs be met along with their physiological needs. The nurse recognizes these needs when telling the patient: *(376)*
   1. "Visiting hours will be limited so you can rest."
   2. "We will help you do everything so you don't have to worry."
   3. "Let's talk about what you used to do at home during the day."
   4. "A private room can be arranged for you."

17. The patient experienced a CVA (stroke) that left her with severe left-sided paralysis and very limited mobility. To prevent prolonged dorsiflexion, the nurse uses a: *(377)*
    1. foot boot.
    2. bed board.
    3. trapeze bar.
    4. trochanter roll.

18. When assessing the neurovascular status of a patient, an expected finding is: *(377-378)*
    1. capillary refill after 8 seconds.
    2. pulses strong and easily palpated.
    3. loss of sensation peripheral to an affected area.
    4. localized discomfort.

19. The ROM that can be safely performed on the neck includes: (Select all that apply) *(379)*
    1. flexion.
    2. supination.
    3. lateral flexion.
    4. rotation.

20. A contracture is defined as: *(376-377)*
    1. abnormal extension and fixation of a joint.
    2. abnormal flexion and fixation of a joint.
    3. abnormal hyperextension of a joint.
    4. abnormal lateral movements of a joint.

21. When moving or transferring older adults, it is important to avoid pulling them across bed linens because this puts them at risk for: *(383)*
    1. dislocation of a joint.
    2. increased stress to the joints.
    3. abnormal hyperextension of a joint.
    4. shearing or tearing of the skin.

Pain Management, Comfort, Rest, and Sleep

chapter

16

Answer Key: Textbook page references are provided as a guide for answering these questions. A complete answer key was provided for your instructor.

TERMS

Objective

- Define the key terms listed.

1. Define or describe the following.

   a. Endorphin: *(396)* _____

   _____

   b. Gate control theory: *(396)* _____

   _____

   c. Noxious: *(395)* _____

   _____

   d. Patient-controlled analgesia (PCA): *(402)* _____

   _____

   e. Transcutaneous electrical nerve stimulation (TENS): *(398)*_____

   _____

COMFORT AND DISCOMFORT

Objective

- List 10 possible causes of discomfort.

2. Identify at least 10 different causes of discomfort that the nurse should be aware of for the patient in the health care or the home environment. *(394)*

_____

_____

_____

_____

DESCRIPTIONS AND THEORIES OF PAIN

Objectives

- Explain McCaffery's description of pain.
- Explain the implications of the gate control theory on the selection of nursing interventions for pain relief.
- Discuss the synergistic relationship of fatigue, sleep disturbance, and depression with perception of pain.

3. McCaffery's description of pain is: *(395)* _____

_____

_____

4. Using the gate control theory of pain, identify the most effective types of nursing interventions. *(396)*

_____

_____

5. Identify how the patient's perception of pain is influenced by factors such as fatigue, sleep disturbance, and depression. *(395)*

_____

_____

ASSESSMENT OF PAIN

Objectives

- Identify subjective and objective data in pain assessment.
- Discuss the concept of making pain assessment the fifth vital sign.
- Explain several scales used to identify intensity of pain.

6. What is the difference between acute and chronic pain? *(396)* _____

_____

_____

7. Identify at least five objective signs that the patient is experiencing pain. *(408)* _____

_____

_____

8. What different types of pain intensity scales are used to assess a pain for adults and children? *(406-407)*

_____

_____

9. What subjective data may the nurse obtain from the patient regarding his or her pain experience? *(405)*

_____

_____

10. What is the rationale for making pain assessment the fifth vital sign? *(397)*_____

_____

_____

11. Identify examples of cultural and ethnic considerations for pain assessment and management. *(407)*

_____

_____

12. The patient has identified to the nurse that she is experiencing pain. What should the nurse do to fully assess the patient's pain? *(405-408)*

_____

_____

PAIN THERAPY

Objectives

- Discuss pain mechanisms affected by each analgesic group.
- List six methods for pain control.

13. a. Management of pain is required by the _____ (organization). *(397)*

    b. Identify three of the key concepts included in the standards that are applied to health care facilities. *(397)*

    _____

    _____

14. Identify at least five guidelines for individualizing pain therapy. *(408-409)* _____

    _____

    _____

15. Provide two examples of noninvasive pain relief measures. *(399)* _____

    _____

    _____

16. For the following drug classifications, identify an example of a specific medication and how the drug affects the pain mechanism. *(399-401)*

	Drug Example	Pain Relief Mechanism
a. Nonopioids		
b. Opioids		
c. Adjuvant medication		

Multiple Choice

17. The patient had a surgical procedure this morning and is requesting pain medication. The nurse assesses the patient's vital signs and decides to withhold the medication based on the finding of: *(400)*
    1. pulse = 90/min.
    2. respirations = 8/min.
    3. blood pressure = 130/80 mm Hg.
    4. temperature = 99° F rectally.

18. The visiting nurse is working with a patient who has arthritis. The patient has no known allergies to any medications, so the nurse anticipates that the physician will prescribe: *(399)*
    1. propoxyphene (Darvon).
    2. diphenhydramine (Benadryl).
    3. ibuprofen (Motrin).
    4. morphine (MS Contin).

NURSING INTERVENTION IN PAIN MANAGEMENT

Objectives

- Discuss the responsibilities of the nurse in pain control.
- Identify nursing interventions to control painful stimuli in the patient's environment.

19. What problem(s) can occur if the nurse does not respond to and treat the patient's pain? *(395)*_____

_____

_____

20. What is the role of the nurse in the administration of epidural analgesia? *(403)* _____

_____

_____

21. Identify nursing interventions that may be implemented to reduce or eliminate the patient's pain. *(408)*

_____

_____

22. Several patients on the medical unit are experiencing varying degrees of discomfort. What criteria are used to determine whether the patient is a candidate for PCA? *(402-403)*

_____

_____

23. The nurse wishes to intervene and reduce the discomfort experienced by an older adult patient. What special considerations for pain control does the nurse have to make for a patient in this age group? *(400)*

_____

_____

Multiple Choice

24. The patient is receiving epidural analgesia. The nurse is alert for a complication of this treatment and observes the patient for: *(403)*
    1. diarrhea.
    2. hypertension.
    3. urinary retention.
    4. an increased respiratory rate.

SLEEP AND REST

Objectives

- Describe the differences and similarities between sleep and rest.
- Discuss the sleep cycle, differentiating between non–rapid eye movement (NREM) and rapid eye movement (REM) sleep.

25. Compare and contrast sleep and rest. *(409)* _____

_____

_____

26. Identify and briefly describe the usual phases and stages of the sleep cycle. *(411)* _____

_____

_____

NURSING ASSESSMENT

Objectives

- List six signs and symptoms of sleep deprivation.
- Identify two nursing diagnoses related to sleep problems.

27. The nurse suspects that a patient is experiencing sleep deprivation when observing the following signs and symptoms: *(411-412)*

_____

_____

28. Identify at least two nursing diagnoses related to sleep problems. *(413)* _____

_____

_____

29. For each of the following factors, identify how sleep may be affected and why. *(410)*

	Effect on Sleep	Reason
a. Physical illness		
b. Anxiety		
c. Drugs		
d. Environment		
e. Nutrition		
f. Exercise		

NURSING INTERVENTIONS

Objective

- Outline nursing interventions that promote rest and sleep.

30. The patient is experiencing difficulty sleeping while in the hospital. Identify nursing interventions that may be implemented to promote sleep. *(412)*

_____

_____

Multiple Choice

31. The nurse enters the patient's room at 3:00 AM and finds that the patient is awake and sitting up in a chair. The patient tells the nurse that she is not able to sleep. The nurse should first: *(412)*
    1. obtain an order for a hypnotic.
    2. instruct the patient to return to bed.
    3. provide a glass of warm milk with honey.
    4. ask about ways that have helped her to sleep before.

32. An older adult patient diagnosed with osteoarthritis suffers from chronic pain. Based on the patient's age, which pain medications will the physician most likely avoid? (Select all that apply) *(401)*
    1. Meperidine
    2. Acetaminophen
    3. Morphine sulfate
    4. Nonsteroidal antiinflammatory drugs

Complementary and Alternative Therapies

Answer Key: Textbook page references are provided as a guide for answering these questions. A complete answer key was provided for your instructor.

TERMS

Objective

- Define the key terms listed.

1. Define or describe the following.

    a. Imagery: *(426)*_____

    _____

    b. Meridians: *(423)* _____

    _____

    c. Qi: *(423)* _____

    _____

TYPES OF THERAPIES

Objectives

- Differentiate between complementary and alternative therapies and allopathic (conventional) medicine.
- Describe how herbs differ from pharmaceuticals.
- Explain the scope of practice of chiropractic therapy.
- Describe the principles behind acupuncture and acupressure.
- Explain the difference between acupuncture and acupressure.
- Explain how essential oils may be used to provide aromatherapy.
- Discuss the therapeutic results of yoga.
- Explain the theory of reflexology.
- Describe the possible benefits of magnetic therapy.
- Discuss animal-assisted therapy.
- Describe safe and unsafe herbal therapies.
- Describe the health benefits of t'ai chi.

2. It is estimated that _____% of the population in the United States uses one or more forms of complementary and alternative therapy. *(416)*

3. What are some of the general benefits for the use of complementary and alternative therapies? *(416-417)*

   _____

   _____

4. How do herbs differ from pharmaceutical agents? *(418)* _____

   _____

   _____

5. What are some of the positive and negative aspects of herbal therapy? *(418)* _____

   _____

   _____

6. Identify at least two commonly taken herbs and their uses. *(419-420)*_____

   _____

   _____

7. The patient asks the nurse what the chiropractic doctor will do for him. Describe the role of the chiropractic physician as you would to the patient. *(423)*

   _____

   _____

8. What is the difference between acupuncture and acupressure? What are the principles underlying these therapies? *(423-424)*

   _____

   _____

9. Identify two essential oils used in aromatherapy and their uses. *(422)* _____

   _____

   _____

10. The principle behind reflexology is: *(424-425)* _____

    _____

    _____

11. The patient asks the nurse if "those magnets they sell in the store are really any good?" The nurse responds by telling the patient that magnetic therapy is thought to: *(426)*

_____

_____

12. What are the benefits of the use of imagery? *(426)* _____

_____

_____

13. The patient is preparing to take a yoga class because she has heard that the positive effects include: *(428)*

_____

_____

14. A positive outcome of animal-assisted therapy is: *(427-428)* _____

_____

_____

15. How can older adults benefit from t'ai chi? *(428-429)*_____

_____

_____

NURSING ASSESSMENT AND INTERVENTIONS

Objectives

- Explain why a thorough health history is important for a patient using complementary and alternative therapies.
- List three conditions when therapeutic massage may be contraindicated.

16. The nurse is obtaining a patient's health history. What should the nurse ask the patient about in regard to complementary and alternative therapies, and why is it important to ask? *(417-418)*

_____

_____

17. The patient is asking about including complementary and/or alternative therapies in the treatment regimen. What information should the nurse include in teaching this patient? *(421)*

_____

_____

18. The nurse is preparing the patient for a therapeutic massage. How should the environment be prepared? *(424)*

_____

_____

19. What assessment findings by the nurse will contraindicate the use of a therapeutic massage? *(424)*

_____

_____

20. When is reflexology used with caution or contraindicated for the patient? *(424-425)*_____

_____

_____

21. Patients with the following health problems should be instructed to avoid the use of magnets: *(426)*

_____

_____

22. The nurse is preparing to demonstrate relaxation techniques to the patient. What types of behaviors will the nurse be teaching? *(426-427)*

_____

_____

23. What is the role of the nurse in the use of complementary and alternative therapies? *(429-431)* _____

_____

_____

24. Identify two cultural considerations that arise in relation to complementary and alternative therapies. *(431)*

_____

_____

Multiple Choice

25. The patient has a history of congestive heart failure and receives a prescription for digoxin. The nurse cautions the patient against the use of which of the following herbs? *(419-420)*
    1. Evening primrose oil (*Oenothera biennis*)
    2. Goldenseal (*Hydrastis canadensis*)
    3. St. John's wort (*Hypericum perforatum*)
    4. Kava (*Kava-Kava*)

26. A pregnant patient in the maternal/child clinic asks the nurse if there are herbs that are safe to take during the pregnancy. The nurse responds accurately by telling the patient that the following herb has shown no definitive problems for pregnant women: *(419-420)*
    1. Ginger (*Ginkgo biloba*)
    2. Asian ginseng (*Panax ginseng*)
    3. Echinacea (*Echinacea pallida*)
    4. Chamomile

27. The patient asks why her physician prefers to prescribe medications for her hypertension rather than treating her with only herbal preparations. The most likely reason the physician has made this decision is: *(418-420)*
    1. physicians receive a bonus for the number of prescriptions written.
    2. patients tend to be more compliant when taking prescription medications.
    3. prescription medications are less expensive than herbal preparations.
    4. herbal preparations are not subject to the same testing and manufacturing regulations as pharmaceuticals.

Hygiene and Care of the Patient's Environment

Answer Key: Textbook page references are provided as a guide for answering these questions. A complete answer key was provided for your instructor.

ENVIRONMENT

Objective

- Discuss the therapeutic hospital room environment.

1. What does the nurse need to do to prepare a therapeutic hospital room environment? *(436-437)* _____

   _____

   _____

2. What is the recommended room temperature for an adult patient? What should the nurse keep in mind regarding the room temperature for infants and older adults? *(436)*

   _____

   _____

HYGIENIC CARE

Objectives

- Describe personal hygienic practices.
- Discuss variations of the bath procedure determined by the patient's condition and physician's orders.
- Perform the procedure for the bed bath.
- Perform the procedures for oral hygiene; shaving; hair care; nail care; and eye, ear, and nose care.
- Perform the procedure for perineal care for the male patient and the female patient.
- Perform the procedure for the back rub.

3. Describe the usual daily hygienic care schedule. *(435)* _____

   _____

   _____

4. What factors influence a patient's personal hygiene? *(435)* _____

    _____

    _____

5. For the following patients, identify how bathing may be affected or altered. *(435, 438)*

    a. The patient is extremely fatigued. _____

        _____

    b. The patient is on complete bed rest. _____

        _____

    c. The patient has right-sided paralysis following a cerebrovascular accident (CVA, or stroke). _____

        _____

    d. There is inflammation of the perianal tissue. _____

        _____

    e. The patient is an East Indian Hindu. _____

        _____

    f. The patient is an older adult who is incontinent. _____

        _____

6. Supply examples of nursing actions to achieve the following while giving a bed bath. *(440-448)*

    a. Provision of privacy and patient dignity: _____

        _____

    b. Promotion of warmth: _____

        _____

    c. Reduction in the spread of microorganisms: _____

        _____

7. In preparing to perform a back rub, the nurse will begin at the patient's _____. The
    types of strokes to use are _____. *(447-448)*

8. Oral hygiene for the unconscious patient includes: *(453-454)* _____

    _____

    _____

9. When is shaving the patient with a straight (blade) razor contraindicated? *(455)* _____

_____

_____

10. What equipment is needed to provide hair care for the bed-bound patient? *(455-456)* _____

_____

_____

11. Describe what information is included in a teaching plan on foot care for a patient newly diagnosed with diabetes mellitus. *(470)*

_____

_____

12. The nurse is evaluating the eye care that has been delegated to and is being provided by a new staff member. Identify whether the following actions are appropriate or inappropriate. *(460-461)*

    a. Removing dried secretions with a dampened cotton ball or gauze: _____

    _____

    b. Using soap and water on a washcloth: _____

    _____

    c. Cleansing the eyes from the outer to the inner canthus: _____

    _____

    d. Washing plastic eyeglass lenses with a special cleaning solution: _____

    _____

13. The nurse observes the patient performing the following ear care. Identify which behaviors are incorrect and indicate that teaching is necessary. *(461)*

    a. Cleaning the internal auditory canal with a cotton-tipped swab: _____

    b. Leaving the hearing aid turned off when not in use: _____

14. What aspects of hygienic care should not be delegated to assistive personnel? *(439)* _____

_____

_____

15. Describe what should be included in teaching care of the nose. *(461)* _____

_____

_____

16. When providing perineal care, provide examples of nursing actions to achieve the following. *(457-460)*

    a. Promotion of privacy and minimal embarrassment: _____

    _____

    b. Facilitating the performance of the procedure: _____

    _____

    c. Preventing the spread of microorganisms for the male and female patient: _____

    _____

17. What patient assessment is completed by the nurse just before performing perineal care? *(458)* _____

_____

_____

Multiple Choice

18. The patient in the hospital requires foot care. The nurse should include in the care provided: *(457)*
    1. cutting away corns and calluses.
    2. filing toenails straight across.
    3. instructing the patient to wear loose shoes.
    4. using alcohol for dryness between the toes.

19. The nurse is caring for an older adult patient in the extended care facility. The patient wears dentures, and the nurse will delegate the denture care to the nursing assistant. The nurse instructs the assistant that the patient's dentures should be: *(454)*
    1. cleaned in hot water.
    2. left in place during the night.
    3. brushed with a soft toothbrush.
    4. wrapped in a soft towel when not worn.

20. The nurse is working out the patient assignment with the nursing assistant. In delegating the morning care for the patient, the nurse expects the assistant to: *(439)*
    1. cut the tangles from the patient's hair.
    2. use soap to wash the patient's eyes.
    3. wash the patient's legs with long strokes from the ankle to the knee.
    4. place the unconscious patient in high Fowler's position to provide oral hygiene.

SKIN ASSESSMENT AND SPECIAL CARE

Objectives

- Discuss the procedures for skin care.
- Identify nursing interventions for the prevention and treatment of pressure ulcers.

21. Identify the stages of pressure ulcers. *(449-450)*_____

_____

_____

22. Identify possible risk factors for development of pressure ulcers. *(448-449)*_____

_____

_____

23. How can the nurse prevent the development of pressure ulcers? *(448-449)* _____

_____

_____

24. Identify general guidelines for care of pressure ulcers. *(450)*_____

_____

_____

Multiple Choice

25. The nurse determines, after completing the assessment, that an expected outcome for a patient with impaired skin integrity will be that the skin: *(469-470)*
    1. remains dry.
    2. has increased erythema.
    3. tingles in areas of pressure.
    4. demonstrates increased diaphoresis.

26. While completing the bath, the nurse notices a reddened area on the patient's sacrum. The nurse should first: *(469-470)*
    1. cleanse the skin with alcohol.
    2. wash the area with hot water and soap.
    3. massage the area vigorously.
    4. assess for any other areas of erythema.

BED MAKING

Objectives

- Perform the procedure for making the unoccupied bed.
- Perform the procedure for making the occupied bed.

27. How can the nurse make the bed as clean and comfortable as possible for the patient? *(462-465)* _____

_____

_____

28. What are the principles of medical asepsis as they relate to bed making? *(465)* _____

_____

_____

NURSING INTERVENTION TO ASSIST WITH ELIMINATION

Objective

- Discuss assisting the patient in the use of the bedpan, the urinal, and the bedside commode.

29. What equipment is necessary to assist the patient who is not able to use the bathroom facilities? *(465-467)*

_____

_____

30. How can the nurse assist the patient with elimination? *(466)* _____

_____

_____

31. Identify whether the following characteristics of urine and stool are expected or unexpected. *(466)*

    a. Pink-tinged urine: _____

    b. Urine negative for protein and ketone bodies: _____

    c. Clay-colored stool: _____

    d. Frequency of stool three times per day: _____

32. List at least two nursing diagnoses related to hygienic care. *(469)* _____

_____

_____

Multiple Choice

33. Risk factors for skin impairment include: (Select all that apply) *(448-449)*
    1. adequate hydration.
    2. incontinence.
    3. immobility.
    4. advanced age.

Specimen Collection and Diagnostic Examination

Answer Key: Textbook page references are provided as a guide for answering these questions. A complete answer key was provided for your instructor.

PURPOSE AND GUIDELINES FOR SPECIMEN COLLECTION

Objectives

- Explain the rationales for collection of each specimen listed.
- Discuss guidelines for specimen collection.

1. Identify the rationale for the collection of specimens identified in the chapter. *(479-517)* _____

   _____

   _____

2. Identify the general guidelines for specimen collection and diagnostic examinations. *(478, 494)*_____

   _____

   _____

NURSING ASSESSMENT AND INTERVENTIONS

Objectives

- Identify the role of the nurse when performing a procedure for specimen collection.
- Discuss patient teaching for diagnostic testing.
- Describe appropriate labeling for a collected specimen.
- Discuss the nursing interventions necessary for proper preparation of a patient having a diagnostic examination.
- List the diagnostic tests for which the nurse should determine whether the patient is allergic to iodine.

3. What are the general responsibilities of the nurse in specimen collection? *(493-494)* _____

   _____

   _____

4. Describe the nursing responsibilities in the general preparation of the patient before diagnostic testing. *(477)*

   _____

   _____

5. In addition to the interventions associated with specimen collection or preparation for a diagnostic examination, the nurse should also assess the patient for the following: *(478)*

   _____

   _____

6. Identify considerations for the older adult in regard to specimen collection and diagnostic testing. *(476)*

   _____

   _____

7. a. What procedures require that the patient be assessed for an allergy to iodine? *(478)* _____

   _____

   _____

   b. If the patient does develop an allergic reaction to the dye used in a diagnostic test, what signs and symptoms will be observed? *(478)*

   _____

   _____

   c. What is the treatment for this allergic reaction? *(478)* _____

   _____

   _____

8. The nurse is performing a gastric secretion analysis. For this procedure, identify the following: *(501-502)*

   a. Specimen is obtained by _____.

   b. The amount of specimen to obtain for analysis is _____.

   c. To perform the analysis, the nurse applies _____ to the slide.

   d. A positive monitor is indicated by _____.

   e. A negative monitor is indicated by _____.

9. Identify at least four diagnostic procedures that require the patient to remain on nothing-by-mouth status (NPO) beforehand. *(479-493)*

   _____

   _____

10. Proper labeling of specimens requires the following: *(499)* _____

_____

_____

11. a. During a bronchoscopy, the most important observation is the patient's _____
   _____. *(481-482)*

   b. Following the bronchoscopy, the patient needs to be assessed for _____
   _____. *(481-482)*

12. For the following diagnostic tests, identify at least one preprocedural and one postprocedural nursing intervention that should be implemented. *(479-493)*

		Preprocedure	Postprocedure
a.	Arteriography		
b.	Barium enema		
c.	Bone scan		
d.	Cardiac catheterization		
e.	Colonoscopy		
f.	Glucose tolerance		
g.	Intravenous pyelogram		
h.	Liver biopsy		
i.	Lumbar puncture		
j.	Magnetic resonance imaging		
k.	Paracentesis		
l.	Ultrasound		

13. Of the following specimen collections, which ones are usually possible to delegate to assistive personnel? *(516)*
    a. Urine and stool _____
    b. Gastric secretion analysis _____
    c. Venipuncture _____
    d. Sputum specimen by suctioning _____
    e. Blood glucose _____
    f. Wound cultures _____

Multiple Choice

14. The nurse is using a commercially prepared tube for the collection of an aerobic wound specimen for culture. After collecting the specimen with the swab, the nurse should: *(502, 505)*
    1. place the swab into the collection tube, close it tightly, and keep the specimen warm until it is sent to the laboratory.
    2. take the swab and mix it with the special color-changing reagent in the collection tube.
    3. place the swab into the collection tube and add the liquid culture medium.
    4. crush the ampule at the end of the tube and put the tip of the swab into the solution.

15. Following a lumbar puncture, the patient tells the nurse that he has a headache. The nurse: *(488-489)*
    1. reduces the patient's fluid intake.
    2. places the patient in low Fowler's position.
    3. informs the patient's physician immediately.
    4. instructs the patient to lie flat for up to 12 hours.

16. The patient is to have a thoracentesis performed. The nurse assists the patient to which position for this test? *(492)*
    1. Dorsal recumbent
    2. Supine with the arms held above the head
    3. Sitting up and leaning over a table
    4. Side-lying with the knees drawn up

17. The physician has ordered a magnetic resonance imaging (MRI) study for the patient. The patient is concerned about the procedure and requests information from the nurse. The nurse informs the patient to expect: *(489)*
    1. having nothing to eat or drink for 4 hours before the test.
    2. hearing humming and loud thumping sounds.
    3. minor discomfort to the area being tested.
    4. frequent position changes.

GLUCOSE TESTING

Objectives

- List the proper steps for teaching blood glucose self-monitoring.
- List the nursing responsibilities for the glucose tolerance test.

18. What information is necessary to include in the teaching plan for a newly diagnosed diabetic patient who needs to monitor blood glucose levels? *(498)*

_____

_____

19. a. The patient is scheduled to have a glucose tolerance test. How will you explain this procedure and how to prepare for it to the patient? *(486)*

_____

_____

   b. What are the nurse's responsibilities during the glucose tolerance test? *(486)* _____

_____

_____

Multiple Choice

20. The nurse is teaching the patient how to collect a specimen for blood glucose monitoring. The patient demonstrates correct technique when: *(498)*
   1. using the center of the finger for the puncture.
   2. holding the finger upright after puncture.
   3. vigorously squeezing the fingertip after puncture.
   4. touching only the blood to the pad on the test strip.

URINE AND STOOL SPECIMENS

Objectives

- Discuss the procedure for obtaining stool specimens.
- List the proper steps when obtaining urine specimens.

21. What are the purposes of obtaining stool specimens? *(499-500)* _____

_____

_____

22. How does urine specimen collection differ depending on the test to be done? *(494-496)* _____

_____

_____

23. a. During a 24-hour urine collection, one of the patient's samples is accidentally discarded. What should the nurse do? *(496-497)*

_____

_____

    b. A positive patient outcome for this procedure is: *(496-497)* _____

_____

_____

Multiple Choice

24. Instruction to the patient for collection of a midstream sample includes: *(495)*
    1. use of a clean specimen cup.
    2. collection of 200 mL of urine for testing.
    3. voiding some urine first and then collecting the sample.
    4. washing the perineal area with Betadine before collection.

25. When obtaining a urine specimen from a patient with an indwelling catheter, the nurse should: *(496)*
    1. apply sterile gloves for the procedure.
    2. clamp the drainage tubing for 30 minutes before specimen collection begins.
    3. disconnect the catheter from the drainage tubing and collect the urine in a specimen cup.
    4. insert a small-gauge needle directly into the catheter tubing to draw up the urine.

26. The patient will be catheterized for residual urine. Which of the following demonstrates correct technique for this procedure? *(494)*
    1. Catheterize the patient when the bladder is full.
    2. Obtain an order for an indwelling catheter.
    3. Catheterize the patient within 10 minutes of voiding.
    4. Use clean technique to obtain the sample.

ADDITIONAL SPECIMEN COLLECTION

Objectives

- State the correct procedure for collecting a sputum specimen.
- Identify procedure for performing a phlebotomy.
- Identify procedure for performing the electrocardiogram.

27. The nurse is to perform an electrocardiogram (ECG). Explain the purpose of the test and describe the usual position of the patient and placement of the electrodes. *(516-517)*

_____

_____

28. For the collection of a sputum specimen: *(503-505)*

    a. Identify the steps of the procedure and the rationale for each step. _____

    _____

    _____

    b. Specify what type of collection device or equipment is needed. _____

    _____

    _____

29. Before performing a venipuncture, the nurse selects and assesses the site to be used. What criteria does the nurse use to determine that the site is acceptable? *(509-510)*

    _____

    _____

30. How does the nurse apply aseptic technique during a venipuncture? *(511-512)* _____

    _____

    _____

31. The best time to collect a throat specimen is the following: *(506)* _____

    _____

    _____

32. The specific procedure for determination of bacteremia is the following: *(506-508)* _____

    _____

    _____

Multiple Choice

33. A risk factor to be considered when performing a venipuncture on a patient is: *(507)*
    1. blood glucose level.
    2. platelet count.
    3. diuretic use.
    4. sex.

34. A tourniquet is used when performing a venipuncture. The nurse is aware that the tourniquet should be: *(511)*
    1. tied into a knot.
    2. left in place no more than 1 to 2 minutes.
    3. placed 6 to 8 inches above the selected site.
    4. tight enough to occlude the distal pulse.

DOCUMENTATION

Objective

- Document the patient's condition before, during, and after a laboratory or diagnostic test.

35. After a procedure is completed, what general evaluations of patient status should the nurse perform? *(476-478, 519)*

_____

_____

36. Give an example of how the nurse should document that a specimen has been obtained or a procedure completed. *(477)*

_____

_____

Multiple Choice

37. The patient is suspected to have a urinary tract infection (UTI). The physician has ordered a urine specimen for culture and sensitivity testing. The patient asks the nurse, "What is the purpose of this test?" The nurse's best response is: *(494)*
    1. "This is just a routine test for any patient suspected of having a UTI."
    2. "Your physician must feel that this test is necessary in determining your diagnosis."
    3. "It is best if you speak with your physician if you have questions regarding this test."
    4. "This test will determine the bacteria causing your UTI and the best antibiotic for your physician to prescribe to treat the infection."

38. When performing a Hemoccult slide test to determine the presence of occult blood in a stool specimen, the nurse would be correct in using which of the following interventions? (Select all that apply) *(499-501)*
    1. Using two separate areas of the stool when obtaining the specimen
    2. Obtaining the specimen from the toilet bowl
    3. Performing the test control on the slide immediately after performing the test on the specimen obtained
    4. Documenting a positive result if a blue color appears on or at the edge of the smear after the developer as been applied

Selected Nursing Skills

Answer Key: Textbook page references are provided as a guide for answering these questions. A complete answer key was provided for your instructor.

IRRIGATIONS

Objectives

- Identify the procedure for irrigating the eye and the ear.
- Explain the procedure for external and internal vaginal irrigation (douche).
- Discuss the procedure for nasal irrigation.

1. For an eye and ear irrigation, identify the following: *(525-528)*

	Eye Irrigation	Ear Irrigation
a. Position of patient		
b. Position of irrigating equipment		
c. Flow of solution		
d. Postprocedure care		

2. The nurse is preparing to perform a vaginal irrigation for a patient. *(583-584)*

    a. Perineal care is required before the irrigation if the patient has: _____.

    b. The patient is positioned in bed on a: _____.

    c. The temperature of the irrigating solution is: _____.

    d. Which type of asepsis is used, medical or surgical? _____

    e. While inserting the irrigating nozzle, the nurse should: _____.

3. A nasal irrigation is being performed on a patient by a nursing colleague. Which steps are appropriate? *(529-530)*
    a. Positioning the patient with the head back _____
    b. Informing the patient not to speak or swallow during the procedure _____
    c. Inserting the tip of the irrigating device ½ inch to 1 inch _____
    d. Having the patient blow the nose immediately after the irrigation _____

HOT AND COLD APPLICATIONS

Objective

*   Discuss heat and cold therapy and procedures.

4. Provide examples of the types of heat and cold applications that may be used. *(532-536)*_____

    _____

    _____

5. When is the use of heat or cold therapy contraindicated for a patient? *(533)* _____

    _____

    _____

6. Identify at least four safety measures to be considered when applying heat or cold therapy. *(533)*

    _____

    _____

7. Before a hot moist compress is applied to an open wound, the nurse may apply _____ around the wound to protect the skin. *(533)*

8. What materials can the patient use in the home to make a quick ice pack? *(534)*_____

    _____

    _____

Multiple Choice

9. A cold application is ordered for the patient. The nurse is aware that a positive effect of this treatment is: *(531)*
   1. vasodilation.
   2. local anesthesia.
   3. reduced blood viscosity.
   4. increased capillary permeability.

10. There are principles to consider when using heat and cold therapy for patients. The nurse recognizes that the: *(532)*
    1. application usually lasts only 10 to 20 minutes.
    2. patient should be able to adjust the temperature settings.
    3. patient should be able to move the application around.
    4. application is positioned so that the patient cannot move away from the temperature source.

PARENTERAL THERAPY

Objectives

- Summarize the nurse's responsibilities for the patient receiving intravenous therapy and procedures.
- Explain the nurse's responsibility when administering blood therapy.
- Discuss the complications of intravenous therapy.
- Discuss the complications of blood therapy.

11. Identify three guidelines for monitoring and maintaining intravenous (IV) therapy. *(536)* _____

    _____

    _____

12. Before a venipuncture, what does the nurse have to assess? *(536, 541)* _____

    _____

    _____

13. What documentation is necessary following insertion of an IV device? *(540)* _____

    _____

    _____

14. The patient has an IV infusion. What assessments at the insertion site would indicate that the infusion should be discontinued? *(545-546)*

    _____

    _____

15. For the following situations, what should the nurse do? *(538-554)*

   a. There is less than 100 mL left in the IV bag. _____

   _____

   b. Blood components will be given by IV route to the patient._____

   _____

   c. The nurse is unsuccessful in the venipuncture attempt. _____

   _____

   d. The patient asks if the IV insertion will hurt. _____

   _____

16. What are the priority nursing responsibilities for a blood transfusion? *(546-547)* _____

   _____

   _____

17. a. The nurse determines that the patient is having a transfusion reaction. What signs and symptoms did the patient most likely exhibit to lead the nurse to this determination? *(548)*

   _____

   _____

   b. What should the nurse do first for the patient with a reaction? *(548)* _____

   _____

   _____

18. Most severe transfusion reactions occur as a result of _____. *(548)*

19. The nurse is going to change the dressing of the peripheral IV line. Select all of the following actions that represent correct technique for this procedure. *(549-550)*
   a. Palpate the catheter site after the old dressing is removed. _____
   b. Leave the tape in place that secures the IV catheter to the skin. _____
   c. Discontinue the infusion if there is erythema or edema at the site. _____
   d. Cover the insertion site with tape. _____
   e. Place tape over the transparent dressing. _____
   f. Label the dressing with the date, the time, and the nurse's initials. _____

Multiple Choice

20. Just before IV line insertion, the nurse should: *(538)*
    1. shave the hair from the selected site.
    2. select a proximal site on the upper extremity.
    3. apply a tourniquet 4 to 6 inches above the site to be used.
    4. vigorously massage the extremity to be used.

21. Upon assessment of the IV insertion site, the nurse suspects that the patient has phlebitis. This is based upon the observation of: *(546)*
    1. edema at the site.
    2. erythema along the vein path.
    3. cool skin around the insertion site.
    4. an increase in systemic blood pressure and pulse.

22. A blood transfusion is prepared for the patient. In setting up the IV, the nurse is aware that an acceptable piggyback solution for the set is: *(546-547)*
    1. normal saline.
    2. 5% dextrose in water.
    3. 10% dextrose in water.
    4. Ringer's solution.

OXYGENATION

Objectives

- Discuss nursing interventions and procedures for the patient receiving oxygen.
- Discuss care of (procedures for) a patient with a tracheostomy.
- Differentiate among oropharyngeal, nasopharyngeal, and nasotracheal suctioning.
- Develop nursing diagnoses for the patient on oxygen therapy.

23. Identify at least four safety precautions for oxygen use in the hospital and home environment. *(555-560)*

   _____

   _____

24. The patient is to receive oxygen. What assessments should be made by the nurse? *(556-557)* _____

   _____

   _____

25. When performing tracheostomy care, the nurse is aware of the following. *(562-564)*

   a. Cleansing solution to be used: _____

   b. Rinsing solution to be used: _____

   c. The part that is removed for cleaning: _____

   d. Safety measures: _____

26. What can the nurse do to reduce possible sensory deprivation for the patient with a tracheostomy? *(564)*

_____

_____

27. What criteria are used for the reinflation of a tracheostomy cuff? *(566)*_____

_____

_____

28. In preparing to suction a patient, the nurse implements the following. *(567-569)*

    a. Position of patient, if patient is able:_____

    b. Appropriate vacuum pressure for adult patient: _____

    c. Check the patency of suction catheter tubing by:_____

    d. Lubricant used on tubing: _____

    e. Length of insertion for nasopharyngeal suctioning for adult patient:_____

    f. Suctioning performed for _____ seconds.

29. Identify at least two signs or symptoms of hypoxia. *(556)*_____

_____

_____

30. The patient is to receive oxygen. *(557-559)*

    a. The nurse is aware that the usual flow rate of oxygen via a nasal cannula is: _____.

    b. Comfort measures that should be implemented for the patient receiving oxygen by nasal cannula include: _____.

    c. The usual flow rate for the patient who is to receive oxygen via a face mask is: _____.

Multiple Choice

31. The patient requires suctioning of pulmonary secretions. An appropriate nursing diagnosis for this patient is: *(565)*
    1. fluid volume excess.
    2. ineffective breathing pattern.
    3. diminished respiratory ability.
    4. ineffective airway clearance.

32. The nurse is working in the special care nursery and will be suctioning the airways of infants. For this age group, the pressure of the wall suction should be set at: *(567)*
    1. 5 to 15 mm Hg.
    2. 20 to 40 mm Hg.
    3. 50 to 95 mm Hg.
    4. 100 to 120 mm Hg.

33. Preparation for tracheostomy care in the acute care environment includes: *(562)*
    1. using clean technique and supplies for cleaning.
    2. placing the patient in supine position.
    3. removing and cleaning the outer cannula.
    4. preparing cotton swabs with hydrogen peroxide and saline.

URINARY ELIMINATION

Objective

- Discuss management of the patient with an indwelling catheter:
  - Male catheterization
  - Female catheterization
  - Discontinuing an indwelling catheter
  - Catheter irrigation
  - Urostomy care

34. Identify at least five nursing interventions for patients with urinary drainage systems. *(570, 579)* _____

_____

_____

35. For urinary catheterization of male and female patients, identify the following. *(571-575)*

	Male	**Female**
a. Position of patient		
b. Method of cleansing before insertion		
c. Length of portion of catheter to be inserted		

36. The nurse is inserting a urinary catheter and encounters the following situations. What should be done? *(571-575)*

    a. Resistance is met: _____

    _____

    b. The male patient has an erection: _____

    _____

    c. The catheter is inserted into the vagina: _____

    _____

37. The catheter itself is checked before insertion by doing the following: *(572)* _____

    _____

    _____

38. After catheter removal, the nurse assesses the patient for the following: *(583)* _____

    _____

    _____

39. Describe catheter care for a male and female patient. *(576-577)* _____

    _____

    _____

40. a. The patient who self-catheterizes at home uses _____ technique. *(579-580)*

    b. The nurse teaches this patient the signs and symptoms of a urinary tract infection, which include: *(579-580)*

    _____

    _____

41. What are the different methods of bladder irrigation? *(577-579)* _____

    _____

    _____

42. The patient is receiving continuous bladder irrigation through a three-way indwelling urinary catheter. Prescribed: 350 mL of normal saline irrigating solution infused. There are 475 mL in the urinary drainage bag. What is the patient's urinary output? *(577-579)*

    _____

    _____

43. The primary concern for a patient with a urostomy is: *(595)*_____

_____

_____

44. Identify two nursing diagnoses for a patient with a urinary disorder. *(581)*_____

_____

_____

Multiple Choice

45. The nurse has inserted the catheter into the patient, and while the balloon is being inflated the patient expresses discomfort. The nurse should: *(573)*
    1. remove the catheter and begin the procedure again.
    2. pull back on the catheter to determine tension.
    3. draw fluid back out from the balloon and move the catheter forward.
    4. continue to inflate the balloon since discomfort is expected.

46. The nurse is providing instruction to the nursing assistant on catheter care for the patient. An appropriate instruction is to: *(576-577)*
    1. maintain strong tension on the external catheter tubing.
    2. empty the drainage bag every 24 hours.
    3. keep the drainage bag on the bed or attached to the side rails.
    4. clean from the urinary meatus down the catheter.

47. When inserting a urinary catheter into a female patient, the nurse knows that it should be inserted: *(573)*
    1. 2 to 4 inches.
    2. 4 to 6 inches.
    3. 6 to 8 inches.
    4. 8 to 10 inches.

48. The charge nurse delegates the removal of an indwelling urinary catheter to a new staff member. The charge nurse goes in to observe the procedure and recognizes that correction is required if the new staff member is observed doing which of the following? *(582)*
    1. Explaining that there may be a burning sensation felt with the first voiding
    2. Obtaining a urine specimen from the port
    3. Cutting the catheter near the connection to the drainage bag
    4. Using clean gloves and performing perineal care

BOWEL ELIMINATION

Objectives

- Identify the procedures for promoting bowel elimination:
    - Administering an enema
    - Inserting a rectal tube
    - Performing ostomy and stoma care
    - Removing a fecal impaction
- Describe nursing care required to maintain structure and function of a bowel diversion.

49. How can the nurse promote normal bowel functioning for the patient in a hospital or extended care facility? *(589)*

_____

_____

50. The nurse is observing the patient at home performing colostomy care. What areas require further teaching? *(598)*
    a. The patient says he is not concerned about the swelling of the stoma. _____
    b. Alcohol and skin cream are used around the stoma. _____
    c. The patient is blotting the skin dry around the stoma. _____
    d. The skin barrier and pouch are being changed twice daily. _____
    e. The patient is leaving $\frac{1}{16}$-inch clearance between the stoma and the skin barrier. _____
    f. 750 mL of warm water is prepared for the irrigation. _____
    g. The irrigation cone is pushed forcefully into the stoma to create the fit. _____

51. For the administration of an enema, the nurse is aware of the following parameters. *(593-594)*

    a. Preferred position of patient: _____

    b. Temperature of prepared solution: _____

    c. Maximum volume of solution for an adult patient: _____

    d. Patient instruction for relaxation of external sphincter: _____

    e. Height of fluid container: _____

    f. Length of insertion of tube for adult patient: _____

    g. Patient complaints of cramping: _____

    h. Documentation required: _____

Multiple Choice

52. Before the digital removal of a fecal impaction, the nurse checks the medical record. Because of the possible effect of the digital manipulation, a patient with a history of which of the following will have to be observed especially closely during the procedure? *(595)*
    1. Cardiac disease
    2. Abdominal discomfort
    3. Urinary infection
    4. Diabetes mellitus

ENTERAL THERAPY

Objectives

- Explain nursing interventions for the patient with nasogastric intubation.
- Discuss gastric and intestinal suctioning care.
- Identify the procedure for nasogastric tube removal.

53. What is the purpose of nasogastric (NG) tube insertion? *(583)* _____

_____

_____

54. The nurse is preparing to perform a NG tube insertion and is aware of the following. *(585-587)*

    a. Measurement procedure for insertion: _____

    _____

    b. Position of patient for insertion: _____

    _____

    c. Instructions for patient during insertion: _____

    _____

    d. Most reliable determination of tube placement: _____

    _____

    e. Securing of NG tube: _____

    _____

55. The patient is not able to talk after the NG tube is inserted. The nurse suspects the following: *(587)*

_____

_____

56. You are evaluating the new staff member's performance of an NG tube irrigation. Which actions indicate that further instruction is needed? *(588)*
    a. The nurse draws up 100 mL of tap water for the irrigation. _____
    b. The solution is instilled slowly. _____
    c. The solution is withdrawn and measured. _____
    d. Solution is forced down afterward to clear the tubing. _____

57. The patient is to have gastric or intestinal suctioning applied. Identify the appropriate nursing interventions. *(589-590)*

    a. Pressure to set the wall suction at: _____

    _____

    b. Assessment of the patient: _____

    _____

   c.   Method to determine patency of the Salem sump: _____

               _____

   d.   Abnormalities to report to the physician: _____

               _____

58. While removing the NG tube, the patient begins to gag. The nurse should do the following: *(590)*_____

      _____

      _____

59. A priority nursing diagnosis for the patient with an NG tube is the following: *(585)* _____

      _____

      _____

60. A priority action for the nurse to implement before performing any skill is to check the following: *(524)*

      _____

      _____

61. Identify how the nurse achieves the following actions before, during, and after the performance of a procedure. *(524-525)*

   a.   Identify the patient: _____

               _____

   b.   Reduce the spread of microorganisms: _____

               _____

   c.   Provide privacy:_____

               _____

   d.   Ensure the patient's safety:_____

               _____

62. Although policy and procedure can vary from agency to agency, what are some of the skills that may, in general, be delegated to assistive personnel? *(532, 538, 565, 569, 589, 597)*

      _____

      _____

Multiple Choice

63. The physician has ordered the application of a warm compress to a patient's leg wound. The patient asks, "What is a compress?" The nurse's best response is: *(532)*
    1. "We will be soaking your leg in a warm solution."
    2. "We will be wrapping your leg with a device similar to a heating pad."
    3. "We will be applying a hot water bottle to your leg and then wrap a towel around it to keep the heat application constant."
    4. "We will be applying a sterile, moist gauze dressing to the wound, then wrap it with a warm aqua-thermia pad in order to maintain the warmth of the compress."

64. Upon assessment of a patient's IV site, the nurse determines that the site has become infiltrated. The signs and symptoms that the nurse assessed include: (Select all that apply) *(546)*
    1. warmth at the insertion site.
    2. swelling at and above the insertion site.
    3. redness at the insertion site.
    4. coolness upon palpation of and above the insertion site.

65. The maximum amount of fluid that should be administered to an adult during a tap water enema is: *(593)*
    1. 150 to 250 mL.
    2. 250 to 500 mL.
    3. 500 to 700 mL.
    4. 750 to 1000 mL.

Basic Nutrition and Nutrition Therapy

chapter

21

Answer Key: Textbook page references are provided as a guide for answering these questions. A complete answer key was provided for your instructor.

TERMS

Objective

- Define the key terms listed.

1. Define the following terms.

   a. Anabolism: *(612)* _____

   _____

   b. Basal metabolic rate (BMR): *(631)* _____

   _____

   c. Catabolism: *(612)* _____

   _____

   d. Essential nutrients: *(608)*_____

   _____

   e. Nitrogen balance: *(612)*_____

   _____

   f. Vegan: *(612)*_____

   _____

ESSENTIAL NUTRIENTS

Objectives

- List the six classes of essential nutrients, and identify those that provide energy.
- List the functions and food sources of protein, carbohydrates, and fats.
- List food sources and possible health benefits of dietary fiber.

- Distinguish between saturated, unsaturated, and trans fats and cholesterol; identify current recommendations for dietary intake of fats and cholesterol.
- Discuss key vitamins and minerals, their role in health, and their food sources.

2. Identify the six classes of nutrients and their general function. *(608)*_____

_____

_____

3. What are the calories provided and the recommended percentage of intake for each of the following nutrients? *(608)*

   a. Protein: _____

   b. Carbohydrates:_____

   c. Fats: _____

4. Identify the following for carbohydrates. *(608-609)*

   a. Role in the body: _____

   b. Types:_____

5. Identify an example of a simple and a complex carbohydrate. *(608)* _____

_____

_____

6. What is the difference between these types of fiber? *(609)*

   a. Insoluble fiber: _____

   _____

   b. Water-soluble fiber: _____

   _____

7. What do fats provide for the body? *(610)* _____

_____

_____

8. Identify examples of food sources for the following. *(610)*

   a. Saturated fats:_____

   b. Unsaturated fats: _____

9. In considering food choices, the nurse recognizes that cholesterol is found mainly in _____
_____. *(610-611)*

10. Lipoproteins have been talked about in the news. Which ones are important in cardiovascular disease? *(611)*

_____

_____

11. What is the role of protein in the body? *(611)* _____

_____

_____

12. Define and identify possible food sources for a complete protein. *(612)* _____

_____

_____

13. For the following types of protein-kilocalorie malnutrition states, describe the problem and the signs and symptoms exhibited by the patient. *(612-613)*

a. Kwashiorkor: _____

_____

b. Marasmus: _____

_____

14. What is the general function of vitamins? *(613)* _____

_____

_____

15. What are the two main types of vitamins? *(613)* _____

_____

_____

16. How do minerals differ from vitamins? *(613)* _____

_____

_____

17. For each of the following vitamins, identify a food source, its function in the body, and signs and symptoms of a deficiency and toxicity (if applicable). *(614-615)*

a. Vitamin C: _____

_____

b. Vitamin D: _____

_____

c. Vitamin K: _____

_____

d. Folic acid: _____

_____

e. Niacin: _____

_____

18. The patient tells the nurse that he has heard about antioxidants but is not sure what they are. The nurse responds by telling the patient that antioxidants are: *(613)*

_____

_____

19. For a patient older than 50 years of age, vitamin _____ is recommended. *(615-616)*

20. For each of the following minerals, identify a food source, its function in the body, and signs and symptoms of a deficiency and toxicity (if applicable). *(616-617)*

a. Calcium: _____

_____

b. Potassium: _____

_____

c. Iron: _____

_____

d. Iodine: _____

_____

e. Zinc: _____

_____

21. a. Identify factors that enhance the absorption of iron. *(619)* _____

_____

_____

b. Patients with the greatest risk for iron deficiency anemia are: *(619)* _____.

22. What is the function of water in the body and the recommended daily intake? *(619)*_____

_____

_____

Multiple Choice

23. The vitamin to be used with caution for a patient who is taking anticoagulants is vitamin: *(615)*
    1. A.
    2. D.
    3. K.
    4. B complex.

24. Patients who have an inadequate intake of vitamin C may develop: *(615)*
    1. bleeding gums.
    2. liver damage.
    3. depression.
    4. convulsions.

25. The patient has been diagnosed with pernicious anemia. The nurse expects that the patient will receive: *(616)*
    1. vitamin B_1.
    2. vitamin B_6.
    3. vitamin B_{12}.
    4. niacin.

26. The nurse is working with a patient who requires an increase in complete proteins in the diet. The nurse will recommend the intake of: (Select all that apply) *(612)*
    1. chicken.
    2. eggs.
    3. peanuts.
    4. beans.

27. A patient in the clinic is asking the nurse about vitamin supplements. The nurse cautions the patient about potential toxicity and not to exceed the guidelines for: *(613)*
    1. vitamin A.
    2. vitamin B.
    3. vitamin C.
    4. folic acid.

28. The patient tells the nurse that the ads on television are talking about zinc and its importance. The patient says that he doesn't know anything about zinc and would like to find out what foods have it. The nurse tells the patient that a good source of zinc is: *(616)*
    1. fruit.
    2. liver.
    3. poultry.
    4. cheese.

DIET MODIFICATIONS

Objectives

- Identify standard hospital diets and modifications for texture, consistency, and meal frequency.
- List medical/surgical conditions that require a high-kilocalorie and high-protein diet, and suggest ways to increase kilocalories and protein in the diet.
- Define obesity. List components of an effective weight management program.
- Describe the diet in the management of type 1 and type 2 diabetes mellitus.
- Distinguish among anorexia nervosa, bulimia nervosa, and binge eating disorder.
- List conditions requiring a fat-modified diet, and identify foods and food preparation methods that should be limited.
- Identify medical/surgical conditions requiring modifications in sodium, potassium, protein, or fluid intake, and describe the dietary adjustments necessary in these conditions.

29. Identify what health problems the following diets are used for. *(630-631)*

    a. Soft, and low residue: _____

    b. High kilocalorie: _____

30. What is the body mass index (BMI) used for? Calculate your own BMI. *(632)* _____

    _____

    _____

31. Identify the risks associated with obesity. *(631-632)* _____

    _____

    _____

32. What is the general dietary approach for the obese patient? *(632, 634)* _____

    _____

    _____

33. Identify the similarities among the eating disorders. *(635)* _____

    _____

    _____

34. What physiologic signs and symptoms should the nurse be alert for that may indicate an eating disorder? *(636)*

_____

_____

35. What are the general dietary guidelines for a patient with type 2 diabetes mellitus? *(637-638)* _____

_____

_____

36. The patient with diabetes mellitus is diaphoretic, weak, and breathing shallowly. What should the nurse do? *(639-640)*

_____

_____

37. What is the 15/15 rule for diabetic patients? *(639)* _____

_____

_____

38. Describe dumping syndrome and ways that the patient may avoid it. *(640)* _____

_____

_____

39. Fat-controlled diets are used for patients with _____. *(640)*

40. How is the patient able to modify the intake of the following fats? *(641)*

    a. Eggs:_____

    b. Meats: _____

41. A protein-restricted diet is used for patients with: _____
_____. *(643)*

42. A sodium-restricted diet is used for patients with: _____
_____. *(643)*

43. Identify the dietary modifications for patients with the following health problems. *(645)*

    a. Acquired immunodeficiency syndrome (AIDS): _____

    _____

b. Constipation: _____

_____

c. Hiatal hernia: _____

_____

44. Develop a plan for the distribution of fluids for a patient on a 24-hour 1000-mL fluid restriction. *(644)*

_____

_____

Multiple Choice

45. A patient in the hospital who is placed on a clear liquid diet may have: *(630)*
    1. fruit juice.
    2. gelatin.
    3. sherbet.
    4. strained soup.

46. The nurse recognizes that the diet for a patient diagnosed with diabetes mellitus will be: *(637)*
    1. fat modified.
    2. sodium restricted.
    3. protein restricted.
    4. carbohydrate modified.

47. A patient who is lactose intolerant needs to avoid: *(640)*
    1. meat.
    2. fish.
    3. cheese.
    4. vegetables.

ENTERAL THERAPY

Objective

- Define enteral nutrition and parenteral nutrition and list medical and surgical conditions in which nutrition support may be indicated.

48. What are the indications for the use of enteral feeding? *(646)* _____

_____

_____

49. What are the possible complications of enteral feeding? *(647)* _____

_____

_____

50. What is parenteral nutrition, and when is it used? *(652-653)* _____

_____

_____

51. Complications of parenteral nutrition include the following: *(653)* _____

_____

_____

52. Identify the nursing assessments and interventions for enteral feeding and the following situations. *(648-652)*

   a. Patient assessment before feeding: _____

   _____

   b. Assessment of gastric aspirate: _____

   _____

   c. Gastric residual above 150 mL: _____

   _____

   d. Formula is cold: _____

   _____

   e. Occlusion of the tubing is suspected: _____

   _____

   f. After feeding is given: _____

   _____

   g. Documentation: _____

   _____

53. What is included in the care of a gastrostomy or jejunostomy site? *(652)* _____

_____

_____

54. Positive outcomes for patients with enteral tube feedings are the following: *(646)* _____

_____

_____

Multiple Choice

55. Patients with nasogastric (NG) tubes may develop otitis media. In order to prevent this occurrence, the nurse will: *(647)*
    1. increase fluid intake.
    2. remove and reinsert the tube every 24 hours.
    3. suction the nose and mouth.
    4. turn the patient side to side every 2 hours.

56. A patient on the unit has an NG tube in place with continuous feedings. When the nurse enters the room, the patient says that he is having stomach cramps. The nurse should first: *(651)*
    1. cool the formula.
    2. remove the NG tube.
    3. use a different type of formula.
    4. decrease the administration rate.

NURSING ASSESSMENT AND INTERVENTIONS

Objectives

- Discuss the role of the nurse in promoting good nutrition.
- Explain how to use diet planning guides in the assessment and planning of a diet.
- Discuss changes in nutrient needs throughout the life cycle, and suggest ideas to ensure adequate nutrition during each stage of life.
- Identify the effects of common medications on nutritional status.

57. Identify the role of the nurse in promoting nutrition. *(605)* _____

_____

_____

58. In the MyPyramid guide, the emphasis is on _____. *(605)*

59. Identify the number of daily servings recommended in the pyramid for a 2000-calorie diet: *(605)*

    a. Vegetables: _____

    b. Meat, beans: _____

    c. Milk:_____

60. An active teenage girl asks the nurse how many calories she should have every day and what types of food she should eat. The nurse provides the following information. *(605)*

    a. Calorie intake: _____

    b. Servings of bread: _____

    c. Servings of vegetables: _____

    d. Servings of fruit:_____

    e. Servings of milk: _____

    f. Servings of meat: _____

61. A patient is asking about a vegetarian diet. Explain the positive and negative aspects of this diet for the patient. *(612)*

    _____

    _____

62. There is an increased need for nutrients during pregnancy because: *(619, 621)*_____

    _____

    _____

63. Increased intake of which vitamins is recommended for the pregnant patient? *(620)*_____

    _____

    _____

64. The nurse teaches the pregnant woman to avoid the following foods and lifestyle activities: *(621-623)*

    _____

    _____

65. In teaching a new parent about nutritional guidelines for the infant, the nurse explains that the following foods should be avoided during the first year: *(623)*

    _____

    _____

66. Identify ways to encourage good dietary habits in children. *(626)*_____

    _____

    _____

67. A common nutritional problem in adolescence is that a large part of the diet may be comprised of the following: *(626)*

_____

_____

68. Nursing home residents may have nutritional problems as a result of the following: *(627)* _____

_____

_____

69. You are evaluating the nursing assistant feeding a patient. Which of the following actions indicate a need for correction? *(655-656)*
    a. Offering the patient the bedpan before the meal. _____
    b. Placing the patient in low Fowler's position. _____
    c. Using a straw for liquids. _____
    d. Directing food toward the patient's paralyzed side. _____
    e. Talking with the patient during the feeding. _____

70. Identify at least two foods or fluids that are allowed on each of the following diets. *(630)*

    a. Clear liquid: _____

    b. Full liquid:_____

    c. Soft: _____

Multiple Choice

71. The mother asks the nurse about giving strained fruits to her infant. The nurse tells the mother that this food should be introduced at around: *(623)*
    1. 2 months.
    2. 5 months.
    3. 8 months.
    4. 12 months.

72. The patient is taking a diuretic medication every day. The nurse observes the patient for signs of a decrease in: *(618)*
    1. vitamin K.
    2. vitamin C.
    3. phosphorus.
    4. potassium.

Fluids and Electrolytes

Answer Key: Textbook page references are provided as a guide for answering these questions. A complete answer key was provided for your instructor.

FLUID AND PARTICLE MOVEMENT

Objectives

- List, describe, and compare the body fluid compartments.
- Discuss active and passive transport processes, and give two examples of each.

1. a.   Identify the body fluid compartments in the body. *(661)* _____

   _____

   _____

   b.   Most of the body fluid in an adult is located in the _____compartment. *(661)*

2.   What is the relationship of body weight to fluid? *(660)* _____

   _____

   _____

3.   For the following types of fluids, identify the how the fluid will move when administered to the patient intravenously. *(664)*

   a.   Hypertonic solution: _____

   b.   Hypotonic solution:_____

4.   Provide examples for each of the following processes in the body. *(664-665)*

   a.   Diffusion:_____

   _____

   b.   Filtration:_____

   _____

    c. Osmosis: _____

         _____

    d. Active transport: _____

         _____

5. The minimum hourly urinary output is _____, and the minimum daily output _____. *(662)*

ELECTROLYTES

Objectives

- Discuss the role of specific electrolytes in maintaining homeostasis.
- Describe the cause and effect of deficits and excesses of sodium, potassium, chloride, calcium, magnesium, phosphorus, and bicarbonate.

6. a. The major extracellular electrolyte is _____. *(665)*

    b. The major intracellular electrolyte is _____. *(665)*

7. Identify the most common signs and symptoms of hyponatremia, and nursing interventions for the imbalance. *(666)*

    _____

    _____

8. Identify the most common signs and symptoms of hypokalemia, and nursing interventions for the imbalance. *(668)*

    _____

    _____

9. What are the most serious problems associated with hyperkalemia, and what are the nursing interventions for the imbalance? *(669)*

    _____

    _____

10. The role of calcium in the body is the following: *(669-670)* _____

    _____

    _____

11. a. Identify the most common signs and symptoms of hypocalcemia, and the nursing interventions for the imbalance. *(670-671)*

_____

_____

b. In the illustrations, what assessments are being performed to determine the presence of this imbalance? *(670-671)*

i. _____

ii. _____

i.
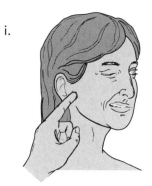

ii.
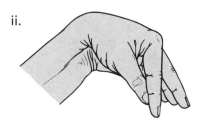

12. Identify possible causes of hypomagnesemia, its common signs and symptoms, and nursing interventions for the imbalance. *(672)*

_____

_____

13. For the following laboratory results, identify the electrolyte imbalance.

a. Serum sodium 127 mEq/L: *(665)* _____

b. Serum potassium 5.6 mEq/L: *(666)* _____

c. Serum calcium 3.8 mEq/L: *(669)* _____

d. Serum magnesium 2.7 mEq/L: *(672)* _____

14. Select all of the following that can contribute to hypokalemia. *(668)*
    a. Vomiting _____
    b. Diarrhea _____
    c. Diuretic use _____
    d. Metabolic acidosis _____
    e. Chemotherapy _____
    f. Deficiency of vitamin D _____
    g. Thyroid surgery _____

Multiple Choice

15. The patient is experiencing hyperkalemia. The nurse anticipates that the treatment will include: *(669)*
    1. intravenous (IV) calcium.
    2. fluid restrictions.
    3. foods high in potassium.
    4. administration of diuretics.

16. Following an auto accident and a significant hemorrhage, the patient was given a large infusion of citrated blood. The patient is assessed for the development of: *(671)*
    1. urinary retention.
    2. poor skin turgor.
    3. increased blood pressure.
    4. positive Chvostek's sign.

17. Good food sources for both calcium and potassium are: *(667, 670)*
    1. meats.
    2. cranberries.
    3. whole grains.
    4. green, leafy vegetables.

ACID-BASE

Objectives

- Differentiate between the roles of the buffers, the lungs, and the kidneys in maintenance of acid-base balance.
- Compare and contrast the four major types of acid-base imbalances.

18. The normal pH range of the blood is _____. *(673)*

19. a. In determining acid-base balance, the base substance that increases or decreases in the blood is _____. *(673-674)*

    b. The acid substance is _____. *(673-674)*

    c. The ratio of these two substances is _____. *(673-674)*

20. What are the three body systems that regulate acid-base balance in the body? *(673-674)* _____

_____

_____

21. a. If carbonic acid increases in the blood, the pH will _____. *(674)*

    b. The respiratory system will respond by _____. *(674)*

22. If the pH of the blood increases, the kidneys will respond by _____. *(674)*

Multiple Choice

23. The patient has experienced a prolonged episode of diarrhea. The nurse is observing the patient for signs of: *(676)*
    1. metabolic acidosis.
    2. metabolic alkalosis.
    3. respiratory acidosis.
    4. respiratory alkalosis.

24. The patient has had emphysema for a number of years. Which of the following arterial blood gas values indicates that the patient is in respiratory acidosis? *(675)*
    1. pH 7.35, $Paco_2$ 40, HCO_3 22
    2. pH 7.40, $Paco_2$ 45, HCO_3 30
    3. pH 7.30, $Paco_2$ 50, HCO_3 24
    4. pH 7.48, $Paco_2$ 55, HCO_3 18

25. While in the delivery room with his wife, the father-to-be begins to develop an anxiety reaction and lightheadedness. Nursing intervention to prevent respiratory alkalosis is: *(676)*
    1. lay him down.
    2. provide nasal oxygen.
    3. have him breathe into a paper bag.
    4. have him cough and deep-breathe.

26. A child has gotten into the medicine cabinet in the home and ingested the remaining contents of an aspirin bottle. The problem that may occur as a result of this ingestion is: *(676)*
    1. metabolic acidosis.
    2. metabolic alkalosis.
    3. respiratory acidosis.
    4. respiratory alkalosis

27. The patient has had continuous gastric suction. The nurse suspects a specific acid-base imbalance that can occur with this treatment. This is confirmed by the following findings: *(677)*
    1. pH elevated, $Paco_2$ normal, and HCO_3 elevated.
    2. pH elevated, $Paco_2$ elevated, and HCO_3 decreased.
    3. pH decreased, $Paco_2$ decreased, and HCO_3 decreased.
    4. pH decreased, $Paco_2$ normal, and HCO_3 decreased.

NURSING

Objectives

- Discuss the role of the nursing process for fluid, electrolyte, and acid-base balances.
- Discuss how the very young, the very old, and the obese patient are at risk for fluid volume deficit.

28. How does body fluid change as an individual ages and grows? *(660-661)* _____

_____

_____

29. Identify at least two considerations for the older adult patient regarding fluid and electrolyte and acid-base balance. *(661)*

_____

_____

30. The nurse is monitoring the patient's intake and output (I&O). What should be counted as part of the output? *(662)*

_____

_____

31. What are the signs and symptoms of respiratory acidosis? *(675)* _____

_____

_____

32. The nurse anticipates that the treatment for respiratory acidosis will include the following: *(675)* _____

_____

_____

33. Identify possible causes of and interventions for metabolic acidosis and alkalosis. *(676-677)* _____

_____

_____

34. Identify possible nursing diagnoses and outcomes for patients experiencing fluid, electrolyte, or acid-base imbalances. *(677)*

_____

_____

35. What are the general nursing interventions that should be implemented for patients with fluid, electrolyte, or acid-base imbalances? *(678)*

_____

_____

Multiple Choice

36. The best way for the nurse to determine the patient's fluid balance is to: *(663)*
    1. assess vital signs.
    2. weigh the patient daily.
    3. monitor IV fluid intake.
    4. check diagnostic test results.

37. For the patient with intracellular dehydration, the nurse anticipates that the patient will receive a(n): *(664)*
    1. hypotonic solution.
    2. hypertonic solution.
    3. isotonic solution.
    4. parenteral feeding.

38. A postoperative patient is receiving an isotonic IV solution. The patient asks the nurse why he is receiving this solution. The nurse's best response is: *(664)*
    1. "This fluid will expand your body's fluid volume that has been lost from your surgery."
    2. "This is a solution that will pull fluid from your cells into your circulatory system."
    3. "This solution will pull fluid from your circulatory system into your cells, where it is needed."
    4. "Since the physician ordered this IV, it would be best if you discussed the reason with your physician."

39. The nurse is aware that electrolytes serve a variety of purposes, including: (Select all that apply) *(665)*
    1. maintenance of normal body metabolism.
    2. regulation of water balance in the body.
    3. regulation of water and electrolyte contents within cells.
    4. formation of hydrochloric acid in gastric juice.

40. The patient has been placed on a low-sodium diet to assist in the treatment of hypertension. The nurse perceives that the patient has understood diet teaching when the patient states: *(665)*
    1. "Cheese is a good between-meal snack for me."
    2. "It is okay for me to eat at my favorite seafood restaurant."
    3. "In order for me to eat enough vegetables, I can prepare canned peas and corn."
    4. "I love cooked frozen broccoli. I'm glad I will still be able to eat it."

41. The nurse realizes that the patient's bicarbonate level is significant in maintaining: *(673)*
    1. electrolyte balance.
    2. fluid balance.
    3. acid-base balance.
    4. serum potassium levels.

Mathematics Review and Medication Administration

Answer Key: Textbook page references are provided as a guide for answering these questions. A complete answer key was provided for your instructor.

CALCULATION

Objectives

- Confidently use basic mathematical skills to solve dosage problems accurately.
- Set up and work problems using the following formula: (desired dose/available dose) = amount.
- Set up and work problems using the proportion method.
- Use "key" equivalents of metric and apothecary measurement systems in dosage problems.
- Convert measurement units within the metric system.
- Convert between measurement units of the metric system and the apothecary system.
- Determine the appropriateness of dosage orders for children by the use of Young's, Clark's, and Fried's rules and the body surface area.

1. For fractions, provide examples of the following. *(682-683)*

   a. Numerator: _____

   b. Denominator: _____

   c. Proper fraction: _____

   d. Improper fraction: _____

   e. Mixed fraction: _____

2. Change the following improper fractions to mixed numbers. *(682)*

   a. $\frac{8}{5} =$ _____

   b. $\frac{12}{7} =$ _____

   c. $\frac{7}{6} =$ _____

   d. $\frac{100}{13} =$ _____

   e. $\frac{30}{4} =$ _____

   f. $\frac{97}{8} =$ _____

3. Change the following mixed numbers to improper fractions. *(682)*

    a. $7\frac{5}{8}$ = _____

    b. $8\frac{1}{5}$ = _____

    c. $15\frac{1}{4}$ = _____

    d. $9\frac{1}{3}$ = _____

    e. $6\frac{5}{7}$ = _____

    f. $25\frac{2}{3}$ = _____

4. Reduce the following fractions to their lowest terms. *(682-683)*

    a. $\frac{4}{8}$ = _____

    b. $\frac{3}{9}$ = _____

    c. $\frac{21}{3}$ = _____

    d. $\frac{15}{30}$ = _____

    e. $\frac{25}{100}$ = _____

    f. $\frac{5000}{1000}$ = _____

    g. $\frac{8}{40}$ = _____

    h. $\frac{4}{16}$ = _____

    i. $\frac{18}{3}$ = _____

    j. $\frac{75}{50}$ = _____

5. Identify which is the largest fraction in the each group. *(683)*

    a. $\frac{6}{14}$ $\frac{8}{14}$ $\frac{13}{14}$: _____

    b. $\frac{3}{4}$ $\frac{4}{5}$ $\frac{7}{8}$: _____

6. Add the following fractions, and reduce the sum to its lowest term. *(683-684)*

    a. $\frac{1}{2} + \frac{5}{2} + \frac{3}{2}$ = _____

    b. $\frac{2}{5} + \frac{1}{3} + \frac{7}{10}$ = _____

    c. $\frac{1}{3} + \frac{1}{5}$ = _____

    d. $\frac{2}{12} + \frac{5}{12} + \frac{9}{12}$ = _____

    e. $2\frac{1}{3} + 5\frac{1}{4}$ = _____

7. Subtract the following fractions, and reduce the answer to its lowest term. *(684)*

    a. $\frac{4}{5} - \frac{1}{5} =$ _____

    b. $\frac{1}{2} - \frac{1}{3} =$ _____

    c. $2\frac{3}{4} - 1\frac{1}{2} =$ _____

    d. $\frac{4}{5} - \frac{1}{7} =$ _____

    e. $\frac{3}{4} - \frac{1}{4} =$ _____

8. Multiply the following fractions, and reduce the product to its lowest term. *(684)*

    a. $\frac{1}{3} \times \frac{3}{12} =$ _____

    b. $2\frac{7}{8} \times 3\frac{1}{3} =$ _____

    c. $\frac{1}{2} \times \frac{1}{5} =$ _____

    d. $\frac{2}{5} \times \frac{1}{7} =$ _____

    e. $41 \times \frac{3}{4} =$ _____

    f. $\frac{6}{5} \times 1\frac{2}{3} =$ _____

9. Divide the following fractions, and reduce the answer to its lowest term. *(685)*

    a. $\frac{1}{2} \div \frac{1}{3} =$ _____

    b. $\frac{21}{4} \div \frac{1}{7} =$ _____

    c. $\frac{5}{8} \div \frac{3}{4} =$ _____

    d. $\frac{5}{3} \div \frac{5}{3} =$ _____

    e. $\frac{3}{10} \div \frac{5}{25} =$ _____

10. Add the following decimals. *(685)*

    a. $5.4 + 6.9 =$ _____

    b. $4.25 + 3.217 =$ _____

    c. $22.1 + 0.75 =$ _____

    d. $4.297 + 1.919 =$ _____

    e. $2.2 + 1.68 =$ _____

    f. $57.629 + 14.22 =$ _____

11. Subtract the following decimals. *(685)*

     a. $0.089 - 0.0057 =$ _____

     b. $2.69 - 1.678 =$ _____

     c. $1.5 - 0.22 =$ _____

     d. $15.6 - 1.2 =$ _____

     e. $75.1 - 24.2 =$ _____

     f. $26 - 6.225 =$ _____

12. Round the following decimals to hundredths and then to tenths. *(686)*

     a. $5.753 =$ _____ _____

     b. $4.215 =$ _____ _____

     c. $3.178 =$ _____ _____

     d. $52.371 =$ _____ _____

     e. $0.604 =$ _____ _____

     f. $152.772 =$ _____ _____

13. Multiply the following decimals. *(686)*

     a. $4.2 \times 5.75 =$ _____

     b. $64.75 \times 22.9 =$ _____

     c. $33.1 \times 25.95 =$ _____

     d. $2.197 \times 0.93 =$ _____

     e. $22.5 \times 50 =$ _____

     f. $154.5 \times 14.2 =$ _____

14. Divide the following decimals, and round to the nearest hundredth. *(686)*

     a. $5.6 \div 6.97 =$ _____

     b. $2.9 \div 0.218 =$ _____

     c. $45.62 \div 1.4 =$ _____

     d. $0.02 \div 0.0007 =$ _____

     e. $75 \div 2.2 =$ _____

     f. $32.7 \div 15.952 =$ _____

15. Convert the following fractions into decimals. *(686)*

    a. ¼ = _____

    b. ½ = _____

    c. ⅕ = _____

    d. ¾ = _____

    e. ⅘ = _____

    f. ⁷⁄₁₂ = _____

16. Convert the following fractions into percents. *(687)*

    a. ⁷⁵⁄₁₀₀ = _____

    b. ⅓ = _____

    c. ⁴²⁄₁₀₀ = _____

    d. ⁵⁄₁₀ = _____

    e. ²⁰⁄₁₀₀ = _____

    f. ³³⁄₁₀₀ = _____

17. In the following ratios, solve for X. *(687)*

    a. $20 : 40 = X : 5$ X = _____

    b. $\frac{1}{150} : 2 = \frac{1}{250} : X$ X = _____

    c. $X : 9 = 4 : 12$ X = _____

    d. $\frac{1}{2} : 2 = \frac{1}{3} : X$ X = _____

    e. $X : 1 = 0.4 : 6$ X = _____

18. Complete the following equivalents. *(689)*

    a. 30 mL = _____ ounces

    b. 1000 mL = _____ L

    c. 1 L = _____ quarts

    d. 500 mL = _____ pints

    e. 60 mg = _____ g

    f. 1 kg = _____ pounds

g. 400 mL = _____ L

h. 2 mcg = _____ mg

i. 4 mg = _____ g

j. 44 pounds = _____ kg

k. 5 mg = _____ mcg

19. What are the differences among Young's rule, Clark's rule, and Fried's rule? *(690-691)* _____

_____

_____

20. Calculate the patient's total fluid intake for breakfast: 8 ounces of milk, 6 ounces of juice, and 10 ounces of coffee. *(689)* _____ mL

21. The prescription is for Tegretol 200 mg po tid. *(687-690)*
    Available—Tegretol 100-mg tablets
    How many tablets should be given per dose? _____

22. The prescription is for Aldomet 250 mg po bid. *(687-690)*
    Available—Aldomet 125-mg tablets
    How many tablets should be given per dose? _____

23. The prescription is for V-Cillin K suspension 500,000 units po. *(687-690)*
    Available—V-Cillin K suspension 200,000 units/5 mL
    How much should be prepared? _____

24. The prescription is for morphine 4 mg IM prn for pain. *(687-690)*
    Available—morphine 10 mg/mL
    The nurse prepares _____ mL.

25. The prescription is for heparin 5000 units subQ. *(687-690)*
    Available—heparin 10,000 units/mL.
    How much should be given? _____

26. The prescription is for Solu-Medrol 50 mg IV. *(687-690)*
    Available—Solu-Medrol 125 mg/2 mL.
    How much is prepared? _____

27. Using Young's rule, identify the dose for a child who is 3 years old when the adult dose is 75 mg. *(690)*
    _____

28. Using Clark's rule, identify the dose for a child who weighs 30 pounds when the adult dose is 50 mg. *(691)* _____

29. Using Fried's rule, identify the dose for a child who is 10 months old when the adult dose is 100 mg. *(691)*

    _____

30. Using the body surface area calculation, identify the dose for a child with a body surface area of 1.1 m^2 when the adult dose is 10 mg. *(691)* _____

Multiple Choice

31. A prescription for codeine gr ½ is written for the patient. The medication is supplied in mg. The nurse should administer: *(687-690)*
    a. 3 g.
    b. 30 g.
    c. 3 mg.
    d. 30 mg.

DRUG ACTION

Objectives

- Explain each phase of drug action.
- Explain the importance of decreased hepatic and renal functioning.

32. Identify the two general types of drug actions. *(692)* _____

_____

_____

33. Describe possible responses that patients may have to medications. *(692-693)* _____

_____

_____

34. Provide two examples of how older adults may respond to medications, and nursing interventions to prevent the occurrence or reduce the severity of these responses. *(694)*

_____

_____

DRUG DOSAGE

Objectives

- Discuss drug dosage.
- Discuss minimal dosage.
- Discuss maximal dosage.
- Discuss toxic dosage.
- Discuss lethal dosage.
- Discuss potentiation.
- Explain the importance of an antagonist counteracting an agonist.
- Describe five factors that affect drug action in patients.

35. What are the terms used to describe drug dosage? *(692)* _____

_____

_____

36. What factors can influence a patient's response to a medication? *(693-694)* _____

_____

_____

37. Provide an example of a drug interaction. *(692)* _____

_____

_____

MEDICATION ORDERS

Objectives

- Describe factors to consider in choosing routes of administration of medication.
- Describe the importance of accurate transcription of medication orders.
- Give the order of priority in the following terms: *stat, ASAP, now,* and *prn.*
- Explain what is meant by a *controlled substance.*
- List three ways medication orders are given.
- Discuss the use of The Joint Commission's abbreviations to prevent medication errors.

38. What is the difference between the trade name and the generic name of a drug? *(695)* _____

_____

_____

39. A medication order should include the following: *(696)* _____

_____

_____

40. Put the following terms in order of priority. *(696)*
    a. prn _____
    b. now _____
    c. stat _____
    d. ASAP _____

41. Provide an example of a controlled substance and the special nursing considerations for storage and administration. *(696)*

_____

_____

42. Identify the different types of medication orders. *(696, 698)* _____

_____

_____

43. Identify the meaning of the following abbreviations. *(699)*

a. bid: _____

b. tid: _____

c. qid: _____

d. pc: _____

44. Provide an example of a form of medication for each of the following routes. *(702, 707, 712)*

a. Enteral: _____

b. Percutaneous: _____

c. Parenteral: _____

NURSING

Objectives

- Discuss the nurse's role and responsibilities in medication administration.
- List the "six rights" of drug administration.
- Discuss "Safety Tips from Nurse-Experts."

45. What are the "six rights" of medication administration? *(698-700)* _____

_____

_____

46. For the following situations, identify what the nurse should do. *(702)*

a. The prescriber's handwriting on the medication order sheet is hard to read. _____

_____

_____

b. One nurse asks another to administer to her patient the medications she has prepared. _____

_____

_____

c. The dosage of the medication prescribed appears high. _____

_____

_____

47. What are some of the guidelines for documentation of medication administration? *(700-701)* _____

_____

_____

48. To prevent errors in the administration of medications, the nurse should do the following: *(701-702)*

_____

_____

49. Identify home health safety information that should be included in a teaching plan for medication administration. *(702)*

_____

_____

50. The nurse is preparing to administer oral medications to the patient. How are the following prepared? *(703-704)*

a. Pills from a multidose vial:_____

_____

b. Tablets in unit-dose packages: _____

_____

51. The nurse is preparing to administer a liquid medication to the patient. *(704-705)*

a. What equipment is needed?_____

_____

b. How is the liquid poured? _____

_____

c. How is the dosage amount checked? _____

_____

52. The site selected for a transdermal patch application should be _____. *(707)*

53. Medication is to be administered via a nasogastric tube. *(705-706)*

a. It is critical for the nurse to check _____.

b. Equipment needed includes_____

_____

c. Medication administration is followed by _____.

54. An example of a sublingual medication is _____. *(712)*

55. For a rectal suppository, the nurse places the patient in _____ position and prepares the suppository for insertion by _____. *(706-707)*

56. The nurse is evaluating the patient's administration of eye drops that are prescribed as gtt ii daily OD. Identify which actions indicate a need for correction: *(709)*
    a. The patient touches the tip of the bottle to the eyelid. _____
    b. One drop is administered to the left eye. _____
    c. The drop is placed in the conjunctival sac. _____

57. In preparing to give ear drops to an adult patient, the nurse will pull the earlobe _____ _____. *(710)*

58. For the following, identify the type of syringe or needle required. *(715-716, 726)*

a. Administration of 0.25 mL of medication: _____

b. An IM injection of 1.5 mL of a nonviscous medication to an average-sized adult: _____

_____

c. Identify the angles of insertion and the types of injections that are administered in the following illustration.

i. _____

ii. _____

iii. _____

i.   ii.   iii.

59. How can needlesticks be prevented? *(718)* _____

_____

_____

60. What information should be included in a teaching plan for a patient who requires a metered-dose inhaler without a spacer? *(713-714)*

_____

_____

61. What sites can be used for a subcutaneous injection? *(724, 726)* _____

_____

_____

62. For a buccal medication, identify which action is correct: *(714-715)*
   a. Placing the medication between the cheek and the gum _____
   b. Following the medication with a glass of water _____

63. Identify the common medications that are used in patient-controlled analgesia (PCA), and the nurse's responsibilities associated with this administration. *(729-730)*

_____

_____

64. What is the procedure for mixing two medications in one syringe? *(720)*_____

_____

_____

65. A microdrip IV set delivers _____ drops/mL. *(730-731)*

66. What are the responsibilities of the nurse in monitoring IV therapy? *(731-732)*_____

_____

_____

67. An IV is prescribed to infuse at 75 mL/hr. The drip factor is 10 gtt/mL. The rate of infusion should be _____ gtt/min. *(731)*

68. An IV is prescribed to infuse at 30 mL/hr with a microdrip set. The rate of infusion should be _____ gtt/min. *(731)*

69. An IV of 1000 mL is to infuse over 6 hours. The drip factor is 15 gtt/mL. The rate of infusion should be _____ gtt/min. *(731)*

70. For an IM injection, identify the following. *(725)*

    a. Preparation of the site: _____

    _____

    b. Action to take if blood is returned on aspiration:_____

    _____

71. What problem does polypharmacy pose for the older adult? *(732)* _____

_____

_____

Multiple Choice

72. An IV of 500 mL D$_5$W is to infuse over 4 hours. The administration set is 15 gtt/mL. How many gtt/min should the infusion run? *(731)*
    1. 19 gtt/min
    2. 24 gtt/min
    3. 31 gtt/min
    4. 42 gtt/min

73. The nurse determines the location for an injection by identifying the greater trochanter of the femur, the anterosuperior iliac spine, and the iliac crest. The injection site being used by the nurse is the: *(722)*
    1. rectus femoris.
    2. ventrogluteal.
    3. dorsogluteal.
    4. vastus lateralis.

74. Upon getting the assignment for the evening, the nurse notices that two patients on the unit have the same last name. The best way to prevent medication errors for these two patients is to first: *(702)*
    1. ask the patients their names.
    2. check the patients' ID bands.
    3. ask another nurse about their identities.
    4. verify their names with the family members.

75. The nurse is working in the newborn nursery and will be giving vitamin K injections to the babies. The site preferred for these injections is the: *(721)*
    1. deltoid.
    2. dorsogluteal.
    3. ventrogluteal.
    4. vastus lateralis.

76. When preparing a narcotic medication, the nurse drops the pill on the floor. The nurse should: *(696)*
    1. discard the medication.
    2. notify the pharmacy.
    3. wipe off the medication and administer it.
    4. have another nurse witness the disposal of the pill.

77. The Z-track technique is used by the nurse when the patient is: *(724)*
    1. extremely obese.
    2. less than 5 years old.
    3. receiving an irritating medication.
    4. having a large dosage of medication given.

78. A Mantoux skin test will be given to the patient. In selecting the site for this intradermal injection, the nurse assesses the: *(724)*
    1. upper outer aspect of the arm.
    2. anterior aspect of the forearm.
    3. middle third of the anterior thigh.
    4. 2-inch diameter around the umbilicus.

79. How does the nurse determine what the drip factor is for an IV set? *(731)*
    1. Ask the primary nurse.
    2. Calculate the IV rate.
    3. Look in a reference book.
    4. Check the IV tubing box.

80. The nurse is observing the patient self-administer medication with a metered-dose inhaler (MDI). What action by the patient requires correction and further instruction? *(713-714)*
    1. Inhaling slowly
    2. Inhaling one puff with each inspiration
    3. Spraying the back of the throat
    4. Using an aerochamber spacer for a better fit

81. The nurse is aware that certain types of medications cannot be crushed for ease in administration. These medications include: (Select all that apply) *(703-704)*
    1. timed-release capsules.
    2. tablets.
    3. sublingual tablets.
    4. enteric-coated tablets.

82. A patient being seen in an outpatient clinic asks the nurse why the hypnotic medication he was prescribed causes him to be awake most of the night. The nurse responds: "Sometimes medications have an unexpected response in an individual." What type of response to a medication is the nurse describing? *(693)*
    1. Synergistic
    2. Antagonist
    3. Idiosyncratic
    4. Potentiative

83. Which route of drug administration will achieve the fastest onset of action? *(712)*
    1. Intradermal
    2. Buccal
    3. Subcutaneous
    4. Enteral

Emergency First Aid Nursing

Answer Key: Textbook page references are provided as a guide for answering these questions. A complete answer key was provided for your instructor.

TERMS

Objective

- Define the key terms as listed.

1. Define the following terms.

a. Cyanosis: *(746)* _____

_____

b. Ecchymosis: *(750)*_____

_____

c. Embolism: *(748)* _____

_____

d. Epistaxis: *(749)* _____

_____

e. Flail chest: *(752)* _____

_____

f. Hematemesis: *(750)* _____

_____

g. Pneumothorax: *(751)* _____

_____

h. Stridor: *(745)* _____

_____

NURSING

Objectives

- List the priorities of assessment to be performed when arriving at a situation requiring first aid.
- Discuss moral, legal, and physical interventions of performing first aid.

2. How are the Good Samaritan laws related to emergency situations? *(738)*_____

_____

_____

3. What is the nursing responsibility in assessment and treatment of a victim in an emergency? *(738-739)*

_____

_____

Multiple Choice

4. You arrive outside of the public library and find a person lying on the ground. The first action to take is to: *(738)*
   1. check if the victim is unconscious.
   2. check the carotid or brachial pulse.
   3. move the victim to a flat, hard surface.
   4. call to have someone activate the emergency medical system (call 911).

CARDIOPULMONARY RESUSCITATION (CPR)

Objectives

- List the reasons cardiopulmonary resuscitation (CPR) should be performed.
- Discuss the legal implications of CPR.
- List the steps in performing one-rescuer and two-rescuer CPR on the adult victim.
- List the steps in performing CPR on the infant and child.

5. When is CPR performed? *(739)*_____

_____

_____

6. What are the "ABCs" for assessing the emergency patient? *(740)* _____

_____

_____

7. a. The nurse opens the patient's airway by doing the following: *(740)* _____

_____

_____

   b. If a neck injury is suspected, the nurse opens the airway by doing the following: *(740)* _____

_____

_____

8. What is the proper rate of mouth-to-mouth ventilation for an adult victim? *(742)* _____

_____

_____

9. For CPR, provide the following information. *(741-742)*

   a. Check the pulse at the: _____ .

   b. If no pulse is found: _____ .

   c. Placement of hands: _____

   d. Depress the sternum for an adult: _____ .

   e. Ratio of compressions to breaths: _____

10. Number the steps for one-rescuer adult CPR in the order that they should be performed. *(742)*
   a. Check for obstruction if unable to ventilate. _____
   b. Determine breathlessness. _____
   c. Reevaluate the victim after four full cycles. _____
   d. Call for help. _____
   e. Position the victim and open the airway. _____
   f. Begin compressions. _____
   g. Determine unresponsiveness. _____
   h. Provide two slow breaths. _____
   i. Determine pulselessness. _____

11. Breaths are given at _____ seconds each to minimize the chance of _____
_____ . *(741)*

12. For pediatric CPR, if help cannot be obtained right away, the rescuer should first _____
_____ . *(743)*

13. For pediatric CPR, identify the following. *(743-744)*

	Infant	Child
a. Where the pulse is checked		
b. Ratio of compressions to breaths		

Multiple Choice

14. For CPR to an adult victim, a single rescuer provides breaths at a rate of: *(742)*
    1. 8 per minute.
    2. 12 per minute.
    3. 20 per minute.
    4. 24 per minute.

AIRWAY

Objectives

- Name the steps in performing the Heimlich maneuver on conscious and unconscious victims.
- Discuss management of airway obstruction in the child and the infant.

15. In a situation involving a possible airway obstruction, the victim is coughing. What should the nurse do? *(744)*

_____

_____

16. a. Describe the procedure for the Heimlich maneuver for a conscious adult victim. *(745)* _____

_____

_____

b. What is the difference in the procedure for an unconscious victim? *(745)* _____

_____

_____

17. How is the airway clearance procedure for an infant different? *(745-746)* _____

_____

_____

Multiple Choice

18. A sign or symptom of a foreign body airway obstruction that necessitates immediate attention is the: *(744-745)*
    1. ability of the victim to speak.
    2. ability of the victim to cough forcefully.
    3. presence of wheezing between coughs.
    4. presence of a high-pitched inspiratory noise.

19. When performing the Heimlich maneuver, the fist should be placed: *(745)*
    1. over the ribs.
    2. over the sternum.
    3. slightly above the navel.
    4. over the xiphoid process.

20. For an unconscious adult victim with a foreign body airway obstruction, a nurse should: *(745)*
    1. apply a series of three quick chest thrusts.
    2. repeat chest thrusts continuously 10 times.
    3. perform finger sweeps between abdominal thrusts.
    4. attempt to ventilate the victim after each abdominal thrust.

SHOCK

Objectives

- Discuss the signs and symptoms of shock.
- List nursing interventions to treat shock.

21. Identify the different types of shock. *(746)* _____

_____

_____

22. What assessments lead the nurse to believe that a victim or patient is in shock? *(746-747)* _____

_____

_____

23. Select all of the following interventions that are appropriate for a victim or patient who is in shock. *(747)*
    a. Establish airway. _____
    b. Control bleeding. _____
    c. Keep the head elevated. _____
    d. Cover the patient. _____
    e. Provide fluids. _____
    f. Administer over-the-counter analgesics. _____

INJURY

Objectives

- Discuss three methods of controlling hemorrhage.
- Define four types of wounds.
- Discuss treatment of wounds.
- Discuss methods of treating three common types of poisonings.
- List the characteristics of assessment of bone, joint, and muscle injuries.
- Discuss emergency care for suspected injuries.

24. If the victim has a suspected head, neck, or spinal injury, the nurse rescuer should: *(760)* _____

_____

_____

25. What are the effects of blood loss on the body? *(747)* _____

_____

_____

26. What are the nursing interventions for a victim or patient who is bleeding? *(748-750)* _____

_____

_____

27. a. Epistaxis is fairly common. What are the nursing interventions for an individual experiencing this
     problem? *(749)*

     _____

     _____

   b. Identify signs and symptoms that are specific to internal bleeding. *(749)* _____

     _____

     _____

28. The individual has a closed wound. What are the appropriate nursing interventions? *(750)* _____

_____

_____

29. For the treatment of the following types of open wounds, provide an example of a specific nursing intervention. *(751)*

    a. Puncture wound: _____

    _____

    b. Avulsion: _____

    _____

30. The victim had an accident and now has a piece of wood protruding from the chest. The nurse should: *(751-752)*

    _____

    _____

31. What interventions should be taken for an individual with a sucking wound to the chest? *(751-752)*

    _____

    _____

32. What is the first action to take when there is a suspected poisoning? *(753-754)*_____

    _____

    _____

33. For the a victim of a poisoning, identify the assessments that may be made for the following body systems. *(753)*

    a. Respiratory: _____

    _____

    b. Neurologic: _____

    _____

    c. Gastrointestinal: _____

    _____

34. The nurse is instructed to provide water to a poisoning victim to dilute the substance ingested. Identify how much water should be given to an adult and how much to a child. *(753-754)*

    _____

    _____

35. The nurse is instructed to give syrup of ipecac to a poisoning victim. Identify the amounts of ipecac that should be given to an adult and to a child. *(753-754)*

_____

_____

36. Vomiting is not induced if an individual has ingested _____. *(753-754)*

37. An employee has been exposed to a chemical that may be absorbed through the skin. The nurse should assist by _____. *(754)*

38. After assessing the ABCs in a victim with a bone injury, the nurse should _____
_____. *(758)*

39. What are the interventions associated with the following acronym? *(759)*

   R   _____

   I   _____

   C   _____

   E   _____

40. Identify areas that should be included in a teaching plan for safety and response to emergency in the home environment. *(765)*

_____

_____

Multiple Choice

41. An appropriate action for a patient having a severe reaction to an insect bite is to first: *(754-755)*
    1. apply a constricting band proximal to the wound.
    2. wash the wound carefully with mild soap and water.
    3. keep the affected part elevated above the level of the heart.
    4. remove the stinger, if visible, with tweezers.

THERMAL INJURY

Objectives

- Define three types of burns.
- Discuss the nursing interventions in the first aid treatment of burns.
- Describe the nursing interventions of heat and cold emergencies.

42. a. What are the signs and symptoms of heat exhaustion? *(756)* _____

_____

_____

   b. A priority nursing action for the victim of heat stroke is: *(756)* _____

_____

_____

43. a. What are the signs and symptoms of hypothermia? *(757)* _____

_____

_____

   b. For the conscious victim with hypothermia, intervention includes: *(757)* _____

_____

_____

44. Describe the three different types of burns. *(759-760)*_____

_____

_____

45. What are the nursing interventions for a patient or victim with a moderate burn? *(760-761)* _____

_____

_____

Multiple Choice

46. An adult patient has severe burns to the anterior and posterior thorax and both upper extremities. Using the rule of nines, how much of the body surface is burned? *(759)*
    1. 18%
    2. 36%
    3. 54%
    4. 63%

TERRORISM AND BIOTERRORISM

Objectives

- Discuss features that should alert you to the possibility of a bioterrorism-related outbreak.
- Discuss high-risk syndromes of bioterrorism.

47. A group of signs and symptoms resulting from a common cause that presents a clinical picture of a disease is known as _____. *(762)*

Multiple Choice

48. The nurse working in a local health department knows that a bioterrorist attack that can occur via food-borne route is: *(762)*
    1. anthrax.
    2. botulism.
    3. plague.
    4. smallpox.

Health Promotion and Pregnancy

Answer Key: Textbook page references are provided as a guide for answering these questions. A complete answer key was provided for your instructor.

TERMS

Objective

- Define the key terms as listed.

1. Define the following terms.

a. Amniocentesis: *(783)* _____

_____

b. Gravida: *(788)* _____

_____

c. Morula: *(769)* _____

_____

d. Para: *(788)* _____

_____

e. Teratogenic agent: *(770)* _____

_____

f. Ectopic pregnancy: *(769)* _____

_____

PHYSIOLOGY

Objectives

- Explain the physiology of conception.
- Discuss the anatomical and physiologic alterations that occur during pregnancy.

2. Fertilization occurs in the _____. The new cell is called the _____. *(768-769)*

3. Enzymes are secreted by the _____ to allow for implantation. Implantation occurs in the _____ of the uterus. *(769)*

4. The embryonic stage of development lasts for _____ weeks. After this initial stage, the embryo is called the _____. *(769-770)*

5. What is the role of the placenta? *(770)* _____

    _____

    _____

6. Identify the usual time that the following developments occur in the mother or the fetus. *(771-780)*

    a. Morning sickness: _____

    b. Genitalia are defined: _____

    c. Swallowing and sucking begin:_____

    d. Stretch marks, redness, and darkening of the skin occur: _____

    e. Surfactant forms in the lungs: _____

7. What is the function of amniotic fluid? *(770, 781)* _____

    _____

    _____

8. What maternal antibodies are usually transferred to the fetus? *(779)* _____

    _____

    _____

9. What is the highest level of the uterus at full term? *(785)* _____

    _____

    _____

10. The usual duration of an uncomplicated pregnancy is _____. This time is divided into _____. *(785)*

Multiple Choice

11. The woman asks the nurse when the baby's heartbeat can be heard. The nurse responds by saying, "The heartbeat can be heard by week _____." *(781)*
    1. 6
    2. 8
    3. 10
    4. 16

12. The very first fetal movements, characterized as "bubbling through a straw" in the stomach, may be experienced at: *(773)*
    1. 4 weeks.
    2. 6 weeks.
    3. 10 weeks.
    4. 18 weeks.

13. The woman has entered her sixteenth week of pregnancy and asks the nurse, "How is the baby growing?" The nurse provides accurate information by informing the mother that the baby will have: *(773)*
    1. development of head hair.
    2. attained a weight of about 27 ounces.
    3. settled into a favorite position.
    4. formed all organs and structures.

HEALTH ASSESSMENT

Objectives

- Differentiate among the presumptive, possible, and positive signs of pregnancy.
- Discuss the common discomforts of pregnancy.
- List the danger signs that might occur during pregnancy.
- Discuss cultural practices and beliefs that may affect ongoing health care during pregnancy.
- Identify the components of antepartal assessment.

14. The mother asks the nurse why she is having such terrible backaches. The nurse responds by telling the woman that: *(780)*

    _____

    _____

15. A basic prenatal examination usually includes: *(786)* _____

    _____

    _____

16. What are the important aspects of genetic counseling? *(785-786)*_____

    _____

    _____

17. An obstetric nursing assessment should include information on the following about the patient: *(786)*

    _____

    _____

18. In determination of pregnancy, identify if the following are presumptive, probable, or positive signs of pregnancy. *(786-787)*

    a. Uterine enlargement: _____

    b. Quickening: _____

    c. Positive pregnancy test: _____

    d. Amenorrhea: _____

    e. Nausea and vomiting: _____

    f. Goodell's sign: _____

    g. Visualization: _____

    h. Breast changes: _____

    i. Hegar's sign: _____

19. The patient had her last menstrual period (LMP) on August 18. Using Naegele's rule, when is the estimated date of birth (EDB)? *(787)*

    _____

    _____

20. What is the usual preparation for an ultrasound? *(782)* _____

    _____

    _____

21. What tests are used to determine the well-being of the fetus? *(781)* _____

    _____

    _____

22. Define the parity of the following woman using the GTPAL system: She has been pregnant four times, delivered three full-term infants, had no abortions or preterm deliveries, and has three living children. *(788)*

    _____

    _____

23. Describe some of the common skin changes that occur during pregnancy. *(783)*_____

_____

_____

24. Psychological aspects that should be considered during the pregnancy are: *(795-796)*_____

_____

_____

Multiple Choice

25. The patient believes that she is pregnant. On examination, Chadwick's sign is found. This is: *(786)*
    1. a sensation of fetal movement.
    2. softening of the cervix.
    3. darkened pigmentation of the cheeks.
    4. purplish discoloration of the vagina, vulva, and cervix.

26. An early amniocentesis is performed to determine: *(783)*
    1. fetal distress.
    2. fetal lung maturity.
    3. presence of intrauterine infection.
    4. presence of biochemical abnormalities.

NURSING

Objectives

- Describe nutritional requirements during pregnancy.
- Identify nursing diagnoses relevant to care of the prenatal patient.

27. What interventions are appropriate for the following maternal discomforts? *(771-780)*

    a. Morning sickness: _____

    _____

    b. Headaches: _____

    _____

    c. Leg cramps:_____

    _____

    d. Indigestion:_____

    _____

28. Identify five drugs that the mother should avoid during pregnancy. *(771-780)* _____

_____

_____

29. Identify the areas of counseling for self-care on the trimester checklist. *(788)* _____

_____

_____

30. What signs and symptoms should the nurse instruct the woman to report during the pregnancy? *(790)*

_____

_____

31. In addition to selected medications, the nurse instructs the woman to avoid the following during the pregnancy. *(771-780)*

_____

_____

32. For the following systems, identify common problems that may develop during pregnancy and interventions to relieve them. *(793)*

   a. Gastrointestinal: _____

   _____

   b. Urinary: _____

   _____

33. a. Identify two common discomforts experienced during the third trimester, and the teaching for self-care for each one. *(792)*

   _____

   _____

   b. Provide examples of complementary and alternative therapies that a woman may use to relieve discomfort. *(792)*

   _____

   _____

34. The usual position of comfort for the woman to sleep or rest is _____. *(794)*

35. What counseling is appropriate regarding sexual activity for the pregnant woman? *(794-795)* _____

_____

_____

36. Identify an example of a cultural or ethnic consideration for pregnancy. *(798)* _____

_____

_____

37. Identify at least three general prenatal nursing interventions. *(800)* _____

_____

_____

38. Formulate a nursing diagnosis, patient outcome, and nursing interventions for a woman experiencing a nonrisk pregnancy. *(798-799)*

_____

_____

_____

_____

Multiple Choice

39. The nurse informs the patient to report which of the following during the pregnancy? *(790)*
    1. Reddened palms
    2. Urinary frequency
    3. Swelling of the face
    4. Dilated capillaries on the skin

40. The patient asks the nurse what can be done specifically about the ptyalism that the physician told her about. The nurse instructs the patient to: *(790)*
    1. eat small, frequent meals.
    2. suck on hard candy.
    3. sit up after eating.
    4. avoid eating spicy foods.

41. Which of the following should be included in a plan for prenatal exercise? *(795)*
    1. Exercise one time per week.
    2. Exercise for 30 minutes, then rest.
    3. Keep moving after exercising.
    4. Reduce exercise sharply 4 weeks before the due date.

42. The pregnant patient has been instructed to count fetal movements (kick count). The patient demonstrates understanding of the procedure if she states: (Select all that apply) *(790)*
    1. "I should count all movements during a 24-hour period."
    2. "I should choose a time of the day when I can sit or lie down quietly to count the movements."
    3. "My baby should move at least 10 times in a 12-hour period."
    4. "I should feel the baby move at least 4 times after I have eaten a meal."

43. After teaching the patient how to perform Kegel exercises, the patient asks the nurse how often she should perform these exercises. The nurse's best response is: *(794)*
    1. "The exercises are most beneficial if you perform them 10 times in a row, at least 3 times a day."
    2. "If you could perform the exercises 100 times in a row you will only have to do them once a day."
    3. "As many times as you think will help you."
    4. "Every patient is different, so we will need to discuss this with your doctor."

Labor and Delivery

Answer Key: Textbook page references are provided as a guide for answering these questions. A complete answer key was provided for your instructor.

IMPENDING LABOR

Objectives

- Explain the five factors that affect the labor process.
- Discuss the signs and symptoms of impending labor.
- Distinguish between true and false labor.

1. Identify the signs of impending labor. *(805-806)* _____

_____

_____

2. Provide a few examples of true versus false labor. *(806)* _____

_____

_____

3. The woman is asking about delivering somewhere other than a hospital. The nurse provides the following information: *(804)*

_____

_____

PROCESS OF LABOR AND DELIVERY

Objectives

- Discuss fetopelvic disproportion.
- Describe the "powers" involved in labor and delivery.
- Identify the mechanisms of labor.
- Identify the stages of labor.

4. The five P's of labor are: *(807)* _____

_____

_____

5. What influence does the passageway have on labor and delivery? *(807-808)*_____

_____

_____

6. What is meant by each of the following? *(809-810)*

   a. Fetal attitude: _____

   _____

   b. Fetal lie: _____

   _____

   c. Fetal presentation: _____

   _____

   d. Fetal position: _____

   _____

7. How is the position of the fetus determined? *(809)*_____

_____

_____

8. a. Identify what the following abbreviations indicate. *(810)*

     i. ROP: _____

     ii. LOA: _____

     iii. LSA: _____

   b. What position is illustrated? _____

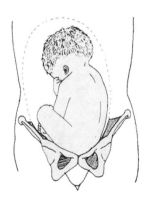

9. a. What is the normal fetal heart rate? _____ *(822)*

    b. What do the following changes in fetal heart rate indicate?

        i. Late deceleration: _____

        ii. Variable deceleration: _____

10. What signs precede the delivery of the placenta, and what is done after the delivery of the placenta? *(817, 819)*

    _____

    _____

11. What is the usual frequency and duration of uterine contractions, and what is their purpose? *(818-819)*

    _____

    _____

12. What position(s) are most effective for the first and second stages of labor? *(818-819)*_____

    _____

    _____

13. Put the following steps in the mechanism of labor in the order in which they occur for vertex positions. *(816)*
    a. Extension _____
    b. Flexion _____
    c. Descent _____
    d. Internal rotation _____
    e. Expulsion _____
    f. Engagement _____
    g. External rotation and restitution _____

Multiple Choice

14. On examination, the patient is found to be 8 cm dilated with contractions every 3 minutes that last for 70 seconds. She also does not want to communicate with the nurse or her coach. This is point in labor is described as: *(818)*
    1. early latent phase.
    2. mid to active phase.
    3. transitional phase.
    4. second stage.

15. A woman who is in the mid to active phase of labor will be expected to have: *(818)*
    1. 2-cm cervical dilation.
    2. contractions every 4 minutes.
    3. a desire to ambulate.
    4. very mild, easily controlled pain.

16. The second stage of labor begins at the: *(818)*
    1. onset of contractions.
    2. rupture of the amniotic sac.
    3. dilation of the cervix to 10 cm.
    4. delivery of the placenta.

17. When coaching the patient through the early or latent phase of labor, the nurse uses the breathing technique of: *(819)*
    1. shallow panting.
    2. slow, deep chest or abdominal breathing.
    3. acceleration through contractions.
    4. holding the breath for 5 seconds and exhaling.

18. The nurse informs the mother that the membranes have ruptured if the results of the nitrazine test are: *(805)*
    1. yellow, pH 4.0.
    2. olive yellow, pH 5.5.
    3. olive green, pH 6.0.
    4. blue green, pH 6.5.

INTERVENTIONS—NURSING AND MEDICAL

Objectives

- Describe the assessment for labor and delivery.
- Explain breathing techniques beneficial for the patient in labor.
- Identify nursing diagnoses relevant to the woman in labor.
- Outline medical interventions related to labor and delivery.
- Discuss nursing interventions related to labor and delivery.

19. The admission assessment to the labor area includes: *(828)* _____

   _____

   _____

20. How is fetal status monitored? *(819-826)* _____

   _____

   _____

21. The nurse suspects fetal distress because of the presence of: *(826)* _____

   _____

   _____

22. The monitor indicates a late deceleration. The patient is positioned: *(822)* _____

_____

_____

23. Identify the interventions for a prolapsed cord. *(838)* _____

_____

_____

24. For regional anesthesia during labor, what are the possible effects on the fetus and the appropriate nursing interventions? *(833)*

_____

_____

25. The patient requires an emergency cesarean section and will be given general anesthesia. The nurse is aware that the adverse effects of this type of anesthesia include: *(833)*

_____

_____

26. The nurse's response to the husband or coach is very important. How can the nurse provide a positive experience for the mother's support person? *(830)*

_____

_____

27. Nursing assessment of a patient's status throughout labor includes: *(835)* _____

_____

_____

28. a. What is the goal of the breathing techniques that are used throughout labor? *(837)* _____

_____

_____

    b. The patient should avoid the following type of breathing during pushing: *(837)* _____

_____

_____

29. Medical intervention during labor includes induction. Why is this implemented, and what methods are used? *(836)*

_____

_____

30. Identify two nursing diagnoses for a woman in labor. *(835)* _____

_____

_____

31. a. Identify a nursing diagnosis for a woman who has had a cesarean delivery. *(838)* _____

_____

_____

    b. Identify a priority goal for a patient with this nursing diagnosis. *(838)* _____

_____

_____

32. What is the purpose of an episiotomy? *(819)* _____

_____

_____

33. For the fourth stage of labor, what are the nursing assessments, and how often are they done? *(819)*

_____

_____

34. Provide at least one example of a medication commonly used for pain relief during labor, possible side effects, and associated nursing interventions. *(820-822)*

_____

_____

35. The baby is assessed after birth and the following are noted: heart rate 124/minute; respiratory effort good, crying; some flexion of the extremities; grimacing; body pink, extremities bluish. Based on this information, what is the Apgar score? *(827)*

_____

_____

36. Care of the baby after birth includes: *(826-827)* _____

_____

_____

37. Complications of a precipitous labor are: *(834)* _____

_____

_____

Multiple Choice

38. The nurse recognizes that which of the following is an acceptable practice in labor and delivery? *(828)*
    1. Maintenance of a full bladder
    2. Maintenance of supine position
    3. Ambulation before membrane rupture
    4. Administration of enemas to a patient with vaginal bleeding

39. The patient is receiving intravenous (IV) Pitocin for the stimulation of labor. The nurse notes that the fetal heart rate (FHR) is dropping below 100/min. The nurse should: *(837)*
    1. stop the infusion.
    2. slow down the infusion.
    3. monitor the FHR for 5 to 10 full cycles of contractions.
    4. do nothing as this is an expected response.

40. Assessment of the amniotic fluid reveals yellow staining. The nurse is aware that this is associated with: *(826)*
    1. intrauterine infection.
    2. fetal hemolytic disease.
    3. abruptio placentae.
    4. meconium passage with a breech birth.

41. A birth plan includes the discussion of possible options related to: (Select all that apply) *(804)*
    1. labor.
    2. delivery.
    3. the postpartum period.
    4. when to plan on becoming pregnant.

42. The patient demonstrates understanding of prenatal class discussions regarding the term "lightening" when she states: *(805)*
    1. "I should be alarmed if I feel like the baby has "dropped" into my pelvis a couple of weeks before my due date."
    2. "During the end of my first trimester I will feel movement of the fetus."
    3. "About 2 weeks before my delivery I can expect to feel the baby settle into my pelvis."
    4. "The presence of meconium is a dangerous sign."

43. The nurse is aware that the pregnant patient will often experience an irregular tightening of the uterus beginning in the first trimester and continuing throughout the pregnancy, known as: *(806)*
    1. restitution.
    2. Braxton-Hicks contractions.
    3. effacement.
    4. engagement.

Care of the Mother and Newborn

chapter

27

Answer Key: Textbook page references are provided as a guide for answering these questions. A complete answer key was provided for your instructor.

POSTPARTUM

Objectives

- Describe postpartum assessment of the mother.
- Identify the physiologic changes that occur in the postpartum period.
- Discuss the psychosocial adaptations that occur postpartum.
- Explain parent-child attachment (bonding).

1. Identify the height of the fundus through the process of involution. *(842)*

   a. Immediately after delivery: _____

   b. 12 hours after delivery: _____

   c. 24 to 48 hours after delivery: _____

   d. 1 week after delivery: _____

   e. 6 weeks after delivery: _____

2. Identify the types of lochia and the characteristics from delivery through the first 14 days after delivery. *(842-843)*

   _____

   _____

3. What type of nonlochia bleeding should be reported right away? *(843)* _____

   _____

   _____

4. What physiologic processes are involved in lactation? *(844)* _____

   _____

   _____

5. Identify the changes that occur in the following body systems after delivery. *(844-846)*

    a. Cardiovascular: _____

        _____

    b. Urinary: _____

        _____

    c. Gastrointestinal: _____

        _____

    d. Endocrine: _____

        _____

    e. Integumentary: _____

        _____

6. Identify postpartum danger signs. *(847)*

    a. Maternal: _____

        _____

    b. Parent-child: _____

        _____

7. What are the basic nutritional needs of the postpartum patient? *(851)* _____

    _____

    _____

8. For hygienic care: *(851-852)*

    a. Following a vaginal delivery, women should avoid _____.

    b. Following a cesarean delivery, women should avoid _____.

9. A slight temperature within 24 hours of delivery is usually indicative of _____. *(853)*

10. After delivery, the mother's sleep and rest is usually disturbed by _____. *(854)*

11. Provide an example of a specific cultural practice that occurs during the postpartum period. *(864)*

    _____

    _____

Multiple Choice

12. The mother has lost a large volume of blood and appears to be in hypovolemic shock following the delivery. The nurse implements an appropriate action by: *(843)*
    1. raising the head of the bed to 80 degrees.
    2. discontinuing the oxytocic agent in the intravenous (IV) infusion.
    3. massaging the uterus firmly and continuously.
    4. providing oxygen by face mask at 8 to 10 L/min.

NEWBORN

Objectives

- Describe the assessment of the normal newborn.
- Identify the physical characteristics of the normal newborn.
- Identify normal reflexes observed in the newborn.
- Explain common variations that may be observed in the newborn.
- Describe the behavioral characteristics of the newborn.
- Discuss nutritional needs and feeding of the newborn.

13. For newborn assessment, specify the normal parameters of the following. *(866-872)*

    a. Relationship of head to chest circumference: _____

    b. Temperature: _____

    c. Pulse: _____

    d. Respirations: _____

    e. Blood pressure: _____

14. Indicate for the following assessment findings whether they are expected (normal) or unexpected. *(866-872)*

    a. Acrocyanosis within the first 7 days: _____

    b. Jaundice within the first 24 hours: _____

    c. Lanugo: _____

    d. Milia: _____

    e. Nevus flammeus: _____

    f. Palpable posterior fontanelle: _____

    g. Low-set ears: _____

    h. Epstein's pearls: _____

    i. Molding: _____

j.   Two-vessel umbilical cord:_____

k.   Syndactyly: _____

l.   Gynecomastia: _____

m.   Asymmetric popliteal folds:_____

15. a.   Identify some of the important safety measures that should be implemented when working with a newborn. *(865)*

_____

_____

b.   To prevent infant abduction, what measures are implemented? *(865)* _____

_____

_____

16. Match the terms in Column A with the appropriate definition or description in Column B. *(870-872)*

Column A
_____   Moro's reflex
_____   Tonic neck reflex
_____   Babinski's reflex
_____   Galant's reflex

Column B
a.   Toes fan out with stroking of the foot.
b.   Trunk is flexed and pelvis swings to the side on which the spine is stimulated.
c.   Change in equilibrium causes flexion and abduction of the extremities.
d.   Arm and leg extend on side of the body toward which the head is turned.

17. What are the daily nutritional and fluid needs of the infant? *(874)* _____

_____

_____

18. For feeding the newborn: *(874)*

a.   What should be done if the baby is allergic to a milk-based formula? _____

_____

_____

b.   What is the purpose of burping the baby?_____

_____

_____

19. How can the nurse reduce the heat loss in a newborn? *(875)* _____

_____

_____

20. Urine and bowel elimination is expected in the newborn within _____ of the delivery. *(876)*

21. Identify the characteristics of the newborn's bowel elimination. *(876)*

   a. Meconium: _____

   _____

   b. Transitional: _____

   _____

   c. Breastfed:_____

   _____

   d. Abnormal:_____

   _____

22. Most newborns sleep _____ hours each day. *(877)*

23. What is the infant's form of communication? *(877)*_____

_____

_____

Multiple Choice

24. The nurse identifies that the mother requires additional teaching if, for the care of the umbilicus, she: *(875)*
   1. gives a tub bath in the first 3 days after delivery.
   2. uses alcohol on the stump daily.
   3. folds the diaper down from the umbilicus.
   4. reports a foul odor or redness from the stump.

25. Care of the circumcision includes: *(875-876)*
   1. removing the yellow crusting right away.
   2. fan-folding the diaper.
   3. applying alcohol to the area.
   4. using petroleum gauze under the Plastibell.

26. An appropriate technique to teach the new mother about the baby's bath is: *(875)*
   1. vigorous removal of the vernix caseosa.
   2. use of plain water on the perineal area.
   3. washing the baby twice daily.
   4. having the bath water at 100° F.

NURSING

Objectives

- Discuss the nursing responsibilities during the postpartum period.
- Explain the importance of teaching personal and infant care.
- Discuss nursing interventions for the circumcised newborn.

27. The nurse assesses the episiotomy for the following: *(845)* _____

_____

_____

28. Before checking the fundus, the nurse asks the patient to _____. *(857)*

29. Before ambulating a patient for the first time after delivery, the nurse should do the following: *(853)*

_____

_____

30. What types of medications are given to the mother and the newborn in the postpartum period? *(855-856)*

_____

_____

31. How can the nurse assess the amount of lochia? *(857)* _____

_____

_____

32. Engorgement is treated as follows. *(857-858)*

     a. Breastfeeding mother: _____

_____

     b. Nonbreastfeeding mother: _____

_____

33. The patient asks the nurse if breastfeeding is really better for the baby. The nurse informs the patient that the benefits of breastfeeding are the following: *(859)*

_____

_____

34. What does the acronym BUBBLE-HE for postpartum assessment mean? *(858)* _____

_____

_____

35. Describe assessment of the fundus during the recovery period for each of the following cases. *(854-857)*

    a. Technique for cesarean delivery: _____

    _____

    b. Atony is noted: _____

    _____

36. The emotional state of the mother changes in the postpartum period. What are the phases that many women go through? *(860-861)*

    _____

    _____

37. What assessment findings would lead the nurse to believe that the patient is having postpartum emotional problems? *(860)*

    _____

    _____

38. Identify two nursing diagnoses and outcomes for the postpartum patient. *(862)* _____

    _____

    _____

39. What behaviors, if observed by the nurse, indicate that the parents are bonding with the infant? *(847)*

    _____

    _____

Multiple Choice

40. The nurse is discussing sexuality with the new mother. Appropriate information to provide is that: *(848)*
    1. menses usually returns in 3 to 5 months.
    2. breastfeeding acts as an effective contraceptive.
    3. ongoing discomfort and bleeding are expected with sexual activity.
    4. resumption of sexual activity should wait until after the first postpartum office visit.

41. In teaching the patient about breastfeeding, the nurse informs the mother to: *(850)*
    1. use only one breast during each feeding.
    2. have the baby nurse for 5 minutes.
    3. put as much of the areolar tissue into the baby's mouth as possible.
    4. pull the breast straight away from the baby's mouth to break the suction seal.

42. The nurse is teaching the patient about the signs and symptoms that should be reported to the health care provider. The patient is instructed to notify the physician if, after 5 days from the delivery date, the patient experiences: *(849)*
    1. a temperature of 99° F.
    2. lochia that is light pink-brown in color.
    3. breast tenderness and redness.
    4. a fundus that feels like a softball.

43. The patient has opted to bottle feed her newborn. The nurse is confident that the patient has understood discharge teaching related to breast engorgement when the patient states: (Select all that apply) *(857)*
    1. "I will most likely not experience breast engorgement if I wear a firm-fitting bra."
    2. "If I experience engorgement, I should use ice to try to get some relief."
    3. "Engorgement will most likely occur about 3 days from my delivery date."
    4. "Breast engorgement is not really very common for most women after delivering their baby."

44. The nurse is caring for an infant that was born at 30 weeks of gestation. The mother asks the nurse, "What is all that hair on my baby's body called?" The correct response is: *(867)*
    1. vernix caseosa.
    2. lanugo.
    3. lochia.
    4. fontanelle.

45. A normal variation in the physical characteristics of a newborn that the parents should not be alarmed in seeing is: (Select all that apply) *(866-872)*
    1. acrocyanosis in an infant that is 5 days old.
    2. the harlequin sign in a 2-day-old infant.
    3. jaundice during the first 24 hours after delivery.
    4. Epstein's pearls on the hard palate of a 2-week-old infant.

Care of the High-Risk Mother, Newborn, and Family with Special Needs

Answer Key: Textbook page references are provided as a guide for answering these questions. A complete answer key was provided for your instructor.

TERMS

Objective

- Define the key terms as listed.

1. Define the following terms.

a. Cerclage: *(890)* _____

_____

b. Erythroblastosis fetalis: *(918)* _____

_____

c. Hydramnios: *(894)* _____

_____

d. Kernicterus: *(918)* _____

_____

e. Tocolytic therapy: *(890)* _____

_____

f. TORCH: *(902)* _____

_____

HIGH-RISK PREGNANCY

Objectives

- List those conditions that increase maternal and fetal risk.
- Discuss bleeding disorders that can occur during pregnancy.
- Identify diagnostic tests used to determine high-risk situations.

- Describe the HELLP syndrome.
- Discuss pregnancy-induced hypertension.
- Identify preexisting maternal health conditions that influence pregnancy.
- List the infectious disease most likely to cause serious complications.
- Discuss the care of the pregnant adolescent.

2. Identify examples of high-risk factors in pregnancy for the following areas. *(883)*

    a. Biophysical:_____

        _____

    b. Psychosocial:_____

        _____

    c. Sociodemographic: _____

        _____

    d. Environmental:_____

        _____

3. Identify factors that place the postpartum mother and infant at risk. *(884)* _____

    _____

    _____

4. For hyperemesis gravidarum, identify the signs and symptoms, medical treatment, and nursing interventions. *(884)*

    a. Signs and symptoms: _____

        _____

    b. Medical treatment:_____

        _____

    c. Nursing interventions: _____

        _____

5. The mother has just had twins, a boy and a girl. This is the result of the fertilization of _____. The term for this is _____. *(885-886)*

6. What are the maternal and the fetal risks in a multifetal pregnancy? *(886)*_____

    _____

    _____

7. Assessment of the presence of a hydatidiform mole is based on: *(886-887)* _____

_____

_____

8. Ninety-five percent of ectopic pregnancies occur in the _____. *(887)*

9. For an ectopic pregnancy, identify the signs and symptoms, the medical treatment, and the nursing interventions. *(888)*

   a. Signs and symptoms: _____

   _____

   _____

   b. Medical treatment:_____

   _____

   _____

   c. Nursing interventions: _____

   _____

   _____

10. A spontaneous abortion may be the result of: *(888-889)*_____

_____

_____

11. The nurse instructs the patient on the treatment for a threatened abortion, which includes: *(889)*_____

_____

_____

12. Treatment for an incompetent cervix usually includes: *(890)* _____

_____

_____

13. a. Diagnosis of placenta previa is made when the patient exhibits: *(891)*_____

_____

_____

b. The nurse instructs the patient to expect that treatment for placenta previa may include: *(891)* _____

_____

_____

14. a. Medical management of abruptio placentae includes: *(892-893)* _____

_____

_____

b. A priority nursing diagnosis and interventions for a patient with abruptio placentae are: *(892-893)*

_____

_____

15. What are the classic signs and symptoms of pregnancy-induced hypertension (PIH)? *(896)* _____

_____

_____

16. Medical management and nursing interventions for PIH usually include: *(897, 899-900)* _____

_____

_____

17. a. The nurse is assessing the postpartum patient and suspects a hemorrhage as a result of observing: *(894-895)*

_____

_____

b. Treatment for postpartum hemorrhage includes: *(894-895)* _____

_____

_____

18. a. What signs and symptoms may be exhibited by the patient who is experiencing disseminated intravascular coagulation (DIC)? *(893-894)*

_____

_____

b. What diagnostic tests are usually performed to determine the presence of DIC? *(893-894)* _____

_____

_____

19. a. In HELLP syndrome, what happens to the platelet, aspartate transaminase (AST), and alanine transaminase (ALT) levels? *(900-901)*

_____

b. What is a priority of care for a patient with HELLP? *(900-901)* _____

_____

20. What complications should the nurse be alert for when the mother is experiencing gestational diabetes? *(905-906)*

_____

_____

21. The patient with gestational diabetes should anticipate that the following diagnostic tests may be performed: *(906)*

_____

_____

22. Postpartum care of the adolescent mother focuses on: *(910-911)* _____

_____

_____

23. A 45-year-old woman is pregnant. She wants the nurse to tell her what complications of pregnancy are more common for women of her age and if the baby is at risk. The nurse recognizes that the risks for an older woman during pregnancy are: *(912)*

_____

_____

Multiple Choice

24. The patient being seen in the obstetrician's office has a missed abortion. The nurse recognizes that this means the patient will have: *(889)*
    1. malodorous bleeding, increased temperature, and cramping.
    2. expelled some, but not all, of the products of conception.
    3. fetal death and cessation of uterine growth.
    4. increased bleeding and a rupture of membranes.

25. The nurse notes that the most appropriate outcome for a woman experiencing hyperemesis gravidarum is: *(885)*
    1. relief of painful uterine contractions.
    2. absence of fetal withdrawal symptoms.
    3. platelets and prothrombin time and partial thromboplastin time (PT/PTT) values within normal limits.
    4. adequate caloric intake for maternal and fetal health.

26. The difference in the diagnosis of placenta previa and abruptio placentae is that abruptio placentae is associated with: *(891-892)*
    1. decreased vaginal bleeding.
    2. sudden uterine pain and rigidity.
    3. occurrence before 20 weeks gestation.
    4. decreased uterine size and poor contractions.

27. The nurse's assignment on the postpartum unit includes patients with the following assessment data. Which patient should the nurse see first? *(896)*
    1. The patient has saturated one feminine pad within the last 2 hours.
    2. The patient has a blood glucose of 160 mg/dL.
    3. The patient had a spontaneous abortion and is experiencing moderate dark bleeding.
    4. The patient has had a continuous headache, upset stomach, and blurred vision.

28. The patient is assessed by the nurse to be hyperglycemic as a result of the patient's: *(906)*
    1. pallor.
    2. hunger.
    3. depressed reflexes.
    4. diaphoretic state.

HIGH-RISK NEWBORN

Objectives

- Discuss the problems created by alcohol and drug abuse.
- Identify concerns related to preterm infants.
- Explain the hemolytic disease of the newborn.

29. How can human immunodeficiency virus and acquired immunodeficiency syndrome (HIV/AIDS) in the mother affect the fetus? *(904)*

_____

_____

30. What are the characteristic physical manifestations of a preterm infant? *(917)* _____

_____

_____

31. a. Signs and symptoms of newborn respiratory distress include: *(917)* _____

_____

_____

    b. Treatment for respiratory distress includes: *(917)*_____

_____

32. a. What is a problem seen in infants who are small for gestational age (SGA)? *(918)*_____

_____

    b. What tool can be used to estimate gestational age? *(918)* _____

_____

33. Hemolytic disease occurs when: *(918)*_____

_____

_____

34. Diagnostic tests that are used to determine possible hemolytic disease are: *(919)*_____

_____

_____

35. Fetal alcohol syndrome (FAS) may result in the newborn experiencing withdrawal symptoms. What will the nurse will observe for? *(921)*

_____

_____

Multiple Choice

36. The nurse recognizes that the chance of a hemolytic disease in the newborn is very low if which of the following findings are present? *(918)*
    1. Mother blood type O, infant blood type A
    2. Mother Rh negative, father Rh negative
    3. Mother Rh negative, infant Rh positive
    4. Mother blood type B, infant blood type A

NURSING

Objective

- Discuss nursing diagnoses related to high-risk conditions of the mother and newborn.

37. Identify the nursing assessment that should take place if the patient experiences bleeding during the pregnancy. *(892)*

_____

_____

38. Identify possible nursing diagnoses for patients experiencing the following complications.

a. Postpartum hemorrhage: *(895)* _____

_____

b. Gestational diabetes: *(906-907)* _____

_____

39. What teaching should be done about the prevention of an infection during pregnancy? *(902)*_____

_____

_____

40. a. What interventions are planned by the nurse for a pregnant patient with a preexisting cardiac condition? *(907-908)*

_____

_____

b. What is the primary difference in cardiopulmonary resuscitation (CPR) technique for the pregnant woman? *(907-908)*

_____

_____

41. Identify a nursing diagnosis that may be formulated for an adolescent patient during her first experience in labor and delivery. *(910)*

_____

_____

42. General nursing interventions for preterm infants include: *(917-918)* _____

_____

_____

43. Identify a nursing diagnosis that may be formulated for a preterm infant. *(917-918)*_____

_____

_____

44. Identify the nursing interventions for a patient with mastitis. *(902)* _____

_____

_____

Multiple Choice

45. The nurse is alert to a significant sign of pregnancy-induced hypertension (PIH), which is: *(896-897)*
    1. edema.
    2. bradycardia.
    3. weight loss.
    4. hypoglycemia.

46. The nurse anticipates that the medication to be given to the patient who is experiencing severe PIH will be: *(897-899)*
    1. meperidine (Demerol).
    2. heparin (Lovenox).
    3. oxytocin (Pitocin).
    4. magnesium sulfate.

47. The nurse is working with an adolescent mother with her first child. A likely nursing diagnosis that is formulated for this patient is: *(910)*
    1. knowledge deficit.
    2. fluid volume deficit.
    3. ineffective parenting.
    4. cardiac output, decreased.

48. The nurse is teaching the pregnant woman about prevention of infection. In discussing toxoplasmosis with the patient, the nurse specifically highlights: *(903)*
    1. hand hygiene after using the bathroom.
    2. vaccination with an attenuated virus.
    3. reduction of sexual relations.
    4. avoidance of cat litter.

49. The nurse suspects that a postpartum patient, being seen for her 6-week postdelivery check-up, is experiencing postpartum depression (PPD) as evidenced by the patient's signs and symptoms of: (Select all that apply) *(921-922)*
    1. showing little interest in her baby.
    2. talking extensively about her labor experience.
    3. discussing her level of fatigue due to getting limited sleep.
    4. stating that she is finding that she has limited maternal feeling towards her baby.

Health Promotion for the Infant, Child, and Adolescent

Answer Key: Textbook page references are provided as a guide for answering these questions. A complete answer key was provided for your instructor.

TERMS

Objective

- Define the key terms as listed.

1. Define the following terms.

a. Anticipatory guidance: *(926)* _____

   _____

b. Botulism: *(935)* _____

   _____

c. Nursing bottle caries: *(936)*_____

   _____

HEALTH PROMOTION

Objectives

- Identify the 10 "Leading Health Indicators" cited in *Healthy People 2010*.
- List three benefits of regular physical activity in children.
- State American Academy of Pediatrics recommendations for immunization administration in healthy infants and children.
- State three strategies to promote dental health.
- Identify six health benefits associated with exercise, activity, and sports.

2. Identify the "Leading Health Indicators" from *Healthy People 2010*. *(926)*_____

   _____

   _____

3. What are the target goals for the following health indicators? *(927)*

   a. Physical activity: _____

   _____

   b. Substance abuse: _____

   _____

   c. Responsible sexual activity: _____

   _____

   d. Immunizations: _____

   _____

4. What are the benefits of physical activity? *(927)* _____

   _____

   _____

5. How can the nurse promote physical activity for children? *(927-928)* _____

   _____

   _____

6. a. What factors contribute to obesity in children and adolescents? *(927)* _____

   _____

   _____

   b. What are the criteria to determine that a child is overweight or obese? *(927)* _____

   _____

   _____

7. The single most preventable cause of death and disease in the United States is _____
   _____. *(929)*

8. Identify social problems associated with substance abuse. *(929)* _____

   _____

   _____

9. What information should be taught about responsible sexual behavior? *(930)* _____

_____

_____

10. What is the newest guideline regarding immunization for children aged 2 to 23 months? *(932)* _____

_____

_____

11. Identify strategies to promote dental health for the following age groups. *(935-936)*

   a. Infant: _____

   _____

   b. Preschooler: _____

   _____

   c. Adolescent: _____

   _____

12. Identify at least one nutritional consideration for the following age groups. *(928)*

   a. Infant: _____

   b. Preschooler: _____

   c. Adolescent: _____

SAFETY MEASURES

Objectives

- State the causes and prevention of accidental poisonings.
- Describe four strategies to prevent aspiration of a foreign body.
- Discuss the proper use of infant safety seats in motor vehicles.
- List 10 safety precautions important in educating parents to prevent environmental injuries to children.

13. Identify measures to teach parents regarding vehicular safety for children. *(930-931)* _____

_____

_____

14. What strategies may be implemented to prevent accidental poisoning? *(936-938)* _____

_____

_____

15. Identify at least five strategies that may be implemented to prevent burns. *(938-939)* _____

_____

_____

16. For the nursing diagnosis *risk for poisoning, related to lack of knowledge of safeguards,* identify at least three interventions or areas for teaching. *(938)*

_____

_____

17. Identify strategies that may be implemented to prevent foreign body aspiration. *(938)*_____

_____

_____

Multiple Choice

18. Of the following, which age group is most at risk for foreign body aspiration? *(938)*
    1. 1 to 5 months
    2. 6 to 12 months
    3. 1 to 2 years
    4. 2 to 4 years

19. The nurse is developing a nutrition plan with the parents of an overweight 12-year-old child. The parents demonstrate an understanding of the plan by stating: (Select all that apply) *(928)*
    1. "Our child's calories from saturated fats should be no more than 7% daily."
    2. "We should not allow our child to drink milk that is less than 2% milk fat."
    3. "Our child should participate in some type of physical activity for at least 60 minutes a day."
    4. "We should be sure our child consumes foods from all the food groups except for grains."

20. Parents should be advised to monitor television shows that their children are viewing since _____ of these transmissions contain violence: *(929-930)*
    1. 21%
    2. 41%
    3. 61%
    4. 81%

Basic Pediatric Nursing Care

chapter

30

Answer Key: Textbook page references are provided as a guide for answering these questions. A complete answer key was provided for your instructor.

TERMS

Objective

- Define the key terms as listed.

1. Define the following terms.

   a. Birth defect: *(941)* _____

   _____

   b. En face position: *(943)* _____

   _____

   c. Mortality: *(952)* _____

   _____

   d. Weaning: *(955)* _____

   _____

HISTORICAL EVENTS

Objectives

- Identify events that had a significant impact on the health care of children in the United States in the twentieth century.
- Discuss the works of Dr. Abraham Jacobi and Lillian Wald.
- Describe the purposes and outcomes of the White House Conferences on Children from 1901 to the 1980s.

2. Identify the activities associated with the following people or events and their impact upon the development of pediatric care. *(941-942)*

   a. Dr. Abraham Jacobi: _____

   _____

   _____

   b. Lillian Wald: _____

   _____

   _____

   c. President Theodore Roosevelt (1909): _____

   _____

   _____

   d. President Franklin Roosevelt (1937): _____

   _____

   _____

   e. President Ronald Reagan (1987): _____

   _____

   _____

ROLE OF THE PEDIATRIC NURSE

Objectives

- Discuss the personal characteristics and professional skills of a pediatric nurse.
- Identify key elements of family-centered care.
- Describe areas in which growth and development principles are used by the pediatric nurse.

3. Identify the main purpose of pediatric nursing. *(943)* _____

   _____

   _____

4. What are the characteristics and role of a pediatric nurse? *(943)* _____

   _____

   _____

5. Identify the key elements in family-centered care. *(944)* _____

_____

_____

6. How are the principles of growth and development used by the nurse? *(946-947)* _____

_____

_____

7. Children with special needs are those children with: *(944)* _____

_____

_____

ASSESSMENT

Objectives

-   Discuss the physical assessment of a child using the head-to-toe method.
-   Describe metabolism and its relationship to nutrition in the child.

8. Identify the guidelines for performing a physical assessment on a child. *(948)* _____

_____

_____

9. a. The temperature of a 6-month-old is higher _____ or lower _____ (check one) than the temperature of an adolescent. *(949-950)*

    b. The preferred method of temperature measurement for a child is _____
    _____. *(949-950)*

10. How does the vision of a child change from infancy to preschool age? *(952)* _____

_____

_____

11. The nurse is teaching the parents about the development of teeth. The nurse instructs the parents that there are _____(number) of primary teeth that are usually all in place by the age of _____ years. The permanent teeth usually appear by age _____. *(952)*

12. The nurse is preparing to auscultate the child's lungs. Describe methods that can be used to have the child assist in this procedure. *(953)*

_____

_____

13. What spinal abnormalities may be found on an assessment of a child or adolescent? *(953-954)*_____

_____

_____

14. a. What is the usual specific gravity of the child's urine? *(954)* _____

_____

_____

  b. What is the usual urinary output for a 6-month-old? *(954)* _____

_____

_____

15. Identify the average time frame for the following foods or nutritional activities to be introduced. *(954-955)*

  a. Whole milk: _____

  b. Solid foods (cereals): _____

  c. Fruits and vegetables: _____

  d. Table food:_____

  e. Weaning: _____

16. Energy requirements for an infant are highest during _____. *(955-956)*

Multiple Choice

17. When assessing the child, the nurse knows that the expected annual rate of growth for a 4-year-old is: *(948)*
    1. 18 to 22 cm.
    2. 14 to 18 cm.
    3. 8 cm.
    4. 5 cm.

18. The temperature measurement site of choice for an infant is: *(950)*
    1. oral.
    2. rectal.
    3. tympanic.
    4. axillary.

19. When measuring the vital signs of a 2-year-old, the nurse expects that they will be close to the average findings for that age, which are: *(950)*
    1. P 110, R 25, BP 94/66.
    2. P 100, R 20, BP 110/80.
    3. P 90, R 22, BP 108/70.
    4. P 70, R 24, BP 120/76.

20. It is expected that the vocabulary for a preschooler will be characterized by: *(956-957)*
    1. three or four familiar words.
    2. 25 to 50 words.
    3. more than 250 words.
    4. full, complete sentences.

21. When measuring the vital signs of a 12-year-old, the nurse expects that they will be close to the average findings for that age, which are: *(950)*
    1. P 114, R 25, BP 94/66.
    2. P 100, R 20, BP 100/80.
    3. P 88, R 20, BP 110/70.
    4. P 70, R 24, BP 120/76.

22. The nurse is reviewing infant development and recognizes that an expected finding for this age group is: *(952)*
    1. having a visual acuity of 20/100 at birth.
    2. enjoying "peek-a-boo" games.
    3. controlling bladder elimination by 10 months.
    4. tripling of birth weight by 6 months.

23. The nurse is preparing to administer medication to a 4-year-old child in the pediatric clinic. The best communication with this child is: *(956-957)*
    1. "This may feel like a pinch."
    2. "Don't move when I give you this."
    3. "Do you want to take this medicine now?"
    4. "I will be coming back to give you a shot."

NURSING INTERVENTIONS

Objectives

- List general strategies to consider when talking with children.
- Outline several approaches for making the hospitalization of children a positive experience for them and their families.
- Discuss pain management in infants and children.
- Explain the needs of parents during their child's hospitalization.
- Discuss common pediatric procedures.
- Discuss administration of pediatric medications.
- Identify each category of age/behavior, accident/hazard, and prevention in the pediatric child.

24. Describe how the nurse would explain the sensations of blood pressure measurement to a child. *(957-958)*

_____

_____

25. Identify strategies that should be used when communicating with children. *(958)*_____

_____

_____

26. What should the nurse do to reduce anxiety for the child and the parents when the child is admitted to the hospital? *(958-959)*

_____

_____

27. Identify an example of an age-related concern or need of a hospitalized child, the child's possible response, and the positive parent or nurse responses. *(961)*

   a. Concern or need: _____

       _____

   b. Child's response: _____

       _____

   c. Parent or nurse response: _____

       _____

28. Pain is often underestimated in children. What can the nurse do to better assess the child's pain? *(960, 962)*

   _____

   _____

29. What methods in addition to pain medication can be used for relief or reduction of the child's pain? *(960, 962)*

   _____

   _____

30. How can the nurse increase the trust and participation of the parents in the care of the hospitalized child? *(963-964)*

   _____

   _____

31. a. The recommended approach for preparing children for procedures is to _____
        _____. *(964-965)*

    b. When is it best to prepare younger children for a procedure? *(964-965)* _____

        _____

32. The nurse is evaluating the bath given to the infant by the adult caregiver. Identify what actions indicate a need for additional teaching. *(965)*
    a. Using soap around the eyes _____
    b. Using a cotton-tipped swab to clean the ear canal _____
    c. Supporting the head while bathing the infant in a tub _____
    d. Washing the extremities after washing the face _____
    e. Washing the perineum in an anterior to posterior direction _____
    f. Retracting the foreskin of the male infant _____

33. How is gavage feeding for the infant provided? *(966-967)* _____

    _____

    _____

34. What are the different types of safety reminder devices that are used for children? *(967-968)* _____

    _____

    _____

35. How can urine be collected from an infant? *(968-969)* _____

    _____

    _____

36. Following a lumbar puncture, what should the nurse do for each of the following patients? *(970)*

    a. Young child: _____

       _____

    b. Adolescent: _____

       _____

37. Delivery of oxygen to a small infant is best provided with: *(970)* _____

    _____

    _____

38. What assessment findings by the nurse would indicate a need for the child's airway to be suctioned? *(971)*

    _____

    _____

39. When suctioning a child, the nurse should: *(971-972)*
    a. Set wall suction pressure at _____.
    b. Insert the tubing _____ (distance).
    c. Suction for _____ seconds.
    d. Suction no more frequently than every _____.

40. When monitoring intake and output for a child who is not toilet-trained, how is the urinary output measured? *(972)*

_____

_____

41. What can the nurse offer that will increase the fluid intake and provide variety for the child? *(972)*

_____

_____

42. The nurse is to administer an intramuscular (IM) injection to a 10-year-old patient. Identify the following parameters. *(974-975)*

   a. Site(s) to use:_____

   b. Needle selection: _____

   c. Pain reduction: _____

43. What intravenous (IV) site is used for children younger than 9 months of age? *(975)* _____

_____

_____

44. For enema administration to each of the following patients, identify the type and amount of solution to use as well as the procedure for tube insertion. *(977)*

	Type of Solution/Amount	Tube Insertion
a. 2 to 4 years old		
b. 11 years old		

45. Identify at least two strategies for administering oral medication to children. *(973)*_____

_____

_____

46. Provide examples of behaviors, accidents or hazards, and preventive measures from at least two different age groups. *(977-979)*

_____

_____

Multiple Choice

47. An older school-age child will be having surgery with anesthesia. The nurse intervenes to reduce anxiety by: *(964)*
    1. showing the child the mask that will be used for the anesthesia.
    2. introducing the child to a peer and having them discuss the procedure.
    3. reassuring the child that only the procedure that is supposed to be done will be completed.
    4. explaining the special type of sleep that will occur with the anesthetic.

48. The nurse is discussing nutritional needs of the toddler with his mother. She asks the nurse how to get him to eat right. The nurse responds appropriately by telling the mother that: *(966)*
    1. food should be left around the house where the child can pick it up when he feels like it.
    2. the child should be restrained in the high chair for meals.
    3. the child should sit at the table for scheduled meals.
    4. meals should be arranged about every 5 hours for the child.

49. A medication is to be administered to a child who has a body surface area (BSA) of 0.94 m². The recommended adult dose is 10 to 20 mg. What is the dosage range that is safe for this child? *(972-973)*
    1. 5.5 to 11 mg
    2. 9.4 to 18.8 mg
    3. 10 to 20 mg
    4. 11 to 22 mg

50. The nurse is confident that health promotion teaching has been successful when the mother of a 3-month-old states: (Select all that apply) *(946)*
    1. "My baby's birth weight should be doubled at the age of 6 months."
    2. "My baby's vision now is about 20/100."
    3. "My baby should enjoy parallel play by the age of 8 months."
    4. "My baby should enjoy toys that bang, shake, or can be pulled."

51. The nurse can calculate the normal systolic blood pressure of a 5 year old by adding: *(951)*
    1. 90 to the age in years.
    2. 83 to double the age in years.
    3. 50 to the age in years.
    4. 20 to triple the age in years.

52. The nurse prepares to give an injection to an infant in the vastus lateralis muscle. The father of the infant asks why the nurse is giving the infant an injection in the leg. The nurse is correct in responding: (Select all that apply) *(974-976)*
    1. "This is the easiest area to expose on the baby."
    2. "This site is a preferred site for infants because it is not close to vessels or nerves."
    3. "We have found in our clinic that this site is the least painful site for injections for infants."
    4. "This leg muscle is the most developed muscle in an infant, so it is a preferred site for injections."

Care of the Child with a Physical Disorder

Answer Key: Textbook page references are provided as a guide for answering these questions. A complete answer key was provided for your instructor.

CARDIOVASCULAR—HEMATOLOGIC—IMMUNE SYSTEM

Objectives

- Describe the etiology/pathophysiology, types of defects, clinical manifestations, diagnostic tests, and medical management of congenital heart defects.
- Describe the etiology/pathophysiology, clinical manifestations, diagnostic tests, medical management, nursing interventions, and patient teaching for children with iron deficiency anemia, sickle cell anemia, and aplastic anemia.
- Discuss the etiology/pathophysiology, clinical manifestations, diagnostic tests, medical management, nursing interventions, patient teaching, and prognosis for children with the coagulation disorders of hemophilia and idiopathic thrombocytopenia purpura.
- Describe the etiology/pathophysiology, clinical manifestations, diagnostic tests, medical management, nursing interventions, patient teaching, and prognosis for children with leukemia.
- Demonstrate an understanding of the etiology, pathophysiology, clinical manifestations, diagnostic tests, medical management, nursing interventions, patient teaching, and prognosis for children with acquired immunodeficiency syndrome (AIDS).
- Discuss the etiology/pathophysiology, clinical manifestations, diagnostic tests, medical management, nursing interventions, patient teaching, and prognosis for children with juvenile rheumatoid arthritis.

1. Identify the four categories of congenital heart disease and an example of a disorder from each category. *(985-992)*

   _____

   _____

2. What are the general clinical manifestations of congenital heart disease? *(987)*_____

   _____

   _____

3. Identify two nursing diagnoses for a child with congenital heart disease. *(987-989)* _____

   _____

   _____

4. What are the four defects found in tetralogy of Fallot? *(990)*_____

    _____

    _____

5. Identify the clinical signs and symptoms associated with tetralogy of Fallot and the medical management for the disorder. *(991)*

    _____

    _____

6. The child has a coarctation of the aorta. The nurse expects that the blood pressure measurement will be: *(992)*

    _____

    _____

7. For the following children, identify the signs and symptoms that may be manifested.

    a. Child with a hemoglobin (Hgb) value of 8 g/dL: *(992)*_____

        _____

        _____

    b. Child with a Hgb value of 4.5 g/dL: *(992)*_____

        _____

        _____

8. a. What is the etiology of iron deficiency anemia? *(992)* _____

        _____

        _____

    b. What information should be provided to the parents of the child who is to receive a liquid iron supplement? *(992)*

        _____

        _____

9. Identify an example of a type of sickle cell crisis and the treatment that should be implemented. *(995)*

    _____

    _____

10. Children who have hemophilia and idiopathic thrombocytopenic purpura (ITP) have similar problems. What common information can be provided to the parents of these children? *(995-997)*

_____

_____

11. Identify a nursing diagnosis for a child with leukemia and nursing interventions that may be implemented. *(998)*

_____

_____

12. Provide the following information regarding HIV infections. *(999-1001)*

    a. The majority of children are infected:_____

    b. The greatest physical threat is:_____

13. The mother of a child with HIV infection asks if the child should receive routine immunizations. The nurse responds by saying: *(1000-1001)*

_____

_____

14. What are the priority nursing diagnoses and outcomes for a child with juvenile rheumatoid arthritis? *(1003)*

_____

_____

Multiple Choice

15. A common sign or symptom of patent ductus arteriosus and septal defects is: *(987, 989-999)*
    1. murmur.
    2. chest pain.
    3. hypotension.
    4. headache.

16. The nurse recognizes that the majority of congenital heart defects are treated with: *(987-992)*
    1. diet.
    2. exercise.
    3. surgery.
    4. medication.

17. Screenings are being conducted on children for blood disorders. The nurse is aware that the most prevalent blood disorder is: *(992)*
    1. hemophilia.
    2. sickle cell anemia.
    3. iron deficiency anemia.
    4. idiopathic thrombocytopenic purpura.

18. The nurse instructs the parents of a child with iron deficiency anemia that iron absorption may be enhanced by: *(993)*
    1. giving the supplement with milk.
    2. giving the supplement with citrus juice or fruits.
    3. offering a chewable form once each day.
    4. waiting until the child has a full stomach to administer.

19. HIV testing for a child who is younger than 18 months of age is done with a: *(1000)*
    1. Western blot test.
    2. reticulocyte test.
    3. polymerase chain reaction (PCR) test.
    4. enzyme-linked immunosorbent assay (ELISA).

RESPIRATORY

Objective

- Discuss the etiology / pathophysiology, clinical manifestations, diagnostic tests, medical management, nursing interventions, patient teaching, and prognosis for children with disorders of the respiratory system, including respiratory distress syndrome, bronchopulmonary dysplasia, pneumonia, sudden infant death syndrome, upper respiratory tract infections, tonsillitis, croup, bronchitis, respiratory syncytial virus, pulmonary tuberculosis, cystic fibrosis, and bronchial asthma.

20. When do the signs and symptoms of respiratory distress syndrome (RDS) become apparent? _____ _____. *(1003)*

21. Treatment for RDS includes: *(1003-1004)* _____

    _____

    _____

22. Identify the common nursing interventions that are implemented for children experiencing respiratory disorders. *(1004-1005)*

    _____

    _____

23. The largest percentage of pneumonia in children is caused by _____ _____. *(1005)*

24. The priority nursing intervention for parents of children with sudden infant death syndrome (SIDS) is: *(1007)*

_____

_____

25. The new parent asks the nurse what the "Back to Sleep" campaign is all about. The nurse explains this campaign: *(1006)*

_____

_____

26. a. Acute pharyngitis is treated with _____. *(1007)*

    b. Diagnosis is based on _____. *(1007)*

    c. Nursing measures include _____. *(1007)*

27. What is a classic sign of croup (laryngotracheobronchitis)? *(1008-1009)* _____

_____

_____

28. What discharge instructions should be provided to the parents of a child who has had a tonsillectomy? *(1008)*

_____

_____

29. Describe the medical treatment for epiglottitis. *(1009)* _____

_____

_____

30. a. What is the pathophysiology involved in cystic fibrosis? *(1011-1012)* _____

    _____

    _____

    b. What is the medical management for this disorder? *(1011-1012)* _____

    _____

    _____

31. One of the most frequent causes of bronchial asthma is _____
_____. *(1013)*

32. For bronchial asthma, identify the following. *(1013-1014)*

    a. Signs and symptoms: _____

         _____

    b. Diagnostic tests: _____

         _____

    c. Medical treatment:_____

         _____

    d. Nursing interventions: _____

         _____

GASTROINTESTINAL

Objective

- Describe the etiology/pathophysiology, clinical manifestations, diagnostic tests, medical management, nursing interventions, patient teaching, and prognosis for children with disorders of the gastrointestinal system, including cleft lip and cleft palate, dehydration, diarrhea, gastroenteritis, constipation, gastroesophageal reflux, hypertrophic pyloric stenosis, intussusception, and Hirschsprung's disease.

33. a. The child is born with a cleft lip and palate. What are the primary problems for this child and the parents? *(1016-1017)*

         _____

         _____

    b. What is included in the postoperative care of the child after a repair of a cleft lip and/or palate? *(1016-1017)*

         _____

         _____

34. Identify the signs and symptoms of dehydration. *(1018)* _____

     _____

     _____

35. Children with gastrointestinal disorders are susceptible to fluid and electrolyte imbalances. Identify the nursing assessments and interventions that should be implemented by the nurse for these children. *(1019-1020)*

     _____

     _____

36. Identify a nursing diagnosis for a child with diarrhea and/or dehydration. *(1019)* _____

_____

_____

37. Identify how the diet may be modified for the following children who are experiencing constipation. *(1020)*

    a. Newborn: _____

        _____

    b. Older infant: _____

        _____

38. The primary sign that is seen in children with hypertrophic pyloric stenosis is _____
    _____. *(1022)*

39. The hallmark sign of intussusception is _____. *(1023)*

40. Treatment for intussusception includes: *(1023-1024)* _____

    _____

    _____

41. A neonate is suspected of having Hirschsprung's disease (megacolon) when _____
    _____. *(1024)*

42. The usual surgical treatment for Hirschsprung's disease (megacolon) involves: *(1024-1025)* _____

    _____

    _____

43. What are general nursing measures that can be implemented for children experiencing gastrointestinal disorders? *(1015-1025)*

    _____

    _____

44. The nurse is aware that cultural practices related to hernias may include: *(1026)* _____

    _____

    _____

Multiple Choice

45. For the child experiencing gastroenteritis with diarrhea, the nurse anticipates that treatment will include: *(1019)*
    1. nothing-by-mouth status (NPO).
    2. oral rehydration.
    3. no solid foods for 48 hours.
    4. traditional BRAT diet.

46. There are several different types of hernias that children may experience. The type of hernia that usually has spontaneous closure by the time the child is 2 years old is: *(1026)*
    1. hiatal.
    2. inguinal.
    3. umbilical.
    4. diaphragmatic.

47. The most severe type of hernia that is found within hours of delivery and requires immediate surgical repair is: *(1026)*
    1. hiatal.
    2. inguinal.
    3. umbilical.
    4. diaphragmatic.

48. The nurse anticipates that a child who is receiving pharmacologic treatment for gastroesophageal reflux will receive: *(1021)*
    1. Compazine (prochlorperazine).
    2. Mylanta (calcium chloride).
    3. Tagamet (cimetidine).
    4. Cerebyx (fosphenytoin).

GENITOURINARY

Objectives

- Discuss the parent teaching necessary to prevent urinary tract infection in infants and children.
- Discuss the etiology/pathophysiology, clinical manifestations, diagnostic tests, medical management, nursing interventions, and patient teaching for children with disorders of the genitourinary system, including nephrotic syndrome, acute glomerulonephritis, and Wilms' tumor.

49. What are the signs and symptoms manifested by the child who has nephritic syndrome (nephrosis)? *(1027)*

    _____

    _____

50. a. Acute glomerulonephritis is most often the result of _____
    _____. *(1028)*

    b. What diagnostic tests are performed to determine the presence of glomerulonephritis? *(1028)* _____

    _____

    _____

51. For acute glomerulonephritis, identify the following. *(1028)*

    a. Signs and symptoms: _____

    _____

    b. Treatment: _____

    _____

52. Wilms' tumor (nephroblastoma) is usually found by the parents when _____
    _____. *(1029)*

53. Treatment for Wilms' tumor includes: *(1029)* _____

    _____

    _____

Multiple Choice

54. The nurse is aware of the disease process and treatment for nephrosis. It is anticipated that treatment for the child will include: *(1027)*
    1. prevention of infection.
    2. increased sodium.
    3. decreased protein.
    4. diuretics.

55. The nurse expects that the treatment for a child with cryptorchidism will include: *(1030)*
    1. circumcision.
    2. fixation of the testes.
    3. extension of the urethra.
    4. bladder neck reconstruction.

ENDOCRINE

Objective

- Discuss the etiology/pathophysiology, clinical manifestations, diagnostic tests, medical management, nursing interventions, and patient teaching for children with disorders of the endocrine system, including hypothyroidism, hyperthyroidism, and diabetes mellitus.

56. What are the signs and symptoms associated with acquired hypothyroidism? *(1030)* _____

    _____

    _____

57. The dietary needs of the child with hyperthyroidism include: *(1031)* _____

_____

_____

58. a. Most children with diabetes mellitus require _____. *(1032-1033)*

    b. A laboratory test that is used to diagnose diabetes mellitus is _____. *(1032-1033)*

59. What information is necessary to include in a teaching plan for a newly diagnosed diabetic child and the parents? *(1033)*

_____

_____

Multiple Choice

60. The nurse recognizes that hyperthyroidism is most common in which one of the following age groups? *(1031)*
    1. Neonates
    2. Toddlers
    3. Preschoolers
    4. Adolescents

MUSCULOSKELETAL

Objective

- Discuss the etiology/pathophysiology, clinical manifestations, diagnostic tests, medical management, nursing interventions, and patient teaching for children with disorders of the musculoskeletal system, including hip dysplasia, Legg-Calvé-Perthes disease, osteomyelitis, talipes, Duchenne's muscular dystrophy, and septic arthritis.

61. In the illustration, identify what the nurse is assessing the infant for. *(1034-1035)* _____

_____

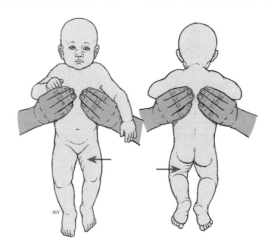

62. Identify the interventions that are important in the care of a cast or corrective device. *(1036)* _____

_____

_____

63. A child with Legg-Calvé-Perthes disease usually exhibits the following: *(1036)* _____

_____

_____

64. a.   What condition is present in the individual in the following illustrations? *(1038)* _____

_____

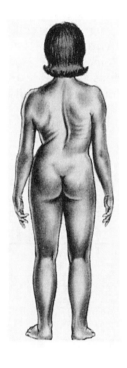 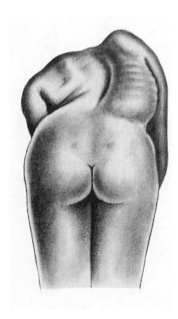

    b.   This condition is most often seen in what age group? *(1038)* _____

    c.   Treatment usually includes: *(1038)* _____

65. The goals of treatment for a child with Duchenne's muscular dystrophy are: *(1039)* _____

_____

_____

Multiple Choice

66. For a child with talipes equinovarus, the nurse explains to the parents that treatment usually includes: *(1038)*
    1. oxygen administration.
    2. medication therapy.
    3. skeletal traction.
    4. cast applications.

NEUROLOGIC

Objectives

- Discuss the etiology/pathophysiology, clinical manifestations, diagnostic tests, medical management, nursing interventions, patient teaching, and prognosis for children with disorders of the nervous system, including meningitis, encephalitis, hydrocephalus, cerebral palsy, seizures, spina bifida, neonatal abstinence syndrome, and neuroblastoma.
- Describe the etiology/pathophysiology, clinical manifestations, diagnostic tests, medical management, nursing interventions, patient teaching, and prognosis for children with lead poisoning.

67. For meningitis, identify the following. *(1040-1042)*

    a. Most common cause:_____

    _____

    b. Classic signs and symptoms: _____

    _____

    c. Diagnostic test:_____

    _____

    d. Medical treatment:_____

    _____

    e. Preventive measure: _____

    _____

68. What are the antenatal factors that may contribute to the development of cerebral palsy? *(1044)* _____

    _____

    _____

69. What are the nursing goals for a child with cerebral palsy? *(1045-1046)* _____

_____

_____

70. Identify whether the following interventions during a child's seizure are appropriate or require correction. *(1046-1047)*
   a. Keeping the side rails padded _____
   b. Moving the child to the bed when the seizure begins _____
   c. Loosening restrictive clothing _____
   d. Turning the child's head to the side _____
   e. Pushing a tongue blade between the teeth _____
   f. Staying with the child throughout the seizure _____

71. Nursing care for a child with a myelomeningocele includes: *(1047)* _____

_____

_____

72. For lead poisoning, identify the following. *(1049-1050)*

   a. Sources of lead:_____

   _____

   b. Prevention: _____

   _____

   c. Screening: _____

   _____

   d. Parent guidelines to reduce lead levels:_____

   _____

INTEGUMENTARY/COMMUNICABLE DISEASE

Objective

- Discuss the etiology/pathophysiology, clinical manifestations, diagnostic tests, medical management, nursing interventions, patient teaching, and prognosis for children with disorders of the integumentary system, including contact dermatitis, diaper dermatitis, eczema, seborrheic dermatitis, acne vulgaris, herpes simplex virus type I, tinea infections, candidiasis, and parasitic infections.

73. Identify some of the common areas for parent teaching for children with contact dermatitis, diaper rash, and eczema. *(1050-1052)*

_____

_____

74. The skin disorder most commonly associated with adolescents is _____ _____. *(1053)*

75. For an adolescent taking Accutane (isotretinoin), there will be specific monitoring for _____ _____ levels. *(1055)*

76. Identify a nursing diagnosis appropriate for a child with an integumentary disorder. *(1054)* _____

_____

_____

77. Identify actions that may be implemented to prevent traumatic injuries. *(1056)* _____

_____

_____

78. For a bacterial infection of the skin, identify an example of a nursing intervention. *(1057)* _____

_____

_____

79. The nurse is presenting information on parasitic infections to parents at a parent-teacher association (PTA) meeting. What information should be included? *(1058)*

_____

_____

80. Which childhood communicable diseases may have cardiac complications? *(1059-1060)* _____

_____

_____

Multiple Choice

81. A possible etiology associated with atopic dermatitis (eczema) is: *(1051-1052)*
    1. food allergy.
    2. bacterial infection.
    3. exposure to poison ivy.
    4. increased sebaceous gland activity.

82. The nurse determines that the child has varicella as a result of observing: *(1059)*
    1. pinpoint red spots with white specks in the buccal cavity.
    2. a pinkish-red maculopapular rash that began on the face.
    3. a rose-pink macular rash on the trunk.
    4. vesicles on an erythematous base.

SENSORY

Objective

- Discuss the etiology/pathophysiology, clinical manifestations, diagnostic tests, medical management, nursing interventions, and patient teaching for children with disorders of the sensory system, including otitis media, refractive errors (myopia, hyperopia), strabismus, periorbital cellulitis, and allergic rhinitis.

83. For otitis media, identify the following. *(1058, 1060-1062)*

    a. Reason for common occurrence in children: _____

    _____

    b. Signs and symptoms: _____

    _____

    c. Nursing interventions: _____

    _____

84. What behaviors usually indicate that a child may be having difficulty with vision? *(1063)*_____

    _____

    _____

85. Children experiencing health deviations and their parents may be referred to community agencies, organizations, and support groups. Identify at least three examples of available community resources. *(983-1066)*

    _____

    _____

86. A symptom of meningitis is _____, which manifests as pain and stiffness in the neck. *(1041)*

87. _____ is a condition caused by a decreased blood supply to the femoral head in children ages 3 to 12 years of age. *(1036)*

Multiple Choice

88. The nurse is assessing a school-age child for signs of scoliosis. Clinical manifestations for this disease include: (Select all that apply) *(1036-1037)*
    1. unequal hip and shoulder height.
    2. scapular and rib prominence.
    3. protrusion of the spine in the lumbar region.
    4. posterior rib hump that is visible when the child bends forward at the waist.

89. The parent of a child with strabismus demonstrates an understanding of the disorder by stating, "If we don't get treatment for this problem, my child may develop: *(1063)*
    1. myopia."
    2. hyperopia."
    3. presbyopia."
    4. amblyopia."

90. The nurse notices that a patient is constantly scratching the skin as a result of atopic dermatitis. The nurse knows that the scratching may lead to: *(1052)*
    1. subluxation.
    2. lichenification.
    3. pica.
    4. priapism.

Care of the Child with a Mental or Cognitive Disorder

chapter

32

Answer Key: Textbook page references are provided as a guide for answering these questions. A complete answer key was provided for your instructor.

TERMS

Objective

- Define the key terms as listed.

1. Define the following terms.

   a. Cognitive impairment: *(1067)* _____

   _____

   b. Failure to thrive: *(1073)* _____

   _____

   c. Intelligence quotient (IQ): *(1067)* _____

   _____

   d. Somatization disorder: *(1077)* _____

   _____

COGNITIVE DISORDERS

Objectives

- Identify six possible causes of cognitive impairment.
- Describe the clinical manifestations of Down syndrome.
- Discuss the appropriate nursing interventions required for caring for a patient with autism.

2. How are cognitive impairments classified? *(1067)* _____

   _____

   _____

3. For cognitive impairments, identify the following. *(1067-1068)*

   a. Possible etiology: _____

   _____

   b. Clinical manifestations: _____

   _____

   c. Diagnostic testing: _____

   _____

   d. Nursing interventions: _____

   _____

4. In 95% of the instances, Down syndrome is the result of _____. *(1069)*

5. Identify the clinical manifestations of Down syndrome. *(1069-1070)*_____

   _____

   _____

6. Medical care for the child with Down syndrome involves: *(1070)* _____

   _____

   _____

7. a. Identify the clinical manifestations of autism. *(1071)*_____

   _____

   _____

   b. Select all of the appropriate interventions for a child with autism. *(1071)*
      i. Encourage the parents to bring in favorite possessions. _____
      ii. Teach the parents about the cure for the disease. _____
      iii. Avoid establishing routines. _____
      iv. Provide brief, concrete communication with the child. _____
      v. Promote increased amounts and frequency of auditory and visual stimulation. _____

CHILD ABUSE

Objective

- State five physical and behavioral indicators that should arouse suspicion of child abuse.

8. Identify the different types of neglect. *(1072)* _____

_____

_____

9. a. What situational factors may contribute to child abuse? *(1072)* _____

_____

_____

   b. What cultural practices may be misinterpreted as abuse? *(1072)* _____

_____

_____

10. What is the role of the nurse regarding child abuse? *(1072-1074)* _____

_____

_____

11. Identify at least one behavioral and one physical indicator for each of the following. *(1073)*

   a. Physical neglect: _____

_____

   b. Physical abuse: _____

_____

   c. Sexual abuse: _____

_____

   d. Emotional neglect and abuse: _____

_____

LEARNING/BEHAVIORAL DISORDERS

Objectives

- Demonstrate an understanding of the medical management and the nursing interventions for the child with a learning disability.
- Describe four nursing interventions for the child with attention deficit hyperactivity disorder.

12. The nurse believes that the child is experiencing school avoidance. What physiologic and psychological assessment findings would lead to that belief? *(1074)*

_____

_____

13. How can the nurse assist and support the parents if the child is experiencing school avoidance? *(1074)*

_____

_____

14. For learning disabilities, identify the following. *(1074-1075)*

a. Possible etiology: _____

_____

b. Clinical signs and symptoms: _____

_____

c. Medical and nursing intervention: _____

_____

15. Management of an attention deficit hyperactivity disorder (ADHD) includes: *(1075-1076)* _____

_____

_____

16. Nursing interventions for a child with ADHD include: *(1076)* _____

_____

_____

MENTAL DISORDERS

Objectives

- Identify six clinical manifestations of depression in children.
- Discuss three nursing interventions for the child who is suicidal.

17. Describe depression and how it is diagnosed. *(1076-1077)* _____

_____

_____

18. In addition to medication, what treatment is provided for children who are depressed? *(1077)*_____

19. Identify a nursing diagnosis for a child who is depressed. *(1077)* _____

20. The nursing interventions for a child who is threatening or has attempted suicide include the following: *(1078-1079)*

21. The occurrence of recurrent abdominal pain (RAP) is mostly associated with: *(1079)* _____

Multiple Choice

22. The nurse anticipates that the child who is depressed will receive which one of the following medications? *(1077)*
    1. Prozac (fluoxetine)
    2. Ritalin (methylphenidate)
    3. Benadryl (diphenhydramine)
    4. Dexedrine (dextroamphetamine)

23. The nurse is alert to careful screening for signs of suicidal thoughts or behaviors. The age group that is most prone to suicide is: *(1077)*
    1. 5 to 7 years.
    2. 8 to 11 years.
    3. 12 to 14 years.
    4. 15 to 19 years.

24. The parents of a child with an IQ of 40 demonstrate an understanding of the child's capabilities by stating: (Select all that apply) *(1067)*
    1. "Our child is considered to have severe cognitive impairment."
    2. "Our child can be taught activities of daily living tasks and perform them on his own."
    3. "Our child is considered to have moderate cognitive impairment."
    4. "Our child will most likely never be able to perform self-care tasks, like bathing, on his own."

25. The school nurse is aware that the incidence of depression among high school girls is approximately: *(1076)*
    1. 15%.
    2. 25%.
    3. 35%.
    4. 45%.

Health Promotion and Care of the Older Adult

Answer Key: Textbook page references are provided as a guide for answering these questions. A complete answer key was provided for your instructor.

OVERVIEW OF AGING

Objectives

- Discuss health and wellness in the aging population of the United States in relation to the aims of *Healthy People 2010*.
- Identify some of the common myths concerning the older adult.
- Describe biological and psychosocial theories of aging.

1. It is estimated that by the year 2030, _____% of the population will be older than 65 years of age. *(1082)*

2. Identify health promotion measures for the older adult. *(1083-1084)* _____

_____

_____

3. There are many myths about older adults. Identify at least two of these myths. *(1086)* _____

_____

_____

4. The screenings that are recommended specifically for men older than age 50 are: *(1084)* _____

_____

_____

5. The first major legislation for financial support of older adults was the _____.
   This legislation established the programs for _____. *(1087)*

6. The two most frequent indicators of elder abuse are _____ and _____
   _____. *(1116-1117)*

7. The main goals of *Healthy People 2010* related to older adults are: *(1085)* _____

_____

_____

8. Erikson's developmental stage for an older adult is _____
_____. *(1086)*

Multiple Choice

9. The theory of aging that presumes the personality of older adults remains the same and behavior becomes more predictable is: *(1086)*
   1. activity theory.
   2. exchange theory.
   3. continuity theory.
   4. programmed aging.

PHYSIOLOGIC CHANGES THAT OCCUR WITH AGING

Objectives

- Describe changes associated with aging for each of the body systems.
- Discuss methods of assessment used for each body system.
- Compare how older adults differ from younger individuals in their response to illness, medications, and hospitalization.
- Discuss changes that occur with aging in intelligence, learning, and memory.

10. Identify at least three changes in the integumentary system that occur with aging. *(1088)* _____

_____

_____

11. Why is the older adult more susceptible to pressure ulcers? *(1089)* _____

_____

_____

12. Identify at least three changes in the gastrointestinal system that occur with aging. *(1090)*_____

_____

_____

13. Why is the older adult more susceptible to the following complications? *(1090-1091)*

   a. Dehydration:_____

   _____

   b. Obesity: _____

   _____

c. Weight loss:_____

_____

14. The older adult may experience problems with oral hygiene, such as _____
_____. *(1091-1092)*

15. a. Identify at least three changes in the urinary system that occur with aging. *(1094-1095)* _____

_____

_____

b. Provide an example of a medication that may be prescribed for urinary incontinence. _____
_____. *(1094-1095)*

16. Identify at least three changes in the cardiovascular system that occur with aging. *(1096)* _____

_____

_____

17. a. Identify at least three changes in the respiratory system that occur with aging. *(1098)*_____

_____

_____

b. A musculoskeletal change that occurs with aging and has an influence on respiratory function is ___
_____. *(1098)*

18. Identify at least three changes in the musculoskeletal system that occur with aging. *(1100)* _____

_____

_____

19. Identify at least three changes in the endocrine system that occur with aging. *(1103)* _____

_____

_____

20. The majority of older adults experience _____ diabetes. *(1103)*

21. Identify at least three changes in the reproductive system that occur with aging. *(1104)* _____

_____

_____

22. Identify the changes that occur with the aging process in the following sensory areas. *(1105)*

   a. Vision: _____

   _____

   b. Hearing:_____

   _____

   c. Taste and smell: _____

   _____

23. An age-related change in the neurologic function of the older adult is _____
   _____. *(1108)*

24. The goals for the patient with Alzheimer's disease are: *(1109-1110)*_____

   _____

   _____

25. What is the difference between a transient ischemic attack (TIA) and a cerebrovascular accident (CVA)? *(1111-1112)*

   _____

   _____

26. What changes occur in the pattern of rest and sleep for the older adult? *(1108-1109)*_____

   _____

   _____

27. Metabolism of medications is decreased in the older adult as a result of: *(1115-1116)*_____

   _____

   _____

Multiple Choice

28. A change that occurs in the integumentary system of the older adult is: *(1088)*
   1. decreased capillary fragility.
   2. increased hair pigmentation.
   3. increased sweat gland function.
   4. decreased vascularity of the dermis.

29. The recommended caloric intake for an average older adult is: *(1090)*
    1. 1000 to 1200 kcal/day.
    2. 1200 to 1500 kcal/day.
    3. 1800 to 2400 kcal/day.
    4. 3000 or more kcal/day.

30. Inadequate arterial circulation to the lower extremities of an older adult is usually evident with the presence of: *(1096-1097)*
    1. edema.
    2. excessive warmth.
    3. bounding pulses.
    4. cramping of the calf muscles.

31. The effects of medications given to older adults may be altered as a result of: *(1115-1116)*
    1. decreased adipose tissue.
    2. increased gastric secretions.
    3. increased total body water.
    4. increased sensitivity of brain receptors.

PSYCHOSOCIAL CHANGES THAT OCCUR WITH AGING

Objectives

- Describe ways finances and housing are major concerns for the older adult.
- Discuss common psychosocial events that occur to the older adult.
- Identify ways to preserve dignity and to increase self-esteem of the older adult.

32. Social reminiscence involves: *(1111)* _____

    _____

    _____

33. Identify the concerns of the older adult related to the following. *(1113-1114)*

    a. Finances: _____

    _____

    b. Housing: _____

    _____

34. Specify whether the following statements are true (T) or false (F). *(1086)*
    a. Cognitive abilities decrease in old age. _____
    b. Medication dosages for older adults may have to be reduced. _____
    c. The majority of older adults reside in nursing homes. _____
    d. A primary factor in the decreased sexual activity of the older adult is the lack of a sexual partner.

    _____

35. Losses experienced by the older adult may include: *(1087)* _____

_____

_____

36. A common response to loss in the older adult is _____. *(1087)*

37. Evaluate whether the following communication is appropriate. *(1120)*
    a. Calling the older woman "Grandma" _____
    b. Addressing the older adult by the first name _____

NURSING INTERVENTIONS

Objectives

- Identify nursing diagnoses appropriate to common health concerns of the older adult.
- Describe appropriate nursing interventions for common health concerns of the older adult.

38. For the following systems, describe the nursing assessment of the older adult. *(1088-1109)*

    a. Integumentary:_____

    _____

    b. Cardiovascular: _____

    _____

    c. Respiratory: _____

    _____

    d. Gastrointestinal:_____

    _____

    e. Urinary:_____

    _____

    f. Musculoskeletal: _____

    _____

    g. Neurologic: _____

    _____

39. Identify nursing interventions that may be implemented for the older adult who is experiencing constipation. *(1093-1094)*

_____

_____

40. What nursing interventions may be implemented for the patient with peripheral vascular disease? *(1097)*

_____

_____

41. Identify a possible nursing diagnosis and interventions for an older adult experiencing respiratory changes. *(1099)*

_____

_____

42. What interventions should be implemented by the nurse to reduce the chance of falls for the older adult in an acute or long-term care setting? *(1114)*

_____

_____

43. How can the nurse promote an older adult's sexuality? *(1105)* _____

_____

_____

44. Measures that should be used by the nurse to promote the patient's vision and hearing are: *(1107)*

_____

_____

45. Reality orientation includes: *(1109)* _____

_____

_____

46. Identify the nursing interventions for the older adult who is taking the following medications. *(1115-1116)*

    a. Antihypertensives: _____

    _____

    b. Diuretics: _____

    _____

c. Opioids and narcotics: _____

_____

47. Upon visiting the patient at home following hospital discharge, the nurse determines that the individual is at risk for the effects of polypharmacy, as evidenced by finding _____ _____. *(1115-1116)*

Multiple Choice

48. For the patient who is experiencing nocturia, the nurse intervenes by: *(1095)*
    1. restraining the patient.
    2. giving diuretics after 7:00 PM.
    3. providing fluids at bedtime.
    4. keeping the call bell within reach.

49. The older adult is experiencing pruritus. The nurse should: *(1089)*
    1. apply water-based lotions.
    2. use an antibacterial soap.
    3. increase the frequency of bathing.
    4. administer regular alcohol rubs.

50. For the older adult patient with dysphagia, the nurse should: *(1092)*
    1. add thickeners to liquids.
    2. feed the patient quickly to reduce fatigue.
    3. place the patient in low Fowler's position for meals.
    4. distract the patient by putting on music or the television.

51. The nurse anticipates that the patient who has osteoporosis will receive: *(1102)*
    1. raloxifene (Evista).
    2. amantadine (Symmetrel).
    3. tacrine (Cognex).
    4. trihexyphenidyl (Artane).

52. The patient is taking a nonsteroidal antiinflammatory agent for arthritis. Appropriate teaching includes instructing the patient to: *(1100)*
    1. take the medication with food.
    2. monitor blood glucose levels.
    3. observe for changes in hearing acuity.
    4. take the medication daily in the early morning.

53. The nurse is performing an admission assessment on a new resident in a long-term care facility. The nurse notes that the resident has kyphosis. This means that the resident an abnormal curvature in the: *(1102)*
    1. cervical spine.
    2. thoracic spine.
    3. lumbar spine.
    4. entire spine.

54. The nurse has been performing patient and family teaching for a male patient who has suffered a stroke. The family demonstrates an understanding of their loved one's condition of difficulty in speaking by stating: *(1112-1113)*
    1. "We hope the aphasia will improve as his condition improves."
    2. "Suffering from dysphasia is going to put him at risk for developing pneumonia."
    3. "Presybyopia is a difficult condition to deal with."
    4. "Having akinesia is going to make care at home very challenging."

55. During the integumentary assessment, the nurse notes that the patient suffers from pruritus. To help the patient with this condition, the nurse should encourage the patient to: (Select all that apply) *(1089)*
    1. avoid antibacterial soap during bathing.
    2. apply water-based lotions after bathing.
    3. bathe or shower daily using only warm water.
    4. be sure to rinse all soap from skin.

Basic Concepts of Mental Health

Answer Key: Textbook page references are provided as a guide for answering these questions. A complete answer key was provided for your instructor.

BASIC CONCEPTS

Objectives

- Describe the mental health continuum.
- Identify defining characteristics of persons who are mentally healthy and those who are mentally ill.
- Describe the parts of personality.
- Describe the factors that influence an individual's response to change.

1. What is the emphasis of mental health nursing? *(1122)* _____

   _____

   _____

2. In relation to treatment of mental illness, identify a major development or historical figure associated with the following time periods or events. *(1123-1125)*

   a. Greco-Roman period: _____

   b. Dark Ages: _____

   c. Late 1700s to 1800s: _____

   d. 1940s: _____

   e. 1970s: _____

   f. Omnibus Budget Reconciliation Act (OBRA):_____

3. What is meant by a *mental health continuum*? *(1125)* _____

   _____

   _____

4. Identify some general characteristics that are associated with mental illness. *(1125)* _____

   _____

   _____

5. For the following theorists, identify the basic concepts of personality development. *(1126)*

   a. Erikson: _____

   b. Freud:_____

6. Identify the following parts of the self. *(1126)*

   a. The part that strives for perfection and morality:_____

   b. The part that demands constant gratification: _____

   c. The part that decides when and how to act: _____

ALTERATIONS IN MENTAL HEALTH

Objectives

- Identify factors that contribute to the development of emotional problems or mental illness.
- Identify barriers to health adaptation.
- Identify sources of stress.
- Identify stages of illness behavior.
- Identify major components of a nursing assessment that focuses on mental health status.
- Identify basic nursing interventions for those experiencing illness or crisis.

7. What are the types and the effects of stressors on a person? *(1127)* _____

   _____

   _____

8. Identify the typical responses to the following types of anxiety. *(1127)*

   a. Mild anxiety:_____

   b. Moderate anxiety: _____

   c. Severe anxiety: _____

   d. Panic: _____

9. Describe how motivation, frustration, conflicts, and coping abilities affect an individual. *(1128)*_____

   _____

   _____

10. What are possible coping responses that may be used by individuals? *(1128)*_____

   _____

   _____

11. Common behaviors seen in illness are: *(1130)* _____

_____

_____

12. Identify examples of nursing diagnoses and patient outcomes that may be used in mental health nursing. *(1130)*

_____

_____

13. a. What are the goals of crisis intervention? *(1131)*_____

_____

_____

   b. Put the following steps of crisis intervention in order. *(1131)*
      i. Implement the plan of interventions. _____
      ii. Begin anticipatory planning. _____
      iii. Assess the situation and the individual involved. _____
      iv. Obtain assistance from significant others. _____

14. What considerations should be made for the older adult in regard to mental health? *(1130)* _____

_____

_____

15. Assessment of the patient's emotional state includes: *(1132)*_____

_____

_____

Multiple Choice

16. The nurse is assessing an individual's use of defense mechanisms. One of the parents has had a bad day at work and comes home and shouts at the children. This is an example of: *(1129)*
   1. projection.
   2. displacement.
   3. identification.
   4. reaction formation.

17. Regressive behavior is identified by the nurse when observing: *(1129)*
   1. the victim of sexual abuse who laughs while telling about the incident.
   2. an adolescent who participates in a lot of competitive sports.
   3. an 80-year-old acts as if an incident of incontinence did not occur.
   4. an 8-year-old begins sucking his thumb and wetting the bed when hospitalized for the first time.

18. An adolescent female patient tells the nurse that she often feels very "uneasy" but can't identify any specific reasons for this feeling. This patient is experiencing: *(1127)*
    1. stress.
    2. anxiety.
    3. crisis.
    4. mental illness.

19. A mentally healthy individual is capable of: (Select all that apply) *(1122)*
    1. adapting successfully to change.
    2. setting realistic goals.
    3. problem solving.
    4. enjoying life's activities.

20. Deinstitutionalization occurred in the 1950s as a result of: *(1124)*
    1. electroconvulsive therapy.
    2. the National Health Act.
    3. insulin shock therapy.
    4. the introduction of psychotherapeutic drugs.

Care of the Patient with a Psychiatric Disorder

Answer Key: Textbook page references are provided as a guide for answering these questions. A complete answer key was provided for your instructor.

MENTAL DISORDERS

Objectives

- List the five axes of *DSM-IV-TR* used to examine and treat mental illnesses.
- Identify and describe the major mental disorders.
- List five warning signs of suicide.

1. What is the difference between neurosis and psychosis? *(1135)* _____

_____

_____

2. What is the purpose of the *Diagnostic and Statistical Manual of Psychiatric Disorders, IV-TR? (1135-1136)*

_____

_____

3. What is the difference between anorexia nervosa and bulimia nervosa? *(1148)* _____

_____

_____

4. For organic mental disorders, what is the difference between delirium and dementia? *(1136)* _____

_____

_____

5. For the following, identify the classification of major mental disorder. *(1136-1139)*

a. Dementia: _____

b. Bizarre behavior, delusions, hallucinations: _____

c. Mood swings with manic episodes: _____

    d.   Irrational fear of a specific object or situation: _____

    e.   Poor impulse control, manipulation of others: _____

6. The inability for a person to experience happiness or joy is known as _____ _____. *(1141)*

7. The patient with schizophrenia suffers from _____, which is characterized by the inability to interpret information being received. *(1140)*

8. _____ often affects patients with schizophrenia, leaving them with a reduced content of speech. *(1140)*

9. The patient with schizophrenia shows little or no nonverbal expression of emotions. The nurse documents this as the patient displaying a _____. *(1141)*

10. _____ is exhibited by a person showing a lack of caring or a state of indifference to the world around him or her. *(1140)*

11. Identify the following types of delusions that are exhibited. *(1140)*

    a.   "The man on the radio is telling me to buy that car." _____

    b.   "That other patient put the idea in my head." _____

    c.   "They are listening to my conversations through the intercom." _____

12. What are the subtypes of schizophrenia? *(1141)* _____

_____

_____

13. Identify the warning signs of suicide. *(1142)* _____

_____

_____

14. What are the signs and symptoms of a panic attack? *(1145)* _____

_____

_____

15. Identify the different types of personality disorders. *(1147)* _____

_____

_____

16. Behavior that indicates a persistent desire to be the opposite sex is termed _____ _____. *(1147)*

TREATMENT

Objectives

- Identify basic interventions for patients experiencing various mental health problems.
- Describe the general care and treatment methods for patients experiencing mental health problems.
- Name two alternative medicines used for mental disorders.

17. What are some of the commonalities in nursing interventions for patients with mental disorders? *(1136-1139)*

_____

_____

18. Identify at least two considerations for older adult patients with mental disorders. *(1140)* _____

_____

_____

19. For a patient with a mood or anxiety disorder, the nurse can decrease stimuli by: *(1138-1139)*_____

_____

_____

20. What are specific treatments for patients who are depressed? *(1143)*_____

_____

_____

21. Identify precautions that should be taken for patients who are suicidal. *(1142)*_____

_____

_____

22. Identify whether the following statements are appropriate when preparing a patient for electroconvulsive therapy (ECT). *(1143)*
    a. Pain will be experienced. _____
    b. Confusion will decrease after a few hours. _____
    c. Grand mal seizures are experienced. _____
    d. Temporary memory loss is experienced after treatment. _____
    e. Most patients are kept in the hospital for 2 to 3 days afterward. _____

23. What medications are typically used for depression? *(1143)* _____

_____

_____

24. Identify possible patient outcomes for an individual who is experiencing depression. *(1144-1145)*_____

_____

_____

25. The patient in the clinic escaped the World Trade Center disaster on September 11, 2001. *(1146)*

   a. The nurse is alert to the possible development of: _____.

   b. Signs and symptoms of this disorder are: _____

_____

_____

26. The patient has come to the physician's office with nausea, vomiting, and stomach pain. The patient tells the nurse that she just got a new job with a lot of responsibilities, many people to supervise, and two projects that are due within the month. The nurse suspects that this patient may be experiencing: *(1148)*

_____

_____

27. The nurse who is working with patients with sexual disorders should first: *(1147)* _____

_____

_____

28. While completing an admission history, the patient asks the nurse not to tell anyone that he wants to end his life. The nurse should respond by: *(1150)*

_____

_____

29. What are the different types of psychotherapy? *(1149-1150)* _____

_____

_____

30. a. For the following, identify examples of medications, side effects, and nursing actions. *(1151-1152)*

   i. Antipsychotics: _____

_____

   ii. Antidepressants: _____

_____

   b. The nurse anticipates that intervention for tardive dyskinesia will include: *(1151-1152)* _____

_____

31. Identify examples of alternative therapies and their uses. *(1154)* _____

_____

_____

32. A serious problem that can occur with selective serotonin reuptake inhibitors (SSRIs) is _____

_____. *(1153)*

Multiple Choice

33. Communication with a patient who is in the manic phase of a bipolar affective disorder should: *(1138)*
    1. reinforce assertive behaviors.
    2. provide focus and consistency.
    3. offer verbal reminders of the day and date.
    4. encourage lengthy expression of thoughts and feelings.

34. The nurse anticipates that the patient with an obsessive-compulsive disorder will receive: *(1151-1152)*
    1. Lithobid (lithium carbonate).
    2. Haldol (haloperidol).
    3. Thorazine (chlorpromazine).
    4. Anafranil (clomipramine).

35. The nurse is aware that a patient who is receiving lithium therapy needs to have an adequate intake of: *(1151-1152)*
    1. calcium.
    2. sodium.
    3. magnesium.
    4. potassium.

36. A patient tells you that he is hearing voices right now that are telling him not to eat. The nurse's best response is: *(1137)*
    1. "What did the voices tell you not to eat?"
    2. "Did the voices say that you couldn't even eat snacks?"
    3. "I don't think that the voices would tell you not to eat anything."
    4. "I don't hear any voices. Tell me what you are experiencing now."

37. The nurse is given the assignment for the day. Based on the report provided, the nurse prioritizes and decides to see which one of the following patients first? *(1142)*
    1. The patient had ECT therapy 30 minutes ago.
    2. The patient has refused to take the prescribed medication.
    3. The patient has said, "I am going to end this suffering."
    4. The patient identified that "voices" told him not to eat the food today.

38. The patient experiencing drug-induced psychosis complains to the nurse while on the behavioral health unit that he has been smelling natural gas in the air for the past 2 days. This patient is experiencing: *(1140)*
    1. delusions.
    2. depression.
    3. mania.
    4. hallucinations.

39. Signs and symptoms of schizophrenia typically include: (Select all that apply) *(1140)*
    1. phobias.
    2. delusions.
    3. mania.
    4. paranoia.

40. Which patient statement would indicate a compulsion? *(1146)*
    1. "I can't stop thinking about my hand towels in the bathroom being out of place on the towel rack."
    2. "I had to drive back home 8 times this morning to be sure I locked my front door."
    3. "Those voices in my head are driving me crazy. Can you make them stop?"
    4. "It terrifies me to think about going fishing this weekend because I know there may be spiders in the boat."

41. Mrs. B. suffers from bipolar disorder and is displaying an outgoing personality, productivity in her work, and great optimism. What phase of bipolar disorder is she experiencing? *(1143)*
    1. Manic
    2. Depressive
    3. Cyclothymic
    4. Hypomanic

42. A wife complains that her husband must be neurotic. What signs and symptoms would you expect the husband to display? (Select all that apply) *(1135)*
    1. Nervousness
    2. Low self-esteem
    3. Psychosis
    4. Phobias

Care of the Patient with an Addictive Personality

Answer Key: Textbook page references are provided as a guide for answering these questions. A complete answer key was provided for your instructor.

ADDICTION

Objectives

- Name two traits attributed to an addictive personality.
- Describe the three stages of dependence.
- Describe one legal effort that has decreased the incidence of substance abuse.

1. What are the four elements of addiction? *(1158)* _____

   _____

   _____

2. a.   An amazing statistic is that _____% of children who begin drinking at or before the age of 14 develop alcoholism. *(1158)*

   b.   _____% of all motor vehicle accident deaths and fatal injuries are associated with alcohol. *(1159)*

3. In relation to drugs, how has federal law influenced the health care provider? *(1159)* _____

   _____

   _____

4. Provide examples of behaviors seen in the early, middle, and late stages of dependence. *(1159)* _____

   _____

   _____

5. Provide examples of the subjective and objective data that typically emerge in the course of completing a nursing assessment that may be indicative of substance abuse. *(1162)*

   _____

   _____

6. What diagnostic tests may be used to determine the possibility of substance abuse? *(1162)* _____

_____

_____

7. Give examples of possible nursing diagnoses and outcomes for addicted patients who have physical and emotional needs. *(1163)*

_____

_____

8. What support groups are available for individuals who are seeking to stop their addictive behavior? *(1164-1165)*

_____

_____

9. The goal of treatment centers is _____. *(1165)*

ALCOHOLISM

Objectives

- Describe three disorders associated with alcoholism.
- Explain the two phases of recovery: detoxification and rehabilitation.

10. a. What are some of the possible contributing factors to alcoholism? *(1160)* _____

_____

_____

   b. A questionnaire that is helpful in determining alcohol abuse is: _____
_____. *(1161)*

11. Alcohol is classified as a _____. *(1160)*

12. One of the reasons that binge drinking by college students is such a hazard is because rapid, large-quantity consumption of alcohol can lead to _____
_____. *(1161)*

13. Identify the electrolyte and nutritional imbalances that may occur with alcoholism and the reason they occur. *(1160-1161)*

_____

_____

14. What complications or problems are associated with fetal alcohol syndrome? *(1161)* _____

_____

_____

15. For the following disorders associated with alcoholism, identify the signs and symptoms and when they usually begin to be seen. *(1161)*

   a. Alcohol withdrawal syndrome:_____

        _____

   b. Delirium tremens: _____

        _____

   c. Korsakoff's psychosis and Wernicke's encephalopathy: _____

        _____

16. Identify the effects that alcohol has on the following body systems. *(1162)*

   a. Gastrointestinal:_____

        _____

   b. Hepatic:_____

        _____

   c. Cardiovascular: _____

        _____

   d. Respiratory: _____

        _____

   e. Musculoskeletal: _____

        _____

17. For the phases of recovery, identify the nursing interventions that should be implemented. *(1163)*

   a. Acute or detoxification:_____

        _____

   b. Rehabilitation: _____

        _____

Multiple Choice

18. A patient has a blood alcohol level of 475 mg/dL (0.475%). The nurse expects that this patient will exhibit: *(1161)*
    1. stupor or coma.
    2. stumbling and blurred vision.
    3. clumsiness and emotional changes.
    4. mild sedation with pleasant, relaxed attitude.

DRUG ABUSE

Objective

- Identify six types of drugs of abuse.

19. Substance abuse affects what part of the brain? *(1160-1161)* _____

    This may alter the person's _____ .

20. Identify the signs and symptoms of central nervous system (CNS) depressants. *(1167)* _____

    _____

    _____

21. Identify at least six commonly abused drugs. *(1166)* _____

    _____

    _____

22. What drugs have been associated with "date rape"? *(1167)* _____

    _____

    _____

23. The most widely abused opioid is_____. *(1167)*

24. For opioids, identify the signs and symptoms of an overdose and withdrawal. *(1167)* _____

    _____

    _____

25. a. What is the use of methadone? *(1167)* _____

    _____

    _____

    b. What drug is being used to obtain better effects than methadone? *(1167)* _____

26. Identify the different types of stimulants. *(1167-1168)* _____

_____

_____

27. What are the signs and symptoms of stimulant use? *(1168)* _____

_____

_____

28. Medications that are used to decrease the craving for cocaine are: *(1168)* _____

_____

_____

29. The nurse is assessing a patient who is suspected of chronic cocaine abuse. The nurse will expect to find: *(1168)*

_____

_____

30. What are the complications of amphetamine use? *(1168)* _____

_____

_____

31. A patient has been abusing a hallucinogen. What serious problems may this patient develop? *(1168-1169)*

_____

_____

32. a. What signs and symptoms may be seen with the use of ecstasy (methylenedioxymethamphetamin, or MDMA)? *(1169)*

_____

_____

b. What makes this drug so dangerous for abuse? *(1169)* _____

_____

_____

33. a. Cannabis is also known as_____. *(1170)*

b. Identify possible effects of its use: *(1170)* _____

_____

_____

34. Identify examples of gateway drugs. *(1158-1170)* _____

_____

_____

35. What are some of the common effects of inhalant use? *(1170-1171)* _____

_____

_____

Multiple Choice

36. A co-worker states that he has had too much caffeine and wants to eliminate it from his diet. He should be advised to drink: *(1168)*
    1. coffee.
    2. cola drinks.
    3. orange juice.
    4. hot chocolate.

37. The patient is quitting smoking cigarettes. The withdrawal from nicotine may result in the patient having: *(1168)*
    1. lethargy.
    2. improved concentration.
    3. decreased heart rate.
    4. decreased appetite.

38. The nurse is working with patients who have abused the following substances. The nurse is *not* anticipating to see withdrawal signs and symptoms with the patient who uses: *(1168-1169)*
    1. cannabis.
    2. CNS stimulants.
    3. CNS depressants.
    4. hallucinogens.

39. A college student who has used marijuana since early high school is diagnosed with amotivational cannabis syndrome. Characteristics of this disorder include: (Select all that apply) *(1170)*
    1. unusual irritability.
    2. frequent mood swings.
    3. depression.
    4. psychosis.

40. Upon admission to a rehabilitation unit, a patient states that he has noticed that he must smoke more marijuana to "get high" than he used to. This patient is exhibiting: *(1170)*
    1. bruxism.
    2. tolerance.
    3. addiction.
    4. withdrawal.

41. Addiction can occur with which of the following substances? (Select all that apply) *(1158-1159)*
    1. Alcohol
    2. Tobacco
    3. Caffeine
    4. Antidepressants

42. Methylenedioxymethamphetamine (MDMA) is an example of which classification of drugs? *(1169)*
    1. Opioids
    2. Amphetamines
    3. Depressants
    4. Hallucinogens

IMPAIRED NURSE

Objective

- Describe steps taken to help the chemically impaired nurse.

43. The chemically impaired nurse may exhibit the same signs and symptoms of abuse as any other individual who is addicted. What are the specific role-related signs or behaviors that may be seen by co-workers? *(1173)*

_____

_____

44. Identify the assistance that is available for the chemically impaired nurse. *(1173)* _____

_____

_____

45. What is the Healthcare Integrity and Protection Data Bank (HIPDB)? *(1173)*_____

_____

_____

Home Health Nursing

Answer Key: Textbook page references are provided as a guide for answering these questions. A complete answer key was provided for your instructor.

TERMS

Objective

- Define the key terms as listed.

1. Define the following terms.

   a. Medicare: *(1187)* _____

   _____

   b. Medicaid: *(1187)*_____

   _____

OVERVIEW AND TRENDS

Objectives

- List at least three types of home health agencies.
- Discuss new developments that are occurring in home health care, including remote electronic monitoring.

2. Identify the historical developments in home health care associated with the following dates. *(1178-1179)*

   a. 1600s: _____

   _____

   b. 1796: _____

   _____

   c. 1893: _____

   _____

d. 1909: _____

_____

e. 1935: _____

_____

f. 1965: _____

_____

g. 1983: _____

_____

3. What special considerations are made by the nurse in regard to the older adult and home care? *(1179)*

_____

_____

4. For the following types of home health agencies, provide an example and state who the agency is governed by. *(1181)*

a. Voluntary: _____

_____

b. Official: _____

_____

c. Proprietary: _____

_____

5. What are some of the regulations that must be followed by home health agencies? *(1179-1180)* _____

_____

_____

6. Identify at least two of the changes that are occurring in home health care. *(1180, 1182)* _____

_____

_____

7. What factors have increased the need for home health care? *(1180, 1182)* _____

_____

_____

8. Discuss telemonitoring in home health care. *(1180)* _____

_____

_____

SERVICES

Objectives

- Describe how home health care differs from community and public health care services.
- List at least four services that may be provided by home health care.
- Describe two major ways home care differs from hospital care.
- Define skilled nursing services.
- Describe the role of the LPN/LVN in the delivery of skilled nursing care.
- Relate the nursing process to home health care practice.
- Relate seven steps to breaking through cultural barriers to communication.

9. Identify the types of services that are provided by home health agencies. *(1182)* _____

_____

_____

10. What is meant by *skilled nursing care*? *(1182)*_____

_____

_____

11. The service goals of home health nursing are: *(1182)* _____

_____

_____

12. The role of the LPN/LVN in home health care is: *(1183)* _____

_____

_____

13. Where do home health care referrals usually come from? *(1185)* _____

_____

_____

14. What are the steps in the home health care process once the patient is referred? *(1185)*_____

_____

_____

15. Identify what is included in the admission of a patient to the home health care agency. *(1185-1186)*_____

_____

_____

16. What type of documentation is used in home health care, and what methods may be used to complete it? *(1186)*

_____

_____

17. The major principles of total quality management or quality improvement are: *(1187)* _____

_____

_____

18. Identify at least two steps that may be taken to break through the cultural barriers to communication. *(1189)*

_____

_____

19. What activities may be delegated to a home health aide? *(1185)*_____

_____

_____

Multiple Choice

20. The home health nurse will refer the patient who requires promotion of independence with the use of a self-help device to the: *(1184)*
    1. social worker.
    2. physical therapist.
    3. home health aide.
    4. occupational therapist.

21. The home health nurse should provide safety information to the patient and family members for home oxygen use. The information should include: (Select all that apply) *(1183)*
    1. the use of petrolatum-based lubricant on the lips is allowed.
    2. "No Smoking" signs should be posted on the front and back doors.
    3. frequent oral hygiene is necessary owing to the drying of mucous membranes.
    4. only wool blankets should be used by the patient.

REIMBURSEMENT

Objectives

- Summarize governmental financing for home health nursing.
- List two sources of reimbursement for home care services.

22. Identify the effect that federal financing has had on home health care since 1997. *(1179)*_____

_____

_____

23. Medicare and Medicaid require that the plan of treatment is: *(1187)* _____

_____

_____

24. What are the Medicare requirements for the following services? *(1184-1185)*

a. Physical therapy: _____

_____

b. Speech therapy: _____

_____

c. Home health aide: _____

_____

Long-Term Care

Answer Key: Textbook page references are provided as a guide for answering these questions. A complete answer key was provided for your instructor.

REGULATIONS AND REIMBURSEMENT

Objectives

- Discuss federal and state regulations related to long-term care.
- Identify the sources of reimbursement for long-term care services.

1. What did the Omnibus Budget Reconciliation Act of 1987 (OBRA) do for long-term care? *(1201)* _____

_____

_____

2. What did OBRA do for the LPN/LVN in long-term care? *(1201)* _____

_____

_____

3. Identify the legal and ethical issues related to long-term care. *(1201)* _____

_____

_____

4. What sources of reimbursement are available for long-term care facilities? *(1201)* _____

_____

_____

5. Describe what is provided under the Program of All-Inclusive Care for the Elderly (PACE). *(1196)*

_____

_____

PATIENTS AND SERVICES

Objectives

- Describe settings of long-term care services.
- Identify patients of long-term care services.
- Define chronic and acute health services.
- Describe goals of long-term care health services.
- Describe long-term care nursing services.
- Describe services available from each type of agency: home health agency, hospice agency, adult day care, assisted living facility, continuing care community, long-term care facility.

6. What are some of the cultural and ethnic considerations for long-term care? *(1194)*_____

_____

_____

7. Identify the different settings for long-term care, and provide an example of each type. *(1194-1199)*

_____

_____

8. For the patient who has a terminal disease, the appropriate referral is to a: *(1196)* _____

_____

_____

9. The patient requires stimulation and supervision while her daughter is at work. What type of setting is recommended? *(1196-1197)*

_____

_____

10. Assisted living offers what types of services for its residents? *(1197)*_____

_____

_____

11. How does a continuing care retirement community differ from an assisted living community? *(1198)*

_____

_____

12. Identify the advantages or benefits associated with subacute care. *(1198)* _____

_____

_____

13. What is the profile of the patient who requires long-term care in an institutional setting? *(1199)*_____

_____

_____

14. Explain how the administration of medications can differ in long-term care facilities. *(1200)*_____

_____

_____

15. What is the purpose of a resident assessment instrument (RAI), and what is involved in the assessment? *(1202)*

_____

_____

16. How does documentation in a long-term care facility differ from that in a hospital setting? *(1202)*_____

_____

_____

17. Identify a nursing diagnosis for a resident in a long-term care facility who has safety needs. *(1203)*_____

_____

_____

18. Identify the usual time frame for the following nursing activities in a long-term care facility. *(1199-1200)*

   a. Making rounds to monitor residents: _____

   b. Reviewing the plan of care: _____

   c. Charting for a resident who has no change in status: _____

19. What are two ethical issues that may arise in relation to long-term care? *(1201)* _____

_____

_____

Multiple Choice

20. The nurse is assisting in training a new certified nurse assistant (CNA) at a long-term care facility. The nurse would be correct in describing activities of daily living (ADLs) as: (Select all that apply) *(1195)*
   1. bathing.
   2. brushing teeth.
   3. exercise.
   4. ambulating.

21. Mr. M. is requiring extensive wound care and intravenous antibiotics due to an infection in his surgical wound. A _____ will best meet his needs. *(1198)*
    1. long-term care facility
    2. subacute unit
    3. residential care facility
    4. hospice unit

22. _____ defines requirements for the quality of care given to residents and covers many aspects of institutional life, including nutrition, staffing, and qualifications required of personnel. *(1201)*
    1. Medicare
    2. HCFA
    3. OBRA
    4. Medicaid

23. The adult children of an elderly couple are concerned about their parents and feel that the parents, at times, need assistance with bathing, dressing, and taking their medication. Both of the parents are alert and oriented at all times. They are mobile, but suffer from arthritis. The setting that the parents would most benefit from would be: *(1197)*
    1. a skilled nursing facility.
    2. a subacute unit.
    3. an adult day care facility.
    4. an assisted living community.

24. The interdisciplinary team at a long-term care facility is meeting to discuss the care plan of one of the residents, Mrs. H. Who should attend this meeting? (Select all that apply) *(1199-1200)*
    1. Mrs. H.
    2. The activities director
    3. The director of nursing
    4. The nursing unit manager

Rehabilitation Nursing

chapter

39

Answer Key: Textbook page references are provided as a guide for answering these questions. A complete answer key was provided for your instructor.

TERMS

Objective

- Define the key terms as listed.

1. Define the following terms.

    a. Interdisciplinary rehabilitation team: *(1209)* _____

    _____

    b. Multidisciplinary rehabilitation team: *(1209)* _____

    _____

    c. Transdisciplinary rehabilitation team: *(1210)* _____

    _____

REHABILITATION NURSING

Objectives

- Define the philosophy of rehabilitation nursing.
- Describe the interdisciplinary rehabilitation team concept and the function of each team member.
- Discuss specialized practice characteristics of the rehabilitation nurse.

2. State the philosophy of rehabilitation nursing. *(1206)* _____

    _____

    _____

3. What are the different needs for rehabilitation? *(1206-1207)* _____

    _____

    _____

4. Identify at least two focus areas related to chronic illness and disability from *Healthy People 2010*. *(1207)*

_____

_____

5. Identify a general goal of rehabilitation. *(1209)* _____

_____

_____

6. a. Who are the members of the rehabilitation team, and what are their roles? *(1210)* _____

_____

_____

   b. Describe the role of the rehabilitation nurse. *(1210)* _____

_____

_____

7. The comprehensive rehabilitation plan has the following characteristics. *(1211)*

   a. The plan is started: _____ .

   b. The plan is reevaluated: _____ .

   c. The plan is developed based upon: _____ .

Multiple Choice

8. Two patients are admitted to a rehabilitation hospital. Both have the same medical condition, but one patient is not able to manage, physically or emotionally, the adaptation that is required. This patient is best described as having a: *(1207)*
   1. disability.
   2. handicap.
   3. chronic illness.
   4. functional limitation.

DISABLING DISORDERS

Objectives

- Discuss two major disabling conditions.
- Provide nursing diagnoses, goals, interventions, and evaluation and outcome criteria for two major disabling conditions.

9. a. Discuss characteristics of chronicity. *(1207)* _____

   _____

   _____

   b. What are two of the major disabling conditions? *(1207)* _____

   _____

   _____

10. Define the following terms. *(1214)*

    a. Quadriplegia: _____

    _____

    b. Paraplegia: _____

    _____

    c. Paresis:_____

    _____

11. For the following problems associated with spinal cord injuries, describe what happens, the signs and symptoms that are seen, and the nursing interventions. *(1217)*

    a. Postural hypotension: _____

    _____

    _____

    b. Heterotopic ossification: _____

    _____

    _____

12. What are the two types of head injuries? *(1217)*_____

    _____

    _____

13. Identify the characteristic rehabilitation needs of patients who have suffered traumatic brain injuries. *(1218-1219)*

    _____

    _____

14. In the rehabilitative assessment of a patient following a traumatic brain injury (TBI), the nurse may expect to find: *(1218)*

_____

_____

15. For patients with a spinal cord injury or a traumatic brain injury, identify possible nursing diagnoses and outcomes. *(1216-1219)*

_____

_____

Multiple Choice

16. The patient experienced a spinal cord injury at the T6–T9 level. The nurse anticipates that the patient should be able to: *(1216)*
    1. assist with activities of daily living (ADLs).
    2. ambulate independently.
    3. drive with hand controls.
    4. control bowel and bladder function.

17. The construction worker sustained an injury to C7 after a fall at a work site. The nurse anticipates that this patient will be: *(1216)*
    1. nonambulatory.
    2. ADL-independent.
    3. independent in bladder care.
    4. returning to prior job responsibilities.

18. The emergency squad brought in the patient following an accident at home. One of the squad members tells the nurse that the patient, according to the spouse, was unconscious for 1½ hours. This head injury is described as: *(1218)*
    1. mild.
    2. moderate.
    3. severe.
    4. catastrophic.

19. The patient has a spinal cord injury above the level of T5. While assisting with hygienic care, the nurse notices that the patient is diaphoretic and shivering, and he states that he has a headache. Upon assessment, it is found that his blood pressure is elevated. The nurse's next action should be to: *(1217)*
    1. position the patient flat.
    2. provide analgesic medication.
    3. check for bladder distention.
    4. cover the patient with blankets.

20. The nurse anticipates that treatment for the patient with a spinal cord injury and deep-vein thrombosis will include: (Select all that apply) *(1217)*
    1. fluid restriction.
    2. assessment for postural hypotension.
    3. application of heat.
    4. prescription of anticoagulants.

ISSUES IN REHABILITATION

Objectives

- Discuss the importance of returning home and preparing for community reentry.
- Recognize the importance and significance of family-centered care in rehabilitation.
- Recognize the uniqueness of pediatric and gerontologic rehabilitation nursing.

21. Differentiate between polytrauma and posttraumatic stress disorder (PTSD). *(1213-1214)* _____

_____

_____

22. Identify the cornerstones of rehabilitation. *(1209)* _____

_____

_____

23. Identify the key elements of family-centered care. *(1212)* _____

_____

_____

24. How are pediatric and gerontologic rehabilitation different from adult rehabilitation? *(1212-1213)* _____

_____

_____

Hospice Care

Answer Key: Textbook page references are provided as a guide for answering these questions. A complete answer key was provided for your instructor.

PHILOSOPHY AND ORGANIZATION

Objectives

- Discuss the philosophy of hospice care.
- Differentiate between palliative care and curative care.
- Name the members of the interdisciplinary team and explain their roles.
- Discuss the role of hospice in families' bereavement period.

1. What was the origin of the concept of hospice care? *(1222)* _____

   _____

   _____

2. The focus and the goals of hospice care are: *(1224)* _____

   _____

   _____

3. Identify the professionals in the core interdisciplinary hospice team and their roles. *(1225)* _____

   _____

   _____

4. What is the purpose of the bereavement team? *(1226)* _____

   _____

   _____

HOSPICE PATIENTS AND COMMON SYMPTOMS

Objectives

- Discuss four criteria for admission to hospice care.
- List three common symptoms related to a terminal illness.

- Discuss the usefulness of pain assessments and when assessments should be completed.
- Develop a care plan with patient goals related to these symptoms.

5. The usual criteria for admission of a patient to hospice are: *(1224)* _____

_____

_____

6. What is included in a pain assessment? *(1228)*_____

_____

_____

7. In addition to assessment, what are the other nursing responsibilities for management of a hospice patient's pain? *(1227-1229)*

_____

_____

8. For pain relief or reduction, identify the types of medications that may be used for the following. *(1227)*

a. Mild to moderate pain: _____

b. Severe pain:_____

c. Long-lasting results: _____

9. In addition to pharmacologic therapy, the nurse recognizes that the following measures may also be implemented to relieve or reduce pain. *(1229)*

_____

_____

10. For the other common symptoms of a terminal illness, identify the nursing interventions. *(1229-1232)*

a. Nausea and vomiting:_____

_____

b. Constipation: _____

_____

c. Anorexia and malnutrition: _____

_____

d. Dyspnea or air hunger: _____

_____

e. Weight loss, dehydration, and weakness: _____

_____

11. An appropriate response for the hospice nurse in determining the patient's spiritual needs is to: *(1222)*

_____

_____

12. Identify signs and symptoms of approaching death and the appropriate nursing interventions. *(1233)*

_____

_____

ISSUES

Objective

- Discuss two ethical issues in hospice care.

13. Identify ethical and legal issues that are associated with hospice care. *(1234)* _____

_____

_____

Multiple Choice

14. The patient asks the nurse what the criteria are for admission to a hospice. The nurse responds correctly when informing the patient that: *(1224)*
    1. a nurse can certify the patient's condition.
    2. the patient must have a prognosis of fewer than 2 to 3 months to live.
    3. the patient and family must understand and be willing to participate in the planning of care.
    4. the patient will agree that life support measures will be performed routinely if needed.

15. The family of a dying patient is feeling physically and emotionally exhausted while taking shifts to care for their loved one 24 hours a day. This family could best benefit from the hospice service of: *(1226)*
    1. respite care.
    2. palliative care consultation.
    3. bereavement counseling.
    4. the hospice ethics committee.

16. The physician orders additional medications as adjuvant therapy to the oral narcotics the terminally ill patient is taking for pain control. Examples of adjuvant medications include: (Select all that apply) *(1228)*
    1. anticholinergics.
    2. anticonvulsants.
    3. pain medication patches.
    4. nonsteroidal antiinflammatory medications.

17. The wife of a terminally ill patient asks the hospice nurse why she gives different amounts of pain medication to her husband rather than the same dose each time. The nurse's best response is: (Select all that apply) *(1229)*
    1. "Determining the right dose of medication is difficult. We must try different amounts to determine a safe dose."
    2. "It is difficult to determine how much pain medication is a safe dose for someone who is dying. I want to be sure we get the right dose."
    3. "Finding the correct dose for pain medication is by trial and error. Every patient is different with how he or she responds to the medication."
    4. "I am titrating his medication amount so that we can best manage his pain while keeping him alert enough to interact with you and your family."

Professional Roles and Leadership

Answer Key: Textbook page references are provided as a guide for answering these questions. A complete answer key was provided for your instructor.

TERMS

Objective

- Define the key terms as listed.

1. Define the following terms.

    a. Advancement: *(1234)*_____

    _____

    b. Burnout: *(1248)*_____

    _____

    c. Endorsement: *(1249)* _____

    _____

    d. Nurse practice act: *(1258)* _____

    _____

    e. Transcribe: *(1261)* _____

    _____

CAREER PLANNING

Objectives

- Discuss the three methods of applying for a job.
- Describe what can be expected from an interview for a new job.
- Discuss career opportunities for the LPN/LVN.
- List the advantages of membership in professional organizations.
- Discuss the place and the nature of telephone manners in professionalism.
- Identify strategies for burnout prevention.

2. Identify the steps in career planning for the nurse. *(1238)* _____

_____

_____

3. What are the guidelines for preparing a letter of application for a position? *(1238)* _____

_____

_____

4. The purpose and components of a good resume are: *(1239)* _____

_____

_____

5. How can the applicant prepare for a successful interview? *(1240)* _____

_____

_____

6. What specific communication techniques should be employed for a successful interview? *(1241)* _____

_____

_____

7. Identify if the interviewer is allowed to ask the interviewee about the following. *(1241)*
    a. Job-related criminal convictions _____
    b. Financial or credit status _____
    c. Marital status _____
    d. Age _____
    e. Educational background _____
    f. Reason for leaving prior employment _____

8. What is usually included in an employment contract? *(1240, 1242)* _____

_____

_____

9. Identify the organizations that represent LPN/LVNs and their major functions. *(1245)* _____

_____

_____

10. What is the purpose of continuing education, and what types are usually offered? *(1245)* _____

_____

_____

11. The LPN/LVN who wants to continue his or her formal professional education should investigate _____
    _____. *(1246)*

12. What types of certification are available to the LPN/LVN? *(1246)*_____

_____

_____

13. Appropriate telephone communication regarding physician's orders involves: *(1260-1261)* _____

_____

_____

14. Identify possible career opportunities for the LPN/LVN. *(1250-1254)* _____

_____

_____

BOARD OF NURSING

Objectives

- Describe the nurse practice act.
- Identify three important functions of a state board of nursing.
- List four reasons a state board of nursing could revoke a nursing license.
- Discuss the computerized adaptive testing (CAT) for the National Council Licensure Examination (NCLEX-PN® and -RN®).
- Discuss the chemically impaired nurse.

15. For the NCLEX-RN® and -PN® examinations, identify the following. *(1247-1248)*

    a. Minimum number of questions: _____

    b. Maximum number of questions: _____

    c. Maximum time allowed:_____

    d. Goal of CAT testing: _____

    e. Average time to receive results:_____

    f. Approval for candidate to take the test given by:_____

    g. Examples of alternate-item format questions:_____

16. Identify the role and functions of a state board of nursing. *(1249-1250)* _____

_____

_____

17. The state board of nursing may revoke a nurse's license for the following reasons: *(1250)* _____

_____

_____

18. What is the purpose of the Nurse Licensing Compact? *(1249)* _____

_____

_____

19. What is the Model Disciplinary Diversion Act? *(1264)* _____

_____

_____

WORK ISSUES

Objectives

- Describe the night shift survival guide.
- Discuss the future of computers in nursing.

20. Identify the type of nursing that the following LPNs/LVNs are involved in. *(1252-1254)*

a. Working in an auto manufacturing plant: _____

b. Working with the terminally ill: _____

c. Working in the community: _____

21. Identify the signs and symptoms of burnout and strategies that may be implemented to prevent this problem. *(1258-1259)*

_____

_____

22. Identify how computers are used to aid nurses in their practice. *(1260)* _____

_____

_____

23. Identify an action that the nurse on the night shift should take for each of the following. *(1243)*

    a. Staying alert at work: _____

    _____

    b. Getting to sleep: _____

    _____

    c. Balancing his or her life with work: _____

    _____

LEADERSHIP

Objectives

- Explain the organizational position and the role of the charge nurse.
- Discuss the guidelines for being an effective leader.
- Discuss styles of leadership that may be used by nurses.
- Discuss the duties of a nurse team leader.
- Discuss mentoring.

24. Identify the type of leadership style that is being described. *(1255-1256)*

    a. Leader relinquishes all control and delegates responsibility to the group: _____

    _____

    b. People-centered approach that allows employees to have more control and participation in decision making:

    _____

    c. Leader retains all authority and responsibility and has one-way communication with the group:

    _____

    d. Takes into account the style of the leader and the characteristics of the group: _____

    _____

25. What is the usual role of a team leader? *(1256)* _____

    _____

    _____

26. Identify the guidelines for effective leadership. *(1257)* _____

_____

_____

27. Principles of time management include: *(1257)* _____

_____

_____

28. The LPN is working with another staff member who has not done what she was supposed to do for the patient. This is not the first time that this has occurred, and the LPN is becoming angry. What should this LPN do? *(1258)*

_____

_____

29. What is the role of a nurse mentor? *(1250)* _____

_____

_____

Multiple Choice

30. There has been an earthquake in the area, and the disaster victims are being brought into the emergency department. In this situation, the type of leadership that is the most effective for the nurse manager is: *(1255-1256)*
    1. democratic.
    2. autocratic.
    3. situational.
    4. laissez-faire.

LEGAL ISSUES

Objectives

- Discuss confidentiality.
- List the three types of physician's orders and discuss the legal aspects of each.
- List three ways the nurse can ensure accuracy when transcribing physician's orders.
- List the pertinent data necessary to compile an effective end-of-shift report.
- Discuss the importance of malpractice insurance.

31. What precautions should be taken by the nurse when transcribing a physician's orders? *(1260-1261)*

_____

_____

32. For the following, identify if the action is appropriate. *(1260-1262)*
    a. The nurse is unsure of the order that is written, but believes that it is appropriate and transcribes it to the medication administration record. _____
    b. The nurse administers a preoperative treatment to a patient the afternoon following the surgery. _____
    c. A discontinued medication is crossed out with a highlighting marker. _____

33. For a change-of-shift report, identify the following. *(1263)*

    a. Purpose:_____

    _____

    b. Methods: _____

    _____

    c. Information to include: _____

    _____

34. Why should the nurse have malpractice insurance? *(1264)* _____

    _____

    _____

35. Identify all of the following actions that are appropriate and maintain patient confidentiality. *(1244)*
    a. Discussing patient information in the cafeteria _____
    b. Copying patient information to review at home _____
    c. Providing information on patient status to the police _____
    d. Keeping information on the password-entry patient data system _____
    e. Giving updates on patient assessment during report _____

Multiple Choice

36. The nurse delegates the task of changing the surgical dressing to the certified nursing assistant (CNA). Which right of delegation is the nurse not following? (Select all that apply) *(1260)*
    1. Task
    2. Direction
    3. Person
    4. Supervision

Skills Performance Checklists

These checklists were developed to assist in evaluating the competence of students in performing the nursing interventions presented in *Foundations of Nursing*. The checklists are perforated for easy removal and reference. Students can be evaluated with a "Satisfactory (S)" or an "Unsatisfactory (U)" performance rating by putting a check in the appropriate column for each step. Specific instruction or feedback can be provided in the "Comments" column. All the checklists have been streamlined to include **only** the critical steps needed to satisfactorily master the skill. They are **not** intended to replace the text, which describes and illustrates each nursing skill in detail.

Student Name_____ Date_____ Instructor's name_____

MEASURING BODY TEMPERATURE

	S	U	Comments
1. Introduce self to patient	❏	❏	_____
2. Identify patient	❏	❏	_____
3. Explain procedure to patient	❏	❏	_____
4. Assess for signs and symptoms of temperature alterations and for factors that influence body temperature	❏	❏	_____
5. Prepare for procedure			
a. Assemble the appropriate thermometer and other necessary supplies	❏	❏	_____
b. Provide privacy	❏	❏	_____
c. Determine whether patient has consumed hot or cold beverage or food or has been smoking	❏	❏	_____
6. Obtaining an oral temperature: electronic thermometer			
a. Follow steps 1 through 5	❏	❏	_____
b. Perform hand hygiene and don clean gloves	❏	❏	_____
c. Remove thermometer pack from charging unit; remove probe from storage well of recording unit	❏	❏	_____
d. Insert probe snugly into probe cover—red probe for rectal readings, blue probe for oral and axillary readings	❏	❏	_____
e. Inspect digital display	❏	❏	_____
f. Request that patient open mouth and gently insert probe correctly; request that patient hold thermometer in place with lips closed	❏	❏	_____
g. Wait for audible signal	❏	❏	_____

		S	U	Comments
h.	Remove probe from patient's mouth and remove probe cover and dispose correctly	❏	❏	_____
i.	Provide for patient comfort	❏	❏	_____
j.	Read and write down reading; return thermometer to storage unit	❏	❏	_____
k.	Perform hand hygiene	❏	❏	_____
l.	Complete procedure by following step 10, a through d	❏	❏	_____

7. Obtaining rectal temperature: electronic thermometer

		S	U	Comments
a.	Follow steps 1 through 5b	❏	❏	_____
b.	Assist patient to the Sims' position	❏	❏	_____
c.	Perform hand hygiene and don clean gloves	❏	❏	_____
d.	Remove thermometer pack from charging unit; make certain correct rectal probe is attached to the unit and slide disposable plastic cover over thermometer probe	❏	❏	_____
e.	Lubricate thermometer probe	❏	❏	_____
f.	Gently spread buttocks and insert thermometer probe appropriately; hold on to thermometer throughout procedure	❏	❏	_____
g.	Hold electronic probe until audible signal occurs; read temperature on digital display	❏	❏	_____
h.	Carefully remove probe from rectum and dispose of plastic cover appropriately	❏	❏	_____
i.	Return probe to storage unit and later return the unit to its charging device	❏	❏	_____
j.	Clean anal area of lubricant and possible feces; remove and dispose of gloves and perform hand hygiene	❏	❏	_____
k.	Assist patient to a position of comfort	❏	❏	_____
l.	Write down reading	❏	❏	_____
m.	Complete procedure by following step 10, a through d	❏	❏	_____

	S	U	Comments
8. Obtaining axillary temperature: electronic thermometer			
a. Follow steps 1 through 5b	❏	❏	_____
b. Perform hand hygiene and don gloves	❏	❏	_____
c. Assist patient to supine or sitting position	❏	❏	_____
d. Expose axilla; make certain the area is clean and dry	❏	❏	_____
e. Prepare electronic thermometer	❏	❏	_____
f. Insert probe into the correct area and position body part correctly	❏	❏	_____
g. Hold electronic probe until audible signal occurs and read digital display	❏	❏	_____
h. Remove probe from patient's axilla; remove probe cover and dispose correctly	❏	❏	_____
i. Return electronic probe to storage well	❏	❏	_____
j. Assist patient to regown and position for comfort	❏	❏	_____
k. Remove gloves and perform hand hygiene	❏	❏	_____
l. Return thermometer to charger base	❏	❏	_____
m. Write down reading	❏	❏	_____
n. Complete procedure by following step 10, a through d	❏	❏	_____
9. Obtaining tympanic temperature: electronic thermometer			
a. Follow steps 1 through 5b	❏	❏	_____
b. Perform hand hygiene	❏	❏	_____
c. Assist patient to an appropriate position	❏	❏	_____
d. Remove hand-held thermometer unit from charging base	❏	❏	_____
e. Slide disposable plastic speculum cover over otoscope-like tip	❏	❏	_____
f. Follow manufacturer's instructions for tympanic probe positioning	❏	❏	_____

		S	U	Comments
(1)	Gently tug ear pinna up and back for an adult; down and back for a child	❏	❏	_____
(2)	Move thermometer gently in a figure-eight fashion	❏	❏	_____
(3)	Fit ear probe snugly into canal	❏	❏	_____
(4)	Point toward the nurse, following manufacturer's positioning recommendations	❏	❏	_____
g.	Depress scan button on hand-held unit and read assessment	❏	❏	_____
h.	Carefully remove sensor from ear and push release button to eject plastic speculum cover, discarding in proper receptacle	❏	❏	_____
i.	Return hand-held unit to charging base	❏	❏	_____
j.	Assist patient to a comfortable position	❏	❏	_____
k.	Perform hand hygiene	❏	❏	_____
l.	Write down reading	❏	❏	_____
m.	Complete procedure by following step 10, a through d	❏	❏	_____
10.	Postprocedure for measuring body temperature			
a.	Compare temperature findings with baseline and normal temperature range for patient's age group	❏	❏	_____
b.	If temperature is abnormal, repeat procedure; if indicated, choose alternate site or instrument for second reading	❏	❏	_____
c.	Record temperature on vital sign flow sheet/graphic sheet/nurse's notes correctly and report abnormal findings to nurse in charge or physician	❏	❏	_____
d.	Do patient teaching	❏	❏	_____

Student Name_____ Date_____ Instructor's name_____

PERFORMANCE CHECKLIST 4-2

OBTAINING A PULSE RATE

	S	**U**	**Comments**
1. Introduce self	❏	❏	_____
2. Identify patient	❏	❏	_____
3. Explain procedure	❏	❏	_____
4. Prepare for procedure			
a. Assemble all necessary supplies	❏	❏	_____
b. Provide privacy	❏	❏	_____
5. Perform hand hygiene and don clean gloves as necessary	❏	❏	_____
6. Implement procedure			
Count pulse for 60 seconds	❏	❏	_____
a. Palpate pulse			
(1) Radial pulse correctly	❏	❏	_____
(2) Ulnar pulse correctly	❏	❏	_____
(3) Brachial pulse correctly	❏	❏	_____
(4) Femoral pulse correctly	❏	❏	_____
(5) Popliteal pulse correctly	❏	❏	_____
(6) Dorsalis pedis pulse correctly	❏	❏	_____
(7) Posterior tibial pulse correctly	❏	❏	_____
b. Determine strength of pulse	❏	❏	_____
7. Write down rate	❏	❏	_____
8. Perform hand hygiene	❏	❏	_____
9. Document rate correctly	❏	❏	_____
10. Follow up by reporting any abnormal pulse rates	❏	❏	_____
11. Do patient teaching	❏	❏	_____

Student Name_____ Date_____ Instructor's name_____

OBTAINING AN APICAL PULSE RATE

	S	U	Comments
1. Introduce self	❏	❏	_____
2. Identify patient	❏	❏	_____
3. Explain procedure	❏	❏	_____
4. Prepare for procedure			
a. Assemble all necessary supplies	❏	❏	_____
b. Provide privacy	❏	❏	_____
5. Perform hand hygiene	❏	❏	_____
6. Implement procedure			
a. Clean stethoscope as recommended	❏	❏	_____
b. Position patient and expose patient's chest as necessary	❏	❏	_____
c. Place stethoscope against patient's chest in correct position	❏	❏	_____
d. Count pulse rate correctly; assist patient to dress	❏	❏	_____
7. Write down pulse rate	❏	❏	_____
8. Perform hand hygiene	❏	❏	_____
9. Document rate correctly	❏	❏	_____
10. Report any abnormal pulse rates	❏	❏	_____
11. Do patient teaching	❏	❏	_____

Student Name_____ Date_____ Instructor's name_____

OBTAINING A RESPIRATORY RATE

	S	U	Comments
1. Introduce self	❏	❏	_____
2. Identify patient	❏	❏	_____
3. Explain procedure	❏	❏	_____
4. Prepare for procedure			
a. Assemble all necessary supplies	❏	❏	_____
b. Provide privacy	❏	❏	_____
c. If patient has been active, wait the recommended time	❏	❏	_____
d. Position patient comfortably	❏	❏	_____
5. Perform hand hygiene	❏	❏	_____
6. Implement procedure			
a. Place fingertip as if to obtain a radial pulse	❏	❏	_____
b. Observe and count respiratory rate correctly	❏	❏	_____
c. Provide comfort	❏	❏	_____
7. Write down rate	❏	❏	_____
8. Perform hand hygiene	❏	❏	_____
9. Document rate correctly	❏	❏	_____
10. Report abnormal rates	❏	❏	_____
11. Do patient teaching	❏	❏	_____

Student Name_____ Date_____ Instructor's name_____

OBTAINING A BLOOD PRESSURE READING

	S	U	Comments
1. Introduce self	❏	❏	_____
2. Identify patient	❏	❏	_____
3. Explain procedure	❏	❏	_____
4. Determine if patient has ingested caffeine or has been smoking and wait the suggested length of time	❏	❏	_____
5. Prepare for procedure			
a. Assemble all necessary supplies; determine correct cuff size	❏	❏	_____
b. Provide privacy	❏	❏	_____
c. Position patient correctly	❏	❏	_____
d. Determine site for blood pressure measurement	❏	❏	_____
6. Perform hand hygiene	❏	❏	_____
7. Implement procedure			
a. Apply cuff correctly	❏	❏	_____
b. Palpate radial artery	❏	❏	_____
c. Inflate cuff, determine approximate systolic pressure	❏	❏	_____
d. Deflate the cuff correctly	❏	❏	_____
e. Palpate the brachial artery and place the stethoscope bell/diaphragm correctly	❏	❏	_____
f. Correctly reinflate cuff	❏	❏	_____
g. Correctly deflate cuff	❏	❏	_____
h. Accurately determine blood pressure reading while listening to Korotkoff sounds	❏	❏	_____
i. Completely deflate and remove the cuff	❏	❏	_____
j. Provide comfort	❏	❏	_____

	S	**U**	**Comments**
8. Write down rate	❏	❏	_____
9. Perform hand hygiene	❏	❏	_____
10. Document reading correctly	❏	❏	_____
11. Report abnormal readings	❏	❏	_____
12. Do patient teaching	❏	❏	_____

Student Name_____ Date_____ Instructor's name_____

MEASURING HEIGHT AND WEIGHT

	S	U	Comments
1. Introduce self	❏	❏	_____
2. Identify patient	❏	❏	_____
3. Explain procedure	❏	❏	_____
4. Prepare for procedure			
a. Assemble supplies	❏	❏	_____
b. Provide privacy	❏	❏	_____
5. Perform hand hygiene	❏	❏	_____
6. Implement procedure			
a. Balance scales at zero and place paper towel for patient to stand on	❏	❏	_____
b. Place paper towel over base of scale where patient will stand, if patient is barefoot	❏	❏	_____
c. Assist patient onto scales correctly	❏	❏	_____
d. Measure height correctly	❏	❏	_____
e. Measure weight correctly	❏	❏	_____
f. Assist patient off scales correctly	❏	❏	_____
g. Provide comfort	❏	❏	_____
7. Write down measurements	❏	❏	_____
8. Perform hand hygiene	❏	❏	_____
9. Document measurements	❏	❏	_____
10. Follow up by reporting measurement	❏	❏	_____

PERFORMANCE CHECKLIST 10-1

CARE OF THE BODY AFTER DEATH

	S	U	Comments
1. Assemble appropriate equipment	❏	❏	_____
2. Perform hand hygiene	❏	❏	_____
3. Don clean gloves	❏	❏	_____
4. Close patient's eyes and mouth as necessary	❏	❏	_____
5. Remove all tubing and other devices from around patient's body unless contraindicated	❏	❏	_____
6. Place patient in supine position (do not place one hand on top of the other); elevate head	❏	❏	_____
7. Replace soiled dressings with clean ones	❏	❏	_____
8. Bathe patient as necessary (place absorbent pad under buttocks)	❏	❏	_____
9. Brush or comb hair	❏	❏	_____
10. Apply clean gown	❏	❏	_____
11. Care for valuables (jewelry) and personal belongings; if wedding band is to remain on the deceased, secure ring to finger with a small strip of tape over ring	❏	❏	_____
12. Allow family to view body and remain in room if family wishes; a sheet or light blanket over the body with only the head and upper shoulders exposed will maintain dignity and respect for the deceased; remove unneeded equipment from the room; provide soft lighting and offer chairs	❏	❏	_____
13. After the family has left the room, attach special label if patient had a contagious disease	❏	❏	_____
14. Close door to room	❏	❏	_____
15. Await arrival of ambulance or transfer to morgue	❏	❏	_____

	S	U	Comments
Some agencies use a shroud to enclose the body before transfer to morgue. If shroud is to be used, enclose body into shroud at this time			
a. The body is in the dorsal recumbent position; arms are straight at the sides; there is a pillow under the head and shoulders	❏	❏	_____
b. Place the body on the shroud	❏	❏	_____
c. Bring the top of the shroud down over the head	❏	❏	_____
d. Fold the bottom of the shroud over the feet	❏	❏	_____
e. Fold the sides over the body, tape or pin the sides together, and attach the identification tag	❏	❏	_____
16. Document procedure and disposition of patient's body as well as belongings and valuables	❏	❏	_____

Student Name_____ Date_____ Instructor's name_____

PERFORMANCE CHECKLIST 11-1

ADMITTING A PATIENT

		S	U	Comments
1.	Perform hand hygiene	❏	❏	_____
2.	Prepare the room			
	a. Care items in place	❏	❏	_____
	b. Bed at proper height and opened	❏	❏	_____
	c. Light on	❏	❏	_____
3.	Greet the patient and family; introduce self, roommate; project interest and concern	❏	❏	_____
4.	Check the ID band and verify its accuracy; in long-term care facilities, the residents do not wear ID bands; a picture of the resident is used for identification purposes	❏	❏	_____
5.	Assess immediate needs	❏	❏	_____
6.	Orient the patient to the unit: lounge and nurses' station	❏	❏	_____
7.	Orient the patient to the room: explain the use of equipment, call light system, bed controls, telephone, and television	❏	❏	_____
8.	Explain hospital routines such as visiting hours, meals, and morning wake-up	❏	❏	_____
9.	Provide privacy, assist to undress as necessary	❏	❏	_____
10.	Properly care for valuables, clothing, and medications	❏	❏	_____
11.	Obtain the patient's health history, and do the initial nursing assessment correctly	❏	❏	_____
12.	Provide for safety: bed in low position, side rails up, call light within easy reach	❏	❏	_____
13.	Begin care as ordered by the physician	❏	❏	_____
14.	Invite the family back into the room if they left earlier	❏	❏	_____
15.	Perform hand hygiene	❏	❏	_____

	S	U	Comments
16. Record the information correctly on the patient's chart according to agency policy	❏	❏	_____
17. Provide the patient and the family time for privacy	❏	❏	_____
18. Do patient teaching	❏	❏	_____

Student Name_____ Date_____ Instructor's name_____

PERFORMANCE CHECKLIST 11-2

TRANSFERRING A PATIENT

	S	U	Comments
1. Perform hand hygiene	❑	❑	_____
2. Check physician's order	❑	❑	_____
3. Inform the patient and family of transfer	❑	❑	_____
4. Notify receiving unit of patient transfer and when to be expected	❑	❑	_____
5. Gather the patient's belongings and necessary care items to accompany the patient	❑	❑	_____
6. Assist in transferring the patient, usually by wheelchair or stretcher	❑	❑	_____
7. Properly introduce patient and family to new unit: nurses and roommate	❑	❑	_____
8. Provide a brief summary of medical diagnoses, treatment care plan, and medications; review medical orders with nurse assuming care. If transfer is to another facility, complete an interagency transfer form correctly	❑	❑	_____
9. Explain equipment, policies, and procedures that are different on the new unit	❑	❑	_____
10. Perform hand hygiene	❑	❑	_____
11. Record condition of patient and means of transfer; the nurse on the new unit should also record an assessment of the patient's condition on arrival	❑	❑	_____
12. Notify other hospital departments of the transfer as necessary, such as diagnostic imaging, laboratory, switchboard, dietary, and business offices	❑	❑	_____
13. For an interagency transfer, dress the patient appropriately; if oxygen is required, a small transport tank may be used; a nurse generally accompanies a critically ill patient who is being transferred	❑	❑	_____

	S	U	Comments
14. If patient is a child, adjust procedure appropriately	❏	❏	_____
15. Do patient teaching	❏	❏	_____

PERFORMANCE CHECKLIST 11-3

Discharging a Patient

	S	U	Comments
1. Perform hand hygiene	❏	❏	_____
2. Verify written discharge order	❏	❏	_____
3. Arrange for patient or family to visit business office as necessary	❏	❏	_____
4. If no discharge order has been written, have patient sign appropriate AMA form	❏	❏	_____
5. Notify the family or person who will be transporting the patient home	❏	❏	_____
6. Make certain patient and family understand instructions for care (medications, special diet, exercise)	❏	❏	_____
7. Gather equipment, supplies, and prescriptions that the patient is to take home	❏	❏	_____
8. Check to see that business office has given a release	❏	❏	_____
9. Assist the patient in dressing and packing items to go home	❏	❏	_____
10. Check clothing and valuables list made on admission according to policy	❏	❏	_____
11. Transfer the patient and belongings via wheelchair to the vehicle; assist patient into the vehicle if needed; as with all procedures, use good communication skills and wish the patient well	❏	❏	_____
12. Perform hand hygiene	❏	❏	_____
13. Chart entire discharge procedure; document the following: teaching, patient's condition, method of discharge	❏	❏	_____
14. If patient is a child, adjust procedure as appropriate	❏	❏	_____

Student Name_____ Date_____ Instructor's name_____

PERFORMING HAND HYGIENE

	S	U	Comments
1. Inspect hands, observing for visible soiling, breaks, or cuts in the skin or cuticles	❏	❏	_____
2. Determine contaminant of hands	❏	❏	_____
3. Assess areas around the hands that are contaminated	❏	❏	_____
4. Explain to the patient the importance of handwashing	❏	❏	_____
5. Remove jewelry (except plain wedding band) and push watch and long sleeves above wrists	❏	❏	_____
6. Adjust the water to appropriate temperature and force	❏	❏	_____
7. Wet hands and wrists, keeping hands lower than elbows	❏	❏	_____
8. Lather hands with liquid soap	❏	❏	_____
9. Perform hand hygiene thoroughly, using a firm, circular motion and friction on back of hands, palms, and wrists; wash each finger individually, paying special attention to areas between fingers and knuckles by interlacing fingers and thumbs and moving hands back and forth, causing friction	❏	❏	_____
10. Wash 1 minute thoroughly, rinse thoroughly, re-lather and wash another minute using a continuous amount of friction	❏	❏	_____
11. Rinse wrists and hands completely, keeping hands lower than elbows	❏	❏	_____
12. Clean fingernails carefully under running water, using fingernails of other hand or blunt end of an orange stick	❏	❏	_____
13. Dry hands thoroughly with paper towels	❏	❏	_____
14. Turn off faucets with a dry paper towel	❏	❏	_____
15. Use hand lotion	❏	❏	_____
16. Inspect hands and nails for cleanliness	❏	❏	_____

	S	U	Comments
17. If hands are visibly soiled, use an alcohol-based waterless antiseptic for routine decontamination of hands in all clinical situations	❏	❏	_____
18. Do patient teaching	❏	❏	_____
19. If contamination continues, technique must be reassessed	❏	❏	_____

Student Name_____ Date_____ Instructor's name_____

GLOVING

	S	U	Comments

Donning Gloves

1. Obtain gloves from dispenser ❏ ❏ _____

2. Inspect gloves for perforation ❏ ❏ _____

3. Don gloves as recommended ❏ ❏ _____

4. Change gloves after direct handling of infectious
material such as wound drainage ❏ ❏ _____

5. Do not touch side rails, tables, or bed stands
with contaminated gloves ❏ ❏ _____

Removing Gloves

6. Remove first glove by grasping outer surface
at palm with other gloved hand and pulling glove
off and inside out; place this glove in other hand ❏ ❏ _____

7. Remove second glove by placing finger under
cuff and turning glove inside out and over other
glove; drop gloves into waste container ❏ ❏ _____

8. Perform hand hygiene ❏ ❏ _____

9. Do patient teaching ❏ ❏ _____

10. If contamination continues, technique must
be reassessed ❏ ❏ _____

Student Name_____ Date_____ Instructor's name_____

GOWNING FOR ISOLATION

	S	U	Comments
1. Remove watch and push up long sleeves	❑	❑	_____
2. Place watch on a paper towel or see-through baggie before taking vital signs	❑	❑	_____
3. Perform hand hygiene	❑	❑	_____
4. Don gown by securely tying gown at neck and waist	❑	❑	_____
5. When finished with patient care, remove gown appropriately	❑	❑	_____
6. Discard soiled gown appropriately	❑	❑	_____
7. Perform hand hygiene	❑	❑	_____
8. Record use of gown in isolation procedure if agency's policy (some agencies charge a daily rate for isolation precautions)	❑	❑	_____
9. Do patient teaching	❑	❑	_____
10. If contamination continues, technique must be reassessed	❑	❑	_____

Student Name_____ Date_____ Instructor's name_____

PERFORMANCE CHECKLIST 12-4

Donning a Mask

	S	U	Comments
1. Obtain a mask	❏	❏	_____
2. Don mask when ready to begin patient care by covering the nose, mouth, and eyes (glasses) with the device; a mask with protective eye shield is worn when the risk of splashing is imminent; secure mask in place with elastic band or by tying the strings behind the head	❏	❏	_____
3. Wear mask for recommended period of time, until it becomes moist but no longer than 20 to 30 minutes	❏	❏	_____
4. Make certain patient feels comfortable and accepted by nurse	❏	❏	_____
5. Remove mask by untying the strings or moving the elastic; make certain not to touch mask	❏	❏	_____
6. Dispose of soiled mask appropriately	❏	❏	_____
7. Perform hand hygiene thoroughly	❏	❏	_____
8. Record use of mask during patient care (some agencies require documentation of specific barriers used)	❏	❏	_____
9. Do patient teaching	❏	❏	_____
10. If contamination continues, technique must be reassessed	❏	❏	_____

Student Name_____ Date_____ Instructor's name_____

Isolation Technique

	S	U	Comments
1. Determine causative microorganism or effectiveness of patient's immune system	❑	❑	_____
2. Recognize mode of transmission and how microorganism exits the body	❑	❑	_____
3. Follow agency policy for specific type of isolation used	❑	❑	_____
4. Provide an environment with adequate equipment and supplies			
a. Private room or isolation with anteroom	❑	❑	_____
b. Place sign stating isolation category	❑	❑	_____
c. Adequate handwashing facilities	❑	❑	_____
d. Special containers for trash, soiled linen, and sharp instruments such as needles	❑	❑	_____
5. Plan time to explain isolation technique to patient, family, and visitors	❑	❑	_____
6. Post card on door of patient's room or wall outside room stating the protective measures in use for patient care	❑	❑	_____
7. Supply the room with designated lined containers for soiled linens and for trash	❑	❑	_____
8. Perform hand hygiene	❑	❑	_____
9. Don gloves and appropriate apparel	❑	❑	_____
10. Assess vital signs, administer medication, administer hygiene, and collect specimens all in the appropriate manner	❑	❑	_____
11. When finished with patient care, remove gloves and apparel per correct protocol	❑	❑	_____
12. Perform hand hygiene	❑	❑	_____
13. Report changes in the patient's health status	❑	❑	_____

	S	U	Comments
14. Record assessments and performance of protective asepsis	❏	❏	_____
15. Determine patient's level of understanding	❏	❏	_____
16. Do patient teaching	❏	❏	_____
17. If contamination continues, technique must be reassessed	❏	❏	_____
18. Additional techniques for acid-fast bacillus (AFB) isolation			
a. Before entering room, apply recommended mask; be sure it fits snugly	❏	❏	_____
b. Explain purpose of AFB to patient, family, and others	❏	❏	_____
c. Offer opportunity for questions	❏	❏	_____
d. Instruct patient to cover mouth with tissue when coughing and to wear disposable surgical mask when leaving room	❏	❏	_____
e. The particulate respirator that the health care worker wears is not to be placed on the patient; the added work of breathing through the respirator is an added stress on an already compromised pulmonary system; simply apply a regular surgical mask			
(1) Provide care	❏	❏	_____
(2) Leave the room and close the door	❏	❏	_____
(3) Remove respiratory protective device	❏	❏	_____
(4) Place reusable device in labeled paper bag for storage, being careful not to crush device (check agency policy for number of times it can be reused)	❏	❏	_____
(5) Perform hand hygiene	❏	❏	_____
(6) Record assessments and performance of patient care	❏	❏	_____

Student Name_____ Date_____ Instructor's name_____

Surgical Hand Hygiene

	S	U	Comments
1. Inspect hands for presence of abrasions, cuts, or open lesions	❑	❑	_____
2. Apply surgical shoe covers, cap or hood, face mask, and protective eyewear	❑	❑	_____
3. Surgical handwashing			
a. Turn on water using knee or foot control and adjust to comfortable temperature	❑	❑	_____
b. Wet hands and arms under running lukewarm water and lather with detergent to 5 cm (2 inches) above elbows (hands need to be above elbows at all times)	❑	❑	_____
c. Rinse hands and arms thoroughly under running water	❑	❑	_____
d. Under running water, clean under nails of both hands with nail pick; discard after use	❑	❑	_____
(1) Wet clean sponge and apply antimicrobial detergent; scrub nails of one hand with 15 strokes; holding sponge perpendicular, scrub palm, each side of thumb and fingers, and posterior side of hand with 10 strokes each	❑	❑	_____
(2) Mentally divide arm into thirds; scrub each third 10 times; entire scrub should last 5 to 10 minutes; rinse sponge and repeat sequence for other arm; a two-sponge method may be substituted (check agency policy)	❑	❑	_____
e. Discard sponge and rinse hands and arms thoroughly; turn off water with foot or knee control and back into room entrance with hands elevated in front of and away from the body	❑	❑	_____

	S	U	Comments
(1) Walk up to sterile tray and lean forward slightly to pick up sterile towel	❏	❏	_____
(2) Dry one hand thoroughly, moving from fingers to elbow; dry in a rotating motion, from cleanest to least clean area	❏	❏	_____
f. Repeat drying method for other hand by carefully reversing towel or using a new sterile towel	❏	❏	_____
g. Discard towel	❏	❏	_____
h. Proceed with sterile gowning	❏	❏	_____
4. Alternate method using alcohol-based antiseptic			
a. Perform hand hygiene with soap and water for 10 to 15 seconds to remove soil	❏	❏	_____
b. Under running water, clean under nails of both hands with nail pick; discard after use and dry hands with a paper towel	❏	❏	_____
c. Apply enough alcohol-based waterless antiseptic to one palm to cover both hands thoroughly; spread the antiseptic over all surfaces of the hands and fingernails; follow product instructions for length of time to rub over hand surfaces; allow to air-dry	❏	❏	_____
d. Repeat process and allow hands to air-dry before applying sterile gloves	❏	❏	_____

Student Name_____ Date_____ Instructor's name_____

PREPARING A STERILE FIELD

	S	U	Comments
1. Prepare sterile field just before planned procedure; supplies are to be used immediately	❑	❑	_____
2. Select clean work surface above waist level	❑	❑	_____
3. Assemble necessary equipment			
a. Sterile drape	❑	❑	_____
b. Assorted sterile supplies	❑	❑	_____
4. Check dates, labels, or condition of package for sterility of equipment	❑	❑	_____
5. Perform hand hygiene thoroughly	❑	❑	_____
6. Place pack containing sterile drape on work surface and open without contamination	❑	❑	_____
7. With fingertips of one hand, pick up folded top edge of sterile drape	❑	❑	_____
8. Gently lift drape up from its outer cover and let it unfold by itself without touching any object; discard outer cover with your other hand	❑	❑	_____
9. With other hand, grasp adjacent corner of drape and hold it straight up and away from your body; now drape can be properly placed while using two hands; the drape must be held away from unsterile surfaces	❑	❑	_____
10. Holding drape, first position the bottom half over intended work surface	❑	❑	_____
11. Allow top half of drape to be placed over work surface last	❑	❑	_____
12. Perform procedure using sterile technique	❑	❑	_____

PERFORMANCE CHECKLIST 12-8

DONNING A STERILE GOWN

	S	U	Comments
1. Don surgical cap, shoe covers, protective eye wear, and mask	❑	❑	_____
2. Perform surgical hand hygiene	❑	❑	_____
2. Ask circulating nurse to open sterile gown and sterile glove packages	❑	❑	_____
3. Don the gown			
a. If available, the scrub nurse will assist by pulling the gown over your extended hands and arms. If there is no assistance from a scrub nurse:			
(1) Pick up the gown touching only the inner surface bellow the neck	❑	❑	_____
(2) Maintain constant control of the folded layers of the gown	❑	❑	_____
(3) While holding the gown at arm's length, allow the gown to unfold from top to bottom; be sure that the gown does not touch the floor	❑	❑	_____
(4) While holding the inside of the gown near the shoulders and below the neckband, slide hands and arms into the sleeves with your fingers stopping at the end of the cuffs	❑	❑	_____
(5) Ask another staff member to grasp the card that is attached to the ties of the gown in order to draw the ties around to the back with the gown overlapping itself; the staff member should now tie the gown, avoiding touching any part of the gown except the ties	❑	❑	_____

Student Name_____ Date_____ Instructor's name_____

PERFORMING OPEN STERILE GLOVING

	S	U	Comments
1. Obtain proper-sized sterile gloves	❏	❏	_____
2. Perform thorough handwashing	❏	❏	_____
3. Remove outer glove package wrapper by carefully separating and peeling apart sides	❏	❏	_____
4. Grasp inner package and lay it on clean, flat surface just above waist level; open package, keeping gloves on wrapper's inside surface	❏	❏	_____
5. Identify right and left gloves; each glove has cuff approximately 2 inches (5 cm) wide; glove dominant hand first	❏	❏	_____
6. With thumb and first two fingers of nondominant hand, grasp edge of glove cuff for dominant hand; touch only glove's inside surface	❏	❏	_____
7. Carefully pull glove over dominant hand, leaving cuff and being sure cuff does not roll up wrist; be sure thumb and fingers are in proper spaces	❏	❏	_____
8. With gloved dominant hand, slip fingers underneath second glove's cuff because the cuff will protect the gloved fingers	❏	❏	_____
9. Carefully pull second glove over nondominant hand; do not allow fingers and thumb of gloved dominant hand to touch any part of exposed nondominant hand; keep thumb of dominant hand abducted back	❏	❏	_____
10. After second glove is on, interlock hands together; cuffs usually fall down after application	❏	❏	_____

Glove Disposal

	S	U	Comments
11. Grasp outside of one cuff with other gloved hand; avoid touching wrist	❏	❏	_____

	S	U	Comments
12. Pull glove off, turning it inside out; discard in receptacle	❏	❏	_____
13. Take fingers of bare hand and tuck inside remaining glove cuff; peel glove off, inside out; discard in receptacle	❏	❏	_____

Student Name_____ Date_____ Instructor's name_____

PREPARING FOR DISINFECTION AND STERILIZATION

	S	U	Comments
1. Prepare equipment and assemble supplies			
a. Disinfectant to use for cleansing	❏	❏	_____
b. Method of sterilization	❏	❏	_____
c. Gloves	❏	❏	_____
d. Running water	❏	❏	_____
e. Scrub brush	❏	❏	_____
f. Cloth wrapper	❏	❏	_____
2. Perform hand hygiene	❏	❏	_____
3. Don gloves	❏	❏	_____
4. Rinse article under cool running water	❏	❏	_____
5. Wash article with detergent	❏	❏	_____
6. Use scrub brush to remove material in grooves	❏	❏	_____
7. Dry article thoroughly	❏	❏	_____
8. Prepare article for sterilization by wrapping it in cloth wrapper	❏	❏	_____
9. Clean work area and put in order	❏	❏	_____
10. Perform hand hygiene	❏	❏	_____
11. Do patient teaching	❏	❏	_____

PERFORMANCE CHECKLIST 13-1

CHANGING A STERILE DRY DRESSING

	S	U	Comments
Prepare for procedure			
1. Refer to medical record, care plan, or Kardex	❏	❏	_____
2. Introduce self	❏	❏	_____
3. Identify patient	❏	❏	_____
4. Explain the procedure	❏	❏	_____
5. Assess need for and provide patient teaching	❏	❏	_____
6. Assemble equipment and complete necessary charges	❏	❏	_____
7. Perform hand hygiene	❏	❏	_____
8. Assess patient	❏	❏	_____
9. Prepare patient for intervention			
a. Close door/pull privacy curtain	❏	❏	_____
b. Raise bed to comfortable working height; lower side rail on side nearest the nurse	❏	❏	_____
c. Position and drape patient as necessary	❏	❏	_____
During the skill			
10. Promote patient involvement as possible	❏	❏	_____
11. Assess patient's tolerance	❏	❏	_____
12. Place refuse container in convenient location away from sterile field	❏	❏	_____
13. Set up sterile field correctly	❏	❏	_____
14. Loosen tape appropriately	❏	❏	_____
15. Don clean gloves	❏	❏	_____
16. Remove dressing and discard correctly	❏	❏	_____
17. Assess status of wound and wound drainage/exudate correctly	❏	❏	_____
18. Remove and discard soiled gloves	❏	❏	_____

	S	U	Comments
19. Perform hand hygiene and don sterile gloves	❏	❏	_____
20. Cleanse wound and surrounding area correctly	❏	❏	_____
21. Use sterile 4 x 4 dressing to dry in same manner or allow antiseptic to air-dry	❏	❏	_____
22. Cleanse drain site appropriately if applicable	❏	❏	_____
23. Apply antibiotic ointment, if ordered, using same techniques as for cleansing	❏	❏	_____
24. Cover wound with appropriately sized dry sterile dressing and use drain dressing, if applicable	❏	❏	_____
25. Secure dressing with appropriate tape, Montgomery straps, or binder	❏	❏	_____

Postprocedure

	S	U	Comments
26. Assist patient to a position of comfort and place needed items within easy reach; be certain patient has a means to call for assistance and knows how to use it	❏	❏	_____
27. Raise side rails and lower bed to lowest position	❏	❏	_____
28. Remove gloves and all protective barriers; dispose of soiled supplies and equipment appropriately	❏	❏	_____
29. Perform hand hygiene after patient contact and after wearing gloves	❏	❏	_____
30. Document and do patient teaching	❏	❏	_____
31. Report any unexpected appearance of wound or drainage or accidental removal of drain within an hour to physician	❏	❏	_____

Student Name_____ Date_____ Instructor's name_____

PERFORMANCE CHECKLIST 13-2

CHANGING A WET-TO-DRY DRESSING

	S	U	Comments
Prepare for procedure			
1. Refer to medical record, care plan, or Kardex	❏	❏	_____
2. Introduce self	❏	❏	_____
3. Identify patient	❏	❏	_____
4. Explain the procedure	❏	❏	_____
5. Assess need for and provide patient teaching during procedure	❏	❏	_____
6. Assemble equipment and complete necessary charges	❏	❏	_____
7. Perform hand hygiene	❏	❏	_____
8. Assess patient	❏	❏	_____
9. Prepare patient for intervention			
a. Close door/pull privacy curtain	❏	❏	_____
b. Raise bed to comfortable working height; lower side rail on side nearest the nurse	❏	❏	_____
c. Position and drape patient as necessary	❏	❏	_____
During the skill			
10. Promote patient involvement as possible	❏	❏	_____
11. Assess patient's tolerance	❏	❏	_____
12. Place waterproof pad appropriately	❏	❏	_____
13. Place refuse container appropriately	❏	❏	_____
14. Set up sterile field	❏	❏	_____
15. Loosen tape correctly	❏	❏	_____
16. Don clean gloves; remove dressing appropriately and discard	❏	❏	_____
17. Assess status of wound and wound exudate/drainage	❏	❏	_____

	S	U	Comments
18. Remove gloves and discard; perform hand hygiene and don sterile gloves	❏	❏	_____
19. Cleanse wound correctly	❏	❏	_____
20. Place 4 x 4 dressing into basin	❏	❏	_____
21. Wring excess solution from dressing, leaving it slightly moist	❏	❏	_____
22. Place dressing over open wound surfaces and press into depressed areas	❏	❏	_____
23. Apply dry dressing over wet dressing	❏	❏	_____
24. Cover with additional dressing as needed	❏	❏	_____
25. Secure with tape or Montgomery straps	❏	❏	_____

Postprocedure

	S	U	Comments
26. Assist patient to a position of comfort and place needed items within easy reach; be certain patient has a means to call for assistance and knows how to use it	❏	❏	_____
27. Raise side rails and lower bed to lowest position	❏	❏	_____
28. Remove gloves and all protective barriers; dispose of soiled supplies and equipment appropriately	❏	❏	_____
29. Perform hand hygiene after patient contact and after wearing gloves	❏	❏	_____
30. Document and do patient teaching	❏	❏	_____
31. Discuss change in dressing procedure with physician as wound surface becomes clean and granulation tissue is evident	❏	❏	_____

PERFORMANCE CHECKLIST 13-3

APPLYING A TRANSPARENT DRESSING

	S	U	Comments
Prepare for procedure			
1. Refer to medical record, care plan, or Kardex	❏	❏	_____
2. Introduce self	❏	❏	_____
3. Identify patient	❏	❏	_____
4. Explain procedure	❏	❏	_____
5. Assess need for and provide patient teaching during procedure	❏	❏	_____
6. Assemble equipment and complete necessary charges	❏	❏	_____
7. Perform hand hygiene	❏	❏	_____
8. Assess patient	❏	❏	_____
9. Prepare patient for intervention			
a. Provide privacy	❏	❏	_____
b. Raise bed to working height and lower nearest side rail	❏	❏	_____
c. Position and drape patient as necessary	❏	❏	_____
During the skill			
10. Promote patient involvement as possible	❏	❏	_____
11. Assess patient's tolerance	❏	❏	_____
12. Place refuse container in convenient location away from contamination	❏	❏	_____
13. Set up sterile field	❏	❏	_____
14. Don clean gloves	❏	❏	_____
15. Loosen tape and remove old dressings	❏	❏	_____
16. Remove soiled gloves and with soiled dressings dispose of in refuse container	❏	❏	_____
17. Assess status of wound	❏	❏	_____

	S	U	Comments
18. Don sterile gloves	❏	❏	_____
19. Cleanse area gently	❏	❏	_____
20. Allow skin surface to dry	❏	❏	_____
21. Apply transparent dressings according to manufacturer's direction	❏	❏	_____
22. Remove soiled gloves and discard; perform hand hygiene	❏	❏	_____

Postprocedure

	S	U	Comments
23. Assist patient to a position of comfort and place needed items within easy reach	❏	❏	_____
24. Raise side rails and lower bed to lowest position	❏	❏	_____
25. Remove gloves and all protective barriers; dispose of soiled supplies and equipment appropriately	❏	❏	_____
26. Perform hand hygiene after patient contact and after wearing gloves	❏	❏	_____
27. Document	❏	❏	_____
28. Report any unexpected appearance of the wound or exudate	❏	❏	_____
29. Do patient teaching	❏	❏	_____

Student Name_____ Date_____ Instructor's name_____

PERFORMING A STERILE IRRIGATION

	S	U	Comments
Prepare for procedure			
1. Refer to medical record, care plan, or Kardex for special interventions	❑	❑	_____
2. Introduce self	❑	❑	_____
3. Identify patient	❑	❑	_____
4. Explain the procedure	❑	❑	_____
5. Assess need for and provide patient teaching during procedure	❑	❑	_____
6. Assemble equipment and complete necessary charges	❑	❑	_____
7. Perform hand hygiene	❑	❑	_____
8. Assess patient	❑	❑	_____
9. Prepare patient for intervention			
a. Close door/pull privacy curtain	❑	❑	_____
b. Raise bed to comfortable working height; lower side rail on side nearest the nurse	❑	❑	_____
c. Position and drape patient as necessary	❑	❑	_____
During the skill			
10. Promote patient involvement as possible	❑	❑	_____
11. Assess patient's tolerance	❑	❑	_____
12. Position waterproof pad appropriately	❑	❑	_____
13. Place refuse container in convenient location away from contamination	❑	❑	_____
14. Set up sterile field	❑	❑	_____
15. Don gown and goggles as appropriate	❑	❑	_____
16. Don clean gloves, remove dressing, and discard appropriately	❑	❑	_____
17. Remove gloves, dispose of in proper receptacle, and perform hand hygiene	❑	❑	_____

	S	U	Comments
18. Assess status of wound and exudate/drainage	❏	❏	_____
19. Place collection basin appropriately	❏	❏	_____
20. Perform hand hygiene and don sterile gloves	❏	❏	_____
21. Cleanse area around wound correctly	❏	❏	_____
22. Fill irrigating syringe with solution; attach soft catheter if irrigating a deep wound with small opening	❏	❏	_____
23. Instill solution gently into wound, holding syringe approximately 1 inch above wound; if using catheter, gently insert into wound opening until slight resistance is met, pull back, and gently instill solution	❏	❏	_____
24. Allow solution to flow from clean area of wound to dirty area	❏	❏	_____
25. Pinch off catheter during withdrawal from wound	❏	❏	_____
26. Refill syringe and continue irrigation until solution returns clear	❏	❏	_____
27. Blot wound edges with sterile dressing	❏	❏	_____
28. Redress wound, if applicable	❏	❏	_____
29. Remove and dispose of gloves	❏	❏	_____
30. Perform hand hygiene	❏	❏	_____

Postprocedure

	S	U	Comments
31. Assist patient to a position of comfort and place needed items within easy reach; be certain patient has a means to call for assistance and knows how to use it	❏	❏	_____
32. Raise side rails and lower bed to lowest position	❏	❏	_____
33. Remove gloves and all protective barriers; dispose of soiled supplies and equipment appropriately	❏	❏	_____
34. Perform hand hygiene after patient contact and after wearing gloves	❏	❏	_____
35. Document and do patient teaching	❏	❏	_____
36. Report immediately any evidence of fresh bleeding, sharp increase in pain, retention of irrigant, or signs of shock to attending physician	❏	❏	_____

Student Name_____ Date_____ Instructor's name_____

Removing Staples or Sutures (Applying Steri-Strips)

	S	U	Comments
Prepare for procedure			
1. Refer to medical record, care plan, or Kardex	❑	❑	_____
2. Introduce self	❑	❑	_____
3. Identify patient	❑	❑	_____
4. Explain the procedure	❑	❑	_____
5. Assess need for and provide patient teaching during procedure	❑	❑	_____
6. Assemble equipment and complete necessary charges	❑	❑	_____
7. Perform hand hygiene	❑	❑	_____
8. Assess patient	❑	❑	_____
9. Prepare patient for intervention			
a. Close door/pull privacy curtain	❑	❑	_____
b. Raise bed to comfortable working height; lower side rail on side nearest the nurse	❑	❑	_____
c. Position and drape patient as necessary	❑	❑	_____
During the skill			
10. Promote patient involvement as possible	❑	❑	_____
11. Assess patient's tolerance, being alert for signs and symptoms of discomfort and fatigue	❑	❑	_____
12. Place refuse container in convenient location away from sterile field	❑	❑	_____
13. Set up sterile field	❑	❑	_____
14. Don clean gloves	❑	❑	_____
15. Remove dressing and soiled gloves; discard appropriately	❑	❑	_____
16. Assess status of wound and drainage on dressing correctly	❑	❑	_____

	S	U	Comments
17. Perform hand hygiene and don sterile gloves	❏	❏	_____
18. Cleanse area correctly	❏	❏	_____

Staple removal

	S	U	Comments
19. Place staple remover under both sides of staple; squeeze handles together and gently remove staples from skin	❏	❏	_____
20. Release handles and discard staple in refuse container	❏	❏	_____
21. Repeat steps 19 and 20 until all staples have been removed	❏	❏	_____
22. Count number of staples removed	❏	❏	_____
23. Notify physician immediately if inadequate wound healing is noted; discontinue removal of all staples	❏	❏	_____

Applying Steri-Strips

	S	U	Comments
24. It is common to see wounds closed with Steri-Strips; these interventions should be followed when applying Steri-Strips			
a. Gently cleanse suture line	❏	❏	_____
b. Carefully inspect the incision	❏	❏	_____
c. When skin is dry, apply Steri-Strips	❏	❏	_____
d. Instruct patient to take showers rather than soak in bathtub according to physician's preference	❏	❏	_____
e. Many physicians request upon removal of sutures that only 1–3 sutures be removed at a time; Steri-Strips are then applied, repeating this action until all sutures are removed and Steri-Strips applied	❏	❏	_____
25. Assess healing status of wound	❏	❏	_____
26. Cleanse area with antiseptic swabs	❏	❏	_____

Removal of intermittent sutures

	S	U	Comments
27. Grasp and elevate knotted end of suture with hemostat or forceps	❏	❏	_____

	S	U	Comments
28. Snip suture at skin level on opposite side, proximal to knot	❏	❏	_____
29. Gently remove entire suture with forceps and discard on sterile gauze	❏	❏	_____
30. Repeat steps 27 to 29 until all sutures have been removed	❏	❏	_____

Removal of continuous sutures including blanket stitch sutures

	S	U	Comments
31. Cut first suture close to skin on side away from knot	❏	❏	_____
32. Remove gently from knotted side with forceps and discard on sterile gauze	❏	❏	_____
33. Snip second suture on same side	❏	❏	_____
34. Repeat steps 31 to 33 until all sutures have been removed	❏	❏	_____
35. Apply sterile dressing or leave open to air as ordered	❏	❏	_____
36. Remove gloves and perform hand hygiene	❏	❏	_____

Postprocedure

	S	U	Comments
37. Assist patient to a position of comfort and place needed items within easy reach; be certain patient has a means to call for assistance and knows how to use it	❏	❏	_____
38. Raise side rails and lower bed to lowest position	❏	❏	_____
39. Remove gloves and all protective barriers; dispose of soiled supplies and equipment appropriately	❏	❏	_____
40. Perform hand hygiene after patient contact and after wearing gloves	❏	❏	_____
41. Document and do patient teaching	❏	❏	_____
42. Report any abnormalities	❏	❏	_____

PERFORMANCE CHECKLIST 13-6

MAINTAINING HEMOVAC OR DAVOL SUCTION AND T-TUBE DRAINAGE

	S	U	Comments
Prepare for procedure			
1. Refer to medical record, care plan, or Kardex	❏	❏	_____
2. Introduce self	❏	❏	_____
3. Identify patient	❏	❏	_____
4. Explain the procedure	❏	❏	_____
5. Assess need for and provide patient teaching	❏	❏	_____
6. Assemble equipment and complete necessary charges	❏	❏	_____
7. Perform hand hygiene	❏	❏	_____
8. Assess patient	❏	❏	_____
Prepare patient for intervention			
9. Close door/pull privacy curtain	❏	❏	_____
10. Raise bed to comfortable working height; lower side rail on side nearest the nurse	❏	❏	_____
11. Position and drape patient as necessary	❏	❏	_____
During the skill			
12. Promote patient involvement as possible	❏	❏	_____
13. Assess patient's tolerance	❏	❏	_____
14. Examine drainage system	❏	❏	_____
15. Don goggles as appropriate	❏	❏	_____
16. Don clean gloves	❏	❏	_____
17. Remove Hemovac/Davol plug labeled "pouring spout;" empty drainage into measuring device, handling device correctly	❏	❏	_____
18. Hold pump of Hemovac tightly compressed and reinsert plug; when caring for a Davol, repump to reestablish suction	❏	❏	_____
19. T-tube maintenance			
a. Remove plug, holding drainage spout over calibrated container	❏	❏	_____

	S	U	Comments
b. Empty drainage into measuring container and replace plug, maintaining sterility	❏	❏	_____
c. Always keep drainage bag below the level of the common bile duct to prevent contamination from backflow; may be fastened to patient's gown. Be very careful to prevent tension on and displacement of T-tube	❏	❏	_____
20. Observe the drainage	❏	❏	_____
21. Measure and record amount of drainage; rinse measuring container	❏	❏	_____
22. Position drainage system on bed and secure system	❏	❏	_____
23. Dispose of drainage and rinse measuring container	❏	❏	_____

Postprocedure

	S	U	Comments
24. Remove gloves and all protective barriers; dispose of soiled supplies and equipment appropriately	❏	❏	_____
25. Perform hand hygiene after patient contact and after wearing gloves	❏	❏	_____
26. Assist patient to a position of comfort and place needed items within easy reach; be certain patient has a means to call for assistance and knows how to use it	❏	❏	_____
27. Raise side rails and lower bed to lowest position	❏	❏	_____
28. If specimen is ordered, label and send to laboratory	❏	❏	_____
29. Perform hand hygiene after patient contact	❏	❏	_____
30. Observe Davol/Hemovac/T-tube every 2–4 hours; measure drainage	❏	❏	_____
31. Document and do patient teaching	❏	❏	_____
32. Report any abnormal characteristics of drainage. Normal amounts of bile drainage vary from 250–500 mL for 24 hours; normal characteristics are thick consistency with greenish-brown color, slightly blood-tinged in the first 24 hours (excessive bile leakage from wound can indicate an occluded system; notify physician)	❏	❏	_____

PERFORMANCE CHECKLIST 13-7

Wound Vacuum-Assisted Closure

	S	U	Comments
Prepare for procedure			
1. Refer to medical record, care plan, or Kardex	❑	❑	_____
2. Introduce self	❑	❑	_____
3. Identify patient	❑	❑	_____
4. Explain procedure and the reason for it	❑	❑	_____
5. Assess need for and provide patient teaching	❑	❑	_____
6. Assemble equipment and complete necessary charges	❑	❑	_____
7. Perform hand hygiene and don clean gloves	❑	❑	_____
8. Assess patient	❑	❑	_____
9. Prepare patient for intervention			
a. Close door and pull privacy curtain	❑	❑	_____
b. Raise bed to a comfortable working height, lower side rail closest to nurse	❑	❑	_____
c. Position and drape patient as necessary	❑	❑	_____
During the skill			
10. Promote patient involvement as possible	❑	❑	_____
11. Assess patient's tolerance	❑	❑	_____
12. Place disposable waterproof bag within work area with top folded down to make a cuff	❑	❑	_____
13. When VAC® is in place, begin by pushing therapy on/off button	❑	❑	_____
a. Keeping tube connection with VAC® unit, disconnect tubes from each other to drain fluids into canister	❑	❑	_____
b. Before lowering, tighten clamps on canister tube	❑	❑	_____

	S	U	Comments
14. With dressing tube unclamped, introduce 10–30 mL of normal saline, if ordered, into tubing to soak underneath foam	❏	❏	_____
15. Gently stretch transparent film horizontally and slowly pull up from the skin	❏	❏	_____
16. Remove old VAC® dressing and observe; discard dressings and remove gloves; perform hand hygiene	❏	❏	_____
17. Apply sterile or clean gloves (new surgical wound calls for sterile technique; chronic wound may use clean technique); irrigate wound with solution ordered by physician; gently blot dry	❏	❏	_____
18. Measure wound as ordered; remove and discard gloves	❏	❏	_____
19. Apply clean gloves or sterile gloves (depending on type of wound)	❏	❏	_____
20. Prepare VAC® foam			
a. Select appropriate foam	❏	❏	_____
b. Using sterile scissors, cut foam to wound size	❏	❏	_____
21. Gently place foam into wound making certain that foam is in contact with entire wound base	❏	❏	_____
22. Apply tubing to foam in the wound	❏	❏	_____
a. For deep wounds, regularly reposition tubing to minimize pressure on wound edges	❏	❏	_____
b. Patients with restricted mobility or sensation must be repositioned frequently so they do not lie on the tubing	❏	❏	_____
23. Apply skin protectant to wound edges	❏	❏	_____
24. Apply wound VAC® dressing			
a. Cover VAC® foam	❏	❏	_____
b. Apply wrinkle-free transparent dressing	❏	❏	_____
c. Secure tubing to transparent film; ensure occlusive seal	❏	❏	_____
25. Secure tubing several centimeters away from dressings	❏	❏	_____

	S	U	Comments
26. Once wound is completely covered, connect tubing from dressing to tubing from canister and VAC® unit			
a. Remove canister from sterile packaging and push into VAC® unit until a click is heard	❏	❏	_____
b. Connect dressing tubing to canister tubing; make certain both clamps are opened	❏	❏	_____
c. Place VAC® unit on level surface or hang from foot of bed	❏	❏	_____
d. Press green-lit power button and set pressure as ordered	❏	❏	_____
27. Discard all dressing material; remove gloves; perform hand hygiene	❏	❏	_____
28. Inspect wound VAC® system to verify that negative pressure is achieved			
a. Verify that display screen reads "therapy on"	❏	❏	_____
b. Be sure clamps are open and tubing is patent	❏	❏	_____
c. Identify air leaks	❏	❏	_____
d. If leak is present, seal with strips of transparent film	❏	❏	_____

Postprocedure

	S	U	Comments
29. Assist patient to a position of comfort and place needed items within easy reach; be certain patient has a means to call for assistance and knows how to use it	❏	❏	_____
30. Raise side rails and lower bed to lowest position	❏	❏	_____
31. Remove gloves and all protective barriers; dispose of soiled supplies and equipment appropriately	❏	❏	_____
32. Perform hand hygiene after patient contact and after wearing gloves	❏	❏	_____
33. Document and do patient teaching	❏	❏	_____
34. Report any unexpected appearance of wound or drainage	❏	❏	_____

PERFORMANCE CHECKLIST 13-8

APPLYING A BANDAGE

	S	U	Comments
Prepare for procedure			
1. Refer to medical record, care plan, or Kardex	❏	❏	_____
2. Introduce self	❏	❏	_____
3. Identify patient	❏	❏	_____
4. Explain the procedure	❏	❏	_____
5. Assess need for and provide patient teaching during procedure	❏	❏	_____
6. Assemble equipment and complete necessary charges	❏	❏	_____
7. Perform hand hygiene	❏	❏	_____
8. Assess patient	❏	❏	_____
9. Prepare patient for intervention			
a. Close door/pull privacy curtain	❏	❏	_____
b. Raise bed to comfortable working height; lower side rail on side nearest the nurse	❏	❏	_____
c. Position and drape patient as necessary	❏	❏	_____
During the skill			
10. Promote patient involvement as possible	❏	❏	_____
11. Assess patient's tolerance	❏	❏	_____
12. Ensure that skin and/or dressing is clean and dry	❏	❏	_____
13. Separate any adjacent skin surfaces	❏	❏	_____
14. Don gloves as necessary	❏	❏	_____
15. Align part to be bandaged appropriately	❏	❏	_____
16. Apply bandage from distal to proximal part	❏	❏	_____
17. Apply bandage correctly			
a. Circular bandage	❏	❏	_____

	S	U	Comments
b. Spiral bandage	❏	❏	_____
c. Spiral-reverse bandage	❏	❏	_____
d. Recurrent (stump) bandage	❏	❏	_____
e. Figure-eight bandage	❏	❏	_____
18. Secure first bandage before applying additional rolls	❏	❏	_____
19. Apply additional rolls without leaving any uncovered areas	❏	❏	_____
20. Assess tension of bandage and circulation of extremity	❏	❏	_____

Postprocedure

	S	U	Comments
21. Assist patient to a position of comfort and place needed items within easy reach; be certain patient has a means to call for assistance and knows how to use it	❏	❏	_____
22. Raise side rails and lower bed to lowest position	❏	❏	_____
23. Remove gloves and all protective barriers; dispose of soiled supplies and equipment appropriately	❏	❏	_____
24. Perform hand hygiene after patient contact and after wearing gloves	❏	❏	_____
25. Document and do patient teaching	❏	❏	_____
26. Report any unexpected outcomes	❏	❏	_____

PERFORMANCE CHECKLIST 13-9

APPLYING A BINDER, ARM SLING, AND T-BINDER

	S	U	Comments
Prepare for procedure			
1. Refer to medical record, care plan, or Kardex	❏	❏	_____
2. Introduce self	❏	❏	_____
3. Identify patient	❏	❏	_____
4. Explain the procedure	❏	❏	_____
5. Assess need for and provide patient teaching during procedure	❏	❏	_____
6. Assemble equipment and complete necessary charges	❏	❏	_____
7. Perform hand hygiene	❏	❏	_____
8. Assess patient	❏	❏	_____
9. Prepare patient for intervention			
a. Close door/pull privacy curtain	❏	❏	_____
b. Raise bed to comfortable working height; lower side rail on side nearest the nurse	❏	❏	_____
c. Position and drape patient as necessary	❏	❏	_____
During the skill			
10. Promote patient involvement as possible	❏	❏	_____
11. Assess patient's tolerance	❏	❏	_____
12. Don gloves as necessary	❏	❏	_____
13. Change dressing if appropriate; cleanse skin if needed	❏	❏	_____
14. Separate skin surfaces or pad bony prominences	❏	❏	_____
15. Apply binder	❏	❏	_____
a. Triangular binder (sling)			
(1) Have patient flex arm at approximately 80-degree angle, depending on purpose of binder	❏	❏	_____

	S	**U**	**Comments**
(2) Place end of triangular binder over shoulder of the uninjured side	❏	❏	_____
(3) Grasp other end of binder and bring it up and over injured arm to shoulder of injured arm	❏	❏	_____
(4) Use square knot to tie two ends together at lateral area of neck on uninjured side	❏	❏	_____
(5) Support wrist well with binder; do not allow it to extend over end of binder	❏	❏	_____
(6) Fold third triangle end neatly around elbow and secure with safety pins	❏	❏	_____
b. T-binder			
(1) Using appropriate binder, place the waistband smoothly under patient's waist; tail(s) should be under patient	❏	❏	_____
(2) Secure two ends of waistband together with safety pin	❏	❏	_____
(3) Single tail—bring the tail up between legs to secure dressing in place; two tails—bring tails up one on each side of penis or large dressing	❏	❏	_____
(4) Bring tails under and over waistband; secure with safety pins	❏	❏	_____
c. Elastic abdominal binder			
(1) Center binder smoothly under appropriate part of patient	❏	❏	_____
(2) Bring ends around patient and overlap away from incision	❏	❏	_____
(3) Secure binder with Velcro or safety pins placed horizontally on abdomen	❏	❏	_____
d. For postsurgical application of scultetus abdominal binder, proceed upward from the bottom, attach each set of tails with safety pins away from incision	❏	❏	_____
16. Note comfort level of patient and smooth binder to prevent wrinkles	❏	❏	_____

Student Name_____ Date_____ Instructor's name_____

	S	U	Comments

Postprocedure

17. Assist patient to a position of comfort and place needed items within easy reach; be certain patient has a means to call for assistance and knows how to use it ❏ ❏ _____

18. Raise side rails and lower bed to lowest position ❏ ❏ _____

19. Remove gloves and all protective barriers; dispose of soiled supplies and equipment appropriately ❏ ❏ _____

20. Perform hand hygiene after patient contact and after wearing gloves ❏ ❏ _____

21. Document and do patient teaching ❏ ❏ _____

22. Report any unexpected outcomes ❏ ❏ _____

Student Name_____ Date_____ Instructor's name_____

Applying Safety Reminder Devices

	S	U	Comments
1. Refer to medical record, care plans, and Kardex; review agency policy	❑	❑	_____
2. Perform hand hygiene	❑	❑	_____
3. Introduce self	❑	❑	_____
4. Identify patient	❑	❑	_____
5. Procedure			
a. Explain procedure	❑	❑	_____
b. Provide privacy and assemble necessary supplies	❑	❑	_____
c. Assess patient for need of SRD (a comprehensive nursing assessment of the patient's potential for injury/treatment related to need for SRD, is crucial before application of SRD)	❑	❑	_____
6. Obtain written permission for application of SRD	❑	❑	_____
7. Apply appropriate type of SRD			
a. Wrist or ankle (extremity) SRD			
(1) If using Kerlix gauze, make a clove hitch correctly (form a figure-eight and pick up loops)	❑	❑	_____
(2) Pad the extremity appropriately	❑	❑	_____
(3) Slip the wrist(s) or ankle(s) through loops directly over the padding; if using a commercially made SRD, wrap the padded portion of the device around affected extremity, thread tie through slit in SRD, and fasten to second tie with a secure knot correctly	❑	❑	_____

389

	S	U	Comments

(4) Secure ends of ties to movable portion of bed frame that moves with the patient when the bed is adjusted, *not to side rails* ❑ ❑ _____

(5) Leave as much slack as possible ❑ ❑ _____

(6) Palpate pulses below the SRD ❑ ❑ _____

b. Elbow SRD

(1) Place SRD over the elbow(s) ❑ ❑ _____

(2) Wrap SRD snugly, tying the SRD at the top. For small infants, tie or pin SRDs to their shirts ❑ ❑ _____

c. Vest

(1) Apply device over the patient's gown ❑ ❑ _____

(2) Put vest on patient with V-shaped opening in the front ❑ ❑ _____

(3) Pull tie at end of vest flap across the chest, and slip tie through slip on opposite side of vest ❑ ❑ _____

(4) Wrap the other end of the flap across patient and secure the straps to frame of bed or behind wheelchair; use the quick-release knot ❑ ❑ _____

(5) Allow enough space between the vest and the patient appropriately (there should be room for a fist in the space between the vest and the patient) ❑ ❑ _____

d. Gait or safety reminder belts

(1) Apply belt over patient's gown ❑ ❑ _____

(2) If patient is ambulating, place belt around the patient's waist ❑ ❑ _____

(3) If the belt does not have a buckle, fasten in slip knot ❑ ❑ _____

8. A quick-release knot rather than a regular knot should be used to secure the safety reminder devices to the bed frame ❑ ❑ _____

9. Secure SRDs so that the patient cannot unfasten them ❑ ❑ _____

	S	U	Comments
10. Apply SRD with gentleness and compassion	❏	❏	_____
11. Perform hand hygiene	❏	❏	_____
12. Document procedure completely and accurately	❏	❏	_____
13. Follow-up			
a. Monitor for skin impairment	❏	❏	_____
b. With the use of extremity SRD, assess extremity distal to SRD at least every 30 minutes	❏	❏	_____
(1) Remove SRD on one extremity at a time at least every 2 hours for 5 minutes	❏	❏	_____
c. Monitor position of SRD, circulation, and skin condition	❏	❏	_____
d. With the use of vest SRD, monitor respiratory status	❏	❏	_____
e. SRD should be removed at least every 2 hours; patient should NOT be left unattended during this time	❏	❏	_____
f. Massage skin beneath SRD; lotion or powder may be applied	❏	❏	_____
g. SRD should be changed when soiled or wet	❏	❏	_____
h. Check frequently for tangled ties or pressure points from knots; adjust SRD device(s) as needed	❏	❏	_____
i. Monitor and document physical and mental status, circulation, and need for SRD; SRDs should be removed when they are no longer needed	❏	❏	_____
j. If SRD use is necessary because of changes in the patient's condition, document the changes and efforts to calm or safeguard the patient without SRD use	❏	❏	_____
k. Assess for any related problems	❏	❏	_____
14. Evaluation			
a. The SRD is adequate and appropriate for the individual patient's condition	❏	❏	_____

		S	U	Comments
b.	SRDs are correctly applied	❏	❏	_____
c.	Quick-release knots are easily released	❏	❏	_____
d.	Related problems, such as to the skin or the musculoskeletal system, are identified	❏	❏	_____
15.	Do patient teaching	❏	❏	_____
16.	Mummy restraint for infants and children (person applying restraint should not be parent or guardian)			
a.	Open a blanket and fold one corner toward center; place infant on blanket with shoulders at fold and feet toward opposite corner	❏	❏	_____
b.	With infant's arm straight down against the body, pull right side of blanket firmly across right shoulder and chest, and secure beneath left side of body	❏	❏	_____
c.	Place left arm straight against body, bring left side of blanket across shoulder and chest, and lock beneath infant's body on right side	❏	❏	_____
d.	Align infant's legs, pull corner of blanket near feet up toward body, and tuck snugly in place or fasten securely with safety pins	❏	❏	_____
e.	Remain with infant while restrained and remove restraint immediately after treatment is complete; if restraint is required for an extended period of time, remove at least every 2 hours and perform range of motion exercise on all extremities	❏	❏	_____

PERFORMANCE CHECKLIST 15-1

Positioning Patients

	S	U	Comments
1. Assess patient's body alignment and comfort level while patient is lying down	❏	❏	_____
2. Assemble equipment and supplies	❏	❏	_____
3. Request assistance as needed	❏	❏	_____
4. Introduce self	❏	❏	_____
5. Identify patient	❏	❏	_____
6. Explain procedure	❏	❏	_____
7. Perform hand hygiene	❏	❏	_____
8. Prepare patient			
a. Close doors	❏	❏	_____
b. Raise level of bed	❏	❏	_____
c. Remove pillows and devices used in previous position	❏	❏	_____
d. Position bed flat or as low as patient is able to tolerate and lower side rail closest to nurse	❏	❏	_____
9. Position patient			
a. Dorsal supine position			
(1) Place patient on back with head flat	❏	❏	_____
(2) Place small rolled towel under lumbar spine	❏	❏	_____
(3) Place pillow under upper shoulders, neck, and head	❏	❏	_____
(4) Place trochanter roll or sandbag along lateral surface of thighs	❏	❏	_____
(5) Place small pillow or roll under back of ankles to elevate heels	❏	❏	_____
(6) Support feet with firm pillows, footboard, or high-top sneakers	❏	❏	_____

	S	U	Comments
(7) Place pillows under pronated forearms, keeping upper arms parallel to patient's body	❏	❏	_____
(8) Place hand rolls in patient's hands	❏	❏	_____
b. Dorsal recumbent			
(1) Lower head of bed	❏	❏	_____
(2) Move patient and mattress to head of bed	❏	❏	_____
(3) Turn patient onto back	❏	❏	_____
(4) Assist patient to raise legs, bend knees, and allow legs to relax	❏	❏	_____
(5) Replace pillow	❏	❏	_____
c. Fowler's			
(1) Move patient and mattress to head of bed	❏	❏	_____
(2) Raise head of bed to 45–60 degrees	❏	❏	_____
(3) Replace pillow	❏	❏	_____
(4) Use footboard	❏	❏	_____
(5) Use pillows to support arms and hands if needed	❏	❏	_____
(6) Place small pillow or roll under ankles	❏	❏	_____
d. Semi-Fowler's			
(1) Move patient and mattress to head of bed and remove pillow	❏	❏	_____
(2) Raise head of bed to 30 degrees	❏	❏	_____
(3) Replace pillow	❏	❏	_____
e. Orthopneic			
(1) Elevate head of bed to 90 degrees	❏	❏	_____
(2) Place pillow between patient's back and mattress	❏	❏	_____
(3) Place pillow on overbed table and assist patient to lean over, placing head on pillow	❏	❏	_____

	S	U	Comments

f. Sims' position

(1) Place patient in supine position ❏ ❏ _____

(2) Place patient in left lateral position, lying partially on the abdomen ❏ ❏ _____

(3) Draw right knee and thigh up near abdomen and support with pillows ❏ ❏ _____

(4) Place patient's left arm along back ❏ ❏ _____

(5) Bring right arm up, flex elbow, and support with pillow ❏ ❏ _____

(6) Allow patient to lean forward to rest on chest ❏ ❏ _____

g. Prone

(1) Assist patient onto abdomen with face to one side ❏ ❏ _____

(2) Flex arms toward the head ❏ ❏ _____

(3) Position pillows for comfort ❏ ❏ _____

h. Knee-chest (genupectoral)

(1) Turn patient onto abdomen ❏ ❏ _____

(2) Assist patient to kneeling position; arms and head should rest on pillow while upper chest rests on bed ❏ ❏ _____

i. Lithotomy

(1) Position patient to lie supine ❏ ❏ _____

(2) Request patient to slide buttocks to the edge at end of examining table ❏ ❏ _____

(3) Lift both legs, have patient bend knees, and place feet in stirrups ❏ ❏ _____

(4) Drape patient appropriately ❏ ❏ _____

(5) May need a small lumbar pillow ❏ ❏ _____

	S	U	Comments
j. Trendelenburg's			
(1) Place patient's head lower than body with body and legs elevated and on an incline (foot of bed may be elevated on blocks); Trendelenburg position is not used to treat shock because of pressure it causes on diaphragm by organs in the abdomen	❏	❏	_____
10. Reassess patient for			
a. Proper body alignment	❏	❏	_____
b. Comfort	❏	❏	_____
c. Skin integrity	❏	❏	_____
d. Respiratory difficulty	❏	❏	_____
e. Tolerance of position	❏	❏	_____
f. Reposition every 2 hours	❏	❏	_____
11. Perform hand hygiene	❏	❏	_____
12. Document appropriate alignment and position of patient	❏	❏	_____
13. Do patient teaching	❏	❏	_____

Student Name_____ Date_____ Instructor's name_____

PERFORMANCE CHECKLIST 15-2

PERFORMING RANGE-OF-MOTION EXERCISES

	S	U	Comments
1. Refer to medical record, care plan, or Kardex for special interventions	❏	❏	_____
2. Assemble equipment	❏	❏	_____
3. Introduce self	❏	❏	_____
4. Identify patient	❏	❏	_____
5. Explain procedure	❏	❏	_____
6. Perform hand hygiene; don clean gloves according to agency policy and guidelines from CDC and OSHA	❏	❏	_____
7. Prepare for procedure by providing privacy and assembling necessary supplies	❏	❏	_____
8. Assist patient to a comfortable position, either sitting or lying down	❏	❏	_____
9. Medicate patient as needed	❏	❏	_____
10. Begin by following exercises in sequence; each movement should be repeated 5 times during exercise period; discontinue if patient complains of pain or if there is resistance or muscle spasm	❏	❏	_____
11. Assist patient in putting each joint through full ROM, appropriately supporting the body part being exercised	❏	❏	_____
a. Neck—Place palm of each hand against side of patient's face, or place one hand under patient's head and one hand on patient's chin; begin by following exercise in sequence; each movement should be repeated 5 times during the exercise period	❏	❏	_____
(1) Bring head forward until chin touches sternum	❏	❏	_____
(2) Return head to straight position and have patient look straight ahead	❏	❏	_____
(3) Bend head backward with chin positioned toward ceiling	❏	❏	_____
(4) Return head to extension	❏	❏	_____

	S	U	Comments
(5) Bend head laterally with ear toward shoulder, first toward right ear then left ear	❏	❏	_____
b. Shoulder—Cup one hand beneath elbow, and grasp wrist with other hand			
(1) Bring arm away from body	❏	❏	_____
(2) Return arm toward side of body	❏	❏	_____
(3) Abduct the arm; continue movement until patient's hand is toward head of bed	❏	❏	_____
(4) Abduct arm to shoulder level	❏	❏	_____
c. Elbow—Support patient's arm by grasping center of forearm with one hand and just above elbow with other hand			
(1) Bend lower arm toward biceps	❏	❏	_____
(2) Straighten lower arm	❏	❏	_____
(3) Hold patient's hand as if to shake hands, and turn palm upward	❏	❏	_____
(4) Continue holding patient's hand, and turn palm of hand downward	❏	❏	_____
d. Wrist—Hold wrist joint with one hand, and hold palm of patient's hand with other hand			
(1) Bend wrist toward lower arm with fingers pointing downward	❏	❏	_____
(2) Return wrist to a straight position	❏	❏	_____
(3) Bend wrist with fingers pointing upward toward ceiling	❏	❏	_____
(4) Extend wrist, and bend it laterally toward ulna side	❏	❏	_____
e. Fingers—Place palm and fingers of one hand directly against back of patient's hand and fingers			
(1) Curve fingers with nurse's fingers to resemble a fist	❏	❏	_____
(2) Straighten all fingers	❏	❏	_____

	S	U	Comments
(3) Using thumb and index finger of one hand, spread fingers apart by moving each one away from nearest finger	❏	❏	_____
(4) Return fingers together until touching each other	❏	❏	_____

f. Thumb—Hold patient's thumb with nurse's thumb and index finger

	S	U	Comments
(1) Manipulate thumb across the palm of hand to touch tip of each finger to tip of patient's thumb	❏	❏	_____
(2) Move thumb away from index finger return thumb toward index finger	❏	❏	_____
(3) Move thumb joint forward and backward	❏	❏	_____

g. Hip—Support under knee joint with one hand, and grasp ankle joint with other hand

	S	U	Comments
(1) Raise leg with knee straight; return leg to bed in straight position	❏	❏	_____
(2) Raise leg and bend knee toward chest to flex to 110–120 degrees; straighten knee and return to bed	❏	❏	_____
(3) Move leg out away from midline	❏	❏	_____
(4) Bring leg back toward other leg	❏	❏	_____
(5) Position legs straight and roll leg outward, toes pointing outward	❏	❏	_____
(6) Position legs straight and roll leg inward, toes pointing toward each other	❏	❏	_____

h. Knee—Support under knee joint with one hand, and grasp ankle joint with the other hand

	S	U	Comments
	❏	❏	_____
(1) Bend knee with calf touching thigh	❏	❏	_____
(2) Straighten knee	❏	❏	_____
(3) Extend knee beyond the normal point of extension	❏	❏	_____
(4) Rotate knee and lower leg toward midline	❏	❏	_____

	S	U	Comments
i. Ankle—Grasp heel in palm of one hand, touching inner aspect of the forearm to the sole of the foot; support top of foot just above ankle with other hand			
(1) Gently press against the sole of the foot with inner arm, toes pointing upward	❏	❏	_____
(2) Press on top of foot to point toes downward	❏	❏	_____
(3) Turn foot away from midline	❏	❏	_____
(4) Turn foot inward	❏	❏	_____
j. Toes—Place fingers over toes; support bottom of foot with hand and bottom of toes with other hand			
(1) Curl toes downward toward bottom of foot	❏	❏	_____
(2) Raise toes to point upward	❏	❏	_____
(3) Spread toes apart	❏	❏	_____
(4) Return toes toward each other	❏	❏	_____
12. Position patient for comfort	❏	❏	_____
13. Adjust bed linens	❏	❏	_____
14. Remove and dispose of gloves and perform hand hygiene	❏	❏	_____
15. Documentation			
a. Report and record abnormal findings	❏	❏	_____
b. Report and record normal findings	❏	❏	_____

PERFORMANCE CHECKLIST 15-3

MOVING THE PATIENT

	S	U	Comments
1. Refer to medical record, care plan, or Kardex for special interventions	❏	❏	_____
2. Assemble equipment	❏	❏	_____
3. Introduce self	❏	❏	_____
4. Identify patient	❏	❏	_____
5. Explain procedure	❏	❏	_____
6. Perform hand hygiene	❏	❏	_____
7. Prepare patient for procedure; close doors; adjust the bed level; medicate patient as needed	❏	❏	_____
8. Arrange for assistance as necessary	❏	❏	_____
9. Lifting and moving patient up in bed			
a. Place patient supine with head flat	❏	❏	_____
b. Face side of bed and provide base of support	❏	❏	_____
c. Place one arm under axilla and opposite arm under shoulder and neck	❏	❏	_____
d. Ask patient to flex knees and push up with feet on count of 3 while assisting	❏	❏	_____
e. Nurses position selves on both sides of patient facing each other and support patient's back with one arm with the second arm under shoulder and neck	❏	❏	_____
f. On count of 3, each nurse moves patient up to head of bed	❏	❏	_____
(1) Roll patient from side to side placing a pull sheet under the patient	❏	❏	_____
(2) One nurse on opposite side of the patient's bed grasps pull sheet firmly with hands near patient's upper arms and hips, rolling the sheet material until hands are close to the patient	❏	❏	_____

	S	U	Comments
(3) Nurses' knees are flexed with body facing the direction of the move	❑	❑	_____
(4) Instruct patient to rest arms on body and to lift head on the count of 3	❑	❑	_____

10. Turning the patient

a. Stand with feet slightly apart and flex knees	❑	❑	_____
b. Place one arm under patient's neck and shoulders and other arm under waist	❑	❑	_____
c. Move patient toward nurse	❑	❑	_____
d. Turn patient on side facing raised side rail	❑	❑	_____
e. Flex one leg over the other, place pad or pillow between legs	❑	❑	_____
f. Align shoulders	❑	❑	_____
g. Support back with pillows if necessary; a "tuck" pillow may be made folding pillow lengthwise	❑	❑	_____

11. Dangling patient

a. Assess pulse and respirations	❑	❑	_____
b. Move patient to side of bed toward nurse	❑	❑	_____
c. Lower bed to lowest position	❑	❑	_____
d. Raise head of bed	❑	❑	_____
e. Support patient's shoulders and help to swing legs around and off bed	❑	❑	_____
f. This may also be accomplished by rolling the patient onto his/her side before sitting up	❑	❑	_____
g. Help patient don slippers; cover legs	❑	❑	_____
h. Assess patient's pulse and respirations	❑	❑	_____

12. Logrolling the patient

a. Enlist assistance of at least one other person	❑	❑	_____
b. Lower head of bed as low as the patient can tolerate	❑	❑	_____
c. Place a pillow between the patient's legs	❑	❑	_____

	S	U	Comments

d. Extend patient's arm over patient's head unless shoulder movement is restricted ❑ ❑ _____

e. Both nurses on the same side of the bed, one places one hand on the patient's shoulder and the other on the hip while the other nurse places one hand to supports the back and the other behind the knees. If a pull sheet is used, hands are placed alternately to provide even support for the length of the rolled sheet ❑ ❑ _____

f. Using a count of 3, turn the patient with a continuous, smooth, coordinated effort ❑ ❑ _____

g. Support the patient with pillows as previously discussed ❑ ❑ _____

13. Transferring the patient from bed to straight chair or wheelchair

a. Lower bed to lowest position ❑ ❑ _____

b. Raise head of bed ❑ ❑ _____

c. Support patient's shoulder, and help patient to sit up and to swing legs around and off of bed ❑ ❑ _____

d. Assist patient to don robe and slippers ❑ ❑ _____

e. Position chair beside bed with seat facing foot of bed

(1) Lock wheels of wheelchair and place at right angle after bed is lowered ❑ ❑ _____

(2) Place straight chair against wall ❑ ❑ _____

f. Stand in front of patient, and place hands at waist level or below and allow patient to use arms and shoulders to facilitate the move ❑ ❑ _____

g. Assist patient to stand and swing around with back toward seat of chair ❑ ❑ _____

h. Help patient to sit down as nurse bends knees ❑ ❑ _____

i. Apply blanket over legs for warmth ❑ ❑ _____

	S	U	Comments

j. If a transfer belt is used, apply after patient is sitting on side of bed and follow these guidelines

   (1) Stand in front of the patient ❏ ❏ _____

   (2) Request patient to hold onto mattress or to place fists on the bed by the thighs ❏ ❏ _____

   (3) Place patient's feet flat on the floor ❏ ❏ _____

   (4) Request patient to lean forward ❏ ❏ _____

   (5) Instruct patient to place his hands on nurse's shoulder ❏ ❏ _____

   (6) Grasp the transfer belt on each side ❏ ❏ _____

   (7) Brace your knees against the patient's knees (block patient's feet with your feet) ❏ ❏ _____

   (8) Request patient to push down on the mattress and to stand on the count of 3. At the same time, lift the patient into a standing position as you straighten your knees ❏ ❏ _____

   (9) Pivot the patient so he can grasp the arm rest of the chair—the back of his legs should be touching the chair ❏ ❏ _____

   (10) Continue to turn the patient until he can grasp the other arm rest ❏ ❏ _____

   (11) As you bend your hips and knees, gradually lower the patient into the chair; the patient can assist by leaning forward and bending his elbows and knees. ❏ ❏ _____

   (12) Make certain the patient's buttocks are up against the back of the chair ❏ ❏ _____

   (13) Cover patient's lap and legs with a blanket ❏ ❏ _____

14. Transferring from bed to stretcher/gurney/back to bed

   a. Position bed flat and raise to the same height as gurney; lower side rails ❏ ❏ _____

	S	U	Comments
b. Cover patient with top sheet or blanket and remove linens without exposing patient	❏	❏	_____
c. Assess for IV line, Foley catheter, tubes, or surgical drains, and position them to avoid tension during the transfer	❏	❏	_____
d. Position the gurney as close to the bed as possible and lock the wheels of the bed and gurney (side rails should be lowered)	❏	❏	_____
e. When patient can assist, stand near side of gurney and instruct patient to move feet, then buttocks, and finally upper body to the gurney bringing cover along; be certain the patient's body is centered on the gurney	❏	❏	_____
f. When patient is unable to assist, place a folded sheet or bath blanket under patient so that it supports patient's head and extends to mid-thighs; roll the sheet or bath blanket close to the patient's body; assist patient to cross arms over chest; two caregivers reach over the bed to patient and two caregivers stand as close to the gurney as possible; a fifth caregiver stands at the foot to transfer the feet. Using a coordinating count of 3, all five caregivers lift the patient to the edge of the bed; with another effort, lift the patient from edge of bed to gurney (roller devices may be used)	❏	❏	_____
15. Perform hand hygiene	❏	❏	_____
16. Assess for appropriate body alignment	❏	❏	_____
17. Document procedure	❏	❏	_____

Student Name_____ Date_____ Instructor's name_____

Using Lifts for Moving Patients

	S	U	Comments
1. Refer to medical record, care plan, or Kardex for special interventions	❑	❑	_____
2. Assemble equipment	❑	❑	_____
a. Hoyer lift			
b. Seat sling attachment			
c. Two cotton blankets			
3. Introduce self	❑	❑	_____
4. Identify patient	❑	❑	_____
5. Explain procedure	❑	❑	_____
6. Perform hand hygiene	❑	❑	_____
7. Prepare for procedure			
a. Close door/pull curtains	❑	❑	_____
b. Adjust bed to working height	❑	❑	_____
c. Medicate patient as needed	❑	❑	_____
8. Secure appropriate number of personnel	❑	❑	_____
9. Place chair near bed	❑	❑	_____
10. Appropriately place canvas seat under patient	❑	❑	_____
11. Slide horseshoe-shaped bar under bed on one side	❑	❑	_____
12. Lower horizontal bar appropriately	❑	❑	_____
13. Fasten hooks on chain to openings in sling	❑	❑	_____
14. Raise head of bed	❑	❑	_____
15. Fold patient's arms over chest	❑	❑	_____
16. Pump lift handle until patient is raised off bed	❑	❑	_____
17. With steering handle, pull lift off bed and down to chair	❑	❑	_____
18. Release valve slowly to lower patient toward chair	❑	❑	_____
19. Close off valve and release straps	❑	❑	_____
20. Remove straps and hydraulic lift	❑	❑	_____

	S	U	Comments
21. Perform hand hygiene	❏	❏	_____
22. Document procedure	❏	❏	_____
a. Evaluate body alignment	❏	❏	_____
b. Evaluate patient's response to movement	❏	❏	_____
23. Do patient teaching	❏	❏	_____

Student Name_____ Date_____ Instructor's name_____

BATHING THE PATIENT AND ADMINISTERING A BACKRUB

	S	U	Comments
1. Refer to medical record, care plan, or Kardex	❏	❏	_____
2. Assemble supplies and complete necessary charges	❏	❏	_____
3. Introduce self	❏	❏	_____
4. Identify patient	❏	❏	_____
5. Explain procedure to patient	❏	❏	_____
6. Perform hand hygiene and don clean gloves as appropriate	❏	❏	_____
7. Assess the patient	❏	❏	_____
8. Prepare patient for intervention			
a. Close door/pull curtain	❏	❏	_____
b. Drape for procedure as appropriate	❏	❏	_____
c. Suggest use of bedpan/urinal/bathroom	❏	❏	_____
d. Arrange supplies	❏	❏	_____
e. Adjust room temperature	❏	❏	_____
f. Raise bed to comfortable working position	❏	❏	_____
9. Bed bath			
a. Lower side rail; position patient on side of bed closest to nurse	❏	❏	_____
b. Loosen top linens from the foot of the bed; place bath blanket over the top linens; remove top linens appropriately	❏	❏	_____
c. Place soiled laundry in laundry bag	❏	❏	_____
d. Assist patient with oral hygiene	❏	❏	_____
e. Remove patient's gown, all undergarments, and jewelry	❏	❏	_____
f. Raise side rail and fill water basin correctly	❏	❏	_____
g. Remove pillow and raise head of bed	❏	❏	_____
h. Form mitt with bath cloth; dip mitt and hand into bath water	❏	❏	_____

		S	U	Comments
i.	Wash around patient's eyes correctly; dry gently	❑	❑	_____
j.	Rinse bath cloth and finish washing face, cleansing ears and neck	❑	❑	_____
k.	Expose arm farthest from nurse; place towel lengthwise under patient's arm; place wash basin on towel and place patient's hands in basin of water; bathe arm; supporting arm, raise it above patient's head to bathe the axilla; rinse and dry well	❑	❑	_____
l.	Do nail care; clean under nails and file smooth; dry thoroughly	❑	❑	_____
m.	Bathe arm closest to nurse as in steps k and l	❑	❑	_____
n.	Cover patient's chest with bath towel; fold bath blanket down to waist and wash chest with circular motion	❑	❑	_____
o.	Fold bath blanket down to pubic area, keeping chest covered with dry towel; wash abdomen, including umbilicus and skin folds; dry thoroughly	❑	❑	_____
p.	Raise side rail; empty basin in proper receptacle	❑	❑	_____
q.	Rinse basin and wash cloth; refill basin correctly	❑	❑	_____
r.	Expose leg farthest away from nurse, keeping perineum covered; place bath towel lengthwise on bed under patient's leg; place wash basin on towel, and place patient's foot in basin	❑	❑	_____
s.	Use long, firm strokes to bathe leg and foot; after soaking, do nail care	❑	❑	_____
t.	Bathe leg and foot closest to nurse as in steps r and s	❑	❑	_____
u.	Raise side rail; make sure patient is covered with bath blanket; change the water; lower side rail; if patient tolerates, position in prone or in Sims' position; place towel lengthwise on bed along back; wash and dry back from neckline down to buttocks	❑	❑	_____
v.	Reposition patient in supine position; provide basin of water, soap, wash cloth, and towel and instruct patient to cleanse perineal area, while providing privacy	❑	❑	_____

	S	U	Comments

w. Make certain patient is covered with blankets; raise side rail; empty basin, and wash and rinse basin; replace basin in bedside stand; place wash cloth in laundry bag for soiled linen ❑ ❑ _____

x. Position patient in Sims' or prone position close to nurse; place towel lengthwise along patient's back; give backrub ❑ ❑ _____

y. Assist patient into clean gown ❑ ❑ _____

z. Place all soiled linen into laundry bag; make certain all bath equipment is clean and replaced as necessary ❑ ❑ _____

aa. Place call light, overbed table, night stand, and telephone within easy reach ❑ ❑ _____

bb. Position patient for comfort and provide warmth ❑ ❑ _____

cc. Remove gloves; discard them in proper receptacle and perform hand hygiene ❑ ❑ _____

10. The partial bed bath differs from the bed bath only in that the patient does not need assistance bathing various anatomic regions. The nurse then helps bathe areas that the patient cannot reach. All steps of the bath are followed, and the same considerations prevail. Supplies are placed within easy reach. Water is changed as noted in the bed bath, and back care, skin care, nail care, and hair care are given. A partial bath, in which the face, neck, axilla, and perineum are washed, is practiced in some agencies ❑ ❑ _____

11. Towel bath

a. Follow steps 1 to 7 ❑ ❑ _____

b. Prepare patient

(1) Remove patient's clothing and excess bedding; place patient on bath blanket, and cover patient with bath blanket ❑ ❑ _____

(2) Cover with plastic any surgical dressing, casts, or areas that should not be wet ❑ ❑ _____

	S	U	Comments
(3) Fan-fold a clean bath blanket at foot of the bed	❏	❏	_____
(4) Place the patient in supine position	❏	❏	_____
c. Prepare towel			
(1) Fold towel in half, top to bottom; fold in half again, side to side; then roll towel-bath towel with bath towel and wash cloth inside, beginning with folded edge	❏	❏	_____
(2) Place rolled-up towel-bath towel in plastic bag with selvage edges toward open end of bag	❏	❏	_____
(3) Draw 2000 mL of water at the correct temperature into plastic pitcher; measure 30 mL of concentrate with a pump; mix 2000 mL of water and concentrate	❏	❏	_____
(4) Pour mixture over towel in plastic bag and close bag	❏	❏	_____
(5) Knead the solution quickly into towel; position plastic bag with open end in sink and squeeze out excess water, giving added wringing twist to selvage edges of towel	❏	❏	_____
d. Bathe patient			
(1) Fold bath blanket down to waist; remove large warm, moist towel from plastic bag and place on patient's right or left chest with open edges up and outward	❏	❏	_____
(2) Open towel to cover entire body while removing top bath blanket; tuck towel-bath towel in and around body	❏	❏	_____
(3) Begin bathing at feet, using gentle, massaging motion	❏	❏	_____
(4) Fold lower part of towel upward away from feet as bathing continues	❏	❏	_____
(5) Place clean bath blanket up over patient as nurse moves upward; leave 3 inches of exposed skin between towel and bath blanket; moisture evaporates quickly	❏	❏	_____

		S	U	Comments
(6)	Wash face, neck, and ears with one of the prepared wash cloths	❏	❏	_____
(7)	Turn patient onto side	❏	❏	_____
(8)	Use smaller prepared bath towel for back care	❏	❏	_____
(9)	Use second wash cloth for perineal care; don disposable gloves (a basin of warm water, soap, wash cloth, and towel may be necessary)	❏	❏	_____
(10)	When bath is completed, remove towel and place with soiled linens in plastic laundry bag	❏	❏	_____
(11)	If top bath blanket is not soiled, fold for reuse	❏	❏	_____
e.	Make occupied bed	❏	❏	_____

12. Tub bath or shower

		S	U	Comments
a.	Follow steps 1 and 3 to 7	❏	❏	_____
b.	Determine whether activity is allowed	❏	❏	_____
c.	Make certain tub or shower appliance is clean; place nonskid mat on tub or shower floor and disposable mat outside of tub or shower	❏	❏	_____
d.	Assemble all items for bathing and complete necessary charges	❏	❏	_____
e.	Assist patient to tub or shower	❏	❏	_____
f.	Instruct patient on how to use call signal; place "in use" sign on tub or shower door if private bath is not being used	❏	❏	_____
g.	If tub is used, fill with warm water at correct temperature; have patient test water, then adjust temperature; instruct patient on use of faucets—which is hot and which is cold; if shower is used, turn water on and adjust temperature	❏	❏	_____
h.	Caution patient to use safety bars; discourage use of bath oil in water; check on patient every 5 minutes; do not allow to remain in tub more than 20 minutes	❏	❏	_____
i.	Return to room when patient signals and offer to wash the patient's back; knock before entering	❏	❏	_____

		S	U	Comments
j.	Assist patient out of tub and with drying; observe patient for signs and symptoms of weakness; if patient complains of weakness, vertigo, or syncope, drain tub before patient gets out and place towel over patient's shoulder	❏	❏	_____
k.	Assist patient into clean gown, robe, and slippers; accompany to room, position for comfort	❏	❏	_____
l.	Make unoccupied bed if patient can tolerate sitting in chair; perform back, hair, nail, and skin care	❏	❏	_____
m.	Return to shower or tub; clean according to agency policy; wear gloves as appropriate; place all soiled linens in laundry bag and return all articles to patient's bedside	❏	❏	_____
n.	Perform hand hygiene	❏	❏	_____
13.	Tepid sponge bath for temperature reduction			
a.	Follow steps 1 to 8	❏	❏	_____
b.	Cover patient with bath blanket, remove gown, and close windows and doors	❏	❏	_____
c.	Test water temperature; place wash cloths in water, then apply wet cloths to each axilla and groin; if patient is in tub, allow to stay in water for 20–30 minutes	❏	❏	_____
d.	Gently sponge an extremity for about 5 minutes; if patient is in tub, gently sponge water over upper torso, chest, and back	❏	❏	_____
e.	Continue sponge bath to other extremities, back, and buttocks for 3–5 minutes each; determine temperature and pulse every 15 minutes	❏	❏	_____
f.	Change water and reapply freshly moistened wash cloths to axilla and groin as necessary	❏	❏	_____
g.	Continue with sponge bath until body temperature falls to slightly above normal; keep body parts that are not being sponged covered; discontinue procedure according to agency policy	❏	❏	_____

		S	U	Comments
h.	Dry patient thoroughly and cover with light blanket or sheet; avoid rubbing the skin too vigorously; leave patient in comfortable position	❏	❏	_____
i.	Return equipment to storage, clean area, and change bed linens as necessary; wash hands	❏	❏	_____

14. Medicated bath

		S	U	Comments
a.	Follow steps 1 to 7	❏	❏	_____
b.	Prepare tub bath	❏	❏	_____
c.	Add agent as ordered	❏	❏	_____
d.	Don gloves as necessary	❏	❏	_____
e.	Assist patient to tub	❏	❏	_____
f.	Allow patient to remain in tub for required time	❏	❏	_____
g.	Assist patient out of tub	❏	❏	_____
h.	Gently pat dry; teach patient not to scratch lesions to avoid further irritation and to prevent infection	❏	❏	_____
i.	Assist patient into gown or pajamas	❏	❏	_____
j.	Assist patient to return to bed, and position for comfort	❏	❏	_____
k.	Remove and dispose of gloves; perform hand hygiene	❏	❏	_____

15. Backrub

		S	U	Comments
a.	Prepare supplies	❏	❏	_____
b.	Follow steps 1 to 7 and provide quiet environment	❏	❏	_____
c.	Lower side rail; position patient with back toward nurse and drape patient with bath blanket after top linens have been fan-folded neatly to the foot of the bed	❏	❏	_____
d.	Warm hands if necessary; warm lotion by holding some in hands; explain that lotion may feel cool	❏	❏	_____
e.	Begin massage by starting in sacral area using circular motion; stroke upwards to shoulders	❏	❏	_____
f.	Use firm, smooth strokes to massage over scapulae; continue to upper arms with one smooth stroke and down along side of back to iliac crest	❏	❏	_____

	S	U	Comments
g. Gently but firmly knead skin by grasping area between thumb and fingers; work across each shoulder and around nape of neck; continue downward along each side to sacrum to increase circulation. Do not break contact with patient's skin	❏	❏	_____
h. With long, smooth strokes, end massage, remove excess lubricant from patient's back with towel, and retie gown; position for comfort; lower bed and raise side rail as needed and place call button within easy reach	❏	❏	_____
i. Place soiled laundry in proper receptacle and perform hand hygiene	❏	❏	_____
16. Assess patient for			
a. Tolerance of activity	❏	❏	_____
b. Level of discomfort	❏	❏	_____
c. Cognitive ability	❏	❏	_____
d. Musculoskeletal function; extent of joint ROM	❏	❏	_____
e. Risk for skin impairment	❏	❏	_____
f. Knowledge of skin hygiene in terms of its importance	❏	❏	_____
g. Vital signs	❏	❏	_____
17. Document			
a. Type of bath	❏	❏	_____
b. Duration of treatment	❏	❏	_____
c. Level of assistance required	❏	❏	_____
d. Condition of skin	❏	❏	_____
e. Vital signs, if applicable	❏	❏	_____
f. Patient's response	❏	❏	_____
g. Patient teaching	❏	❏	_____
18. Report alterations in skin integrity to nurse in charge or physician	❏	❏	_____

PERFORMANCE CHECKLIST 18-2

ADMINISTERING ORAL HYGIENE

		S	U	Comments
1.	Refer to medical record, care plan, or Kardex	❏	❏	_____
2.	Assemble supplies and complete necessary charges	❏	❏	_____
3.	Introduce self	❏	❏	_____
4.	Identify patient	❏	❏	_____
5.	Explain procedure to patient	❏	❏	_____
6.	Perform hand hygiene; don clean gloves	❏	❏	_____
7.	Assess patient			
	a. Integrity of lips, teeth, buccal mucosa, gums, palate, and tongue	❏	❏	_____
	b. Risk of dehydration	❏	❏	_____
	c. Presence of nasogastric or oxygen (O_2) tubes	❏	❏	_____
	d. Chemotherapeutic drugs or radiation therapy to head and neck	❏	❏	_____
	e. Presence of artificial airway	❏	❏	_____
	f. Oral surgery, trauma to mouth	❏	❏	_____
	g. Aging	❏	❏	_____
	h. Diabetes mellitus	❏	❏	_____
	i. Ability to perform own oral care	❏	❏	_____
8.	Prepare patient for intervention			
	a. Close door/pull privacy curtain	❏	❏	_____
	b. Raise bed to comfortable working position	❏	❏	_____
	c. Arrange supplies	❏	❏	_____
	d. If patient can tolerate activity, provide supplies in bathroom and allow privacy	❏	❏	_____

		S	U	Comments
e.	If patient is on bed rest but can tolerate the activity while remaining in bed, arrange overbed table in front of patient; provide supplies and allow patient privacy	❏	❏	_____
f.	Position patient's head toward the nurse if patient is unconscious	❏	❏	_____

9. Oral care

		S	U	Comments
a.	Place towel under patient's face and emesis basin under patient's chin	❏	❏	_____
b.	Carefully separate patient's jaws	❏	❏	_____
c.	Cleanse mouth; clean inner and outer teeth surfaces; swab roof of mouth and inside cheeks; use flashlight for better visualization of oral cavity; gently swab tongue; rinse and repeat cleansing action as necessary	❏	❏	_____
d.	Apply lubricant to lips	❏	❏	_____

10. Cleansing dentures

		S	U	Comments
a.	Fill emesis basin half-full of tepid water	❏	❏	_____
b.	Ask patient to remove dentures and place in emesis basin; if patient is unable to remove own dentures, break suction that holds upper denture in place; with gauze apply gentle downward tug and carefully remove from patient's mouth; next remove lower denture	❏	❏	_____
c.	Cleanse biting surfaces; cleanse outer and inner teeth surfaces; be certain to cleanse under surface of dentures	❏	❏	_____
d.	Rinse dentures thoroughly with tepid water	❏	❏	_____
e.	Replace dentures either in patient's mouth or in container of solution placed in safe location	❏	❏	_____
f.	When reinserting the dentures, replace the upper denture first if patient has both dentures; moisten dentures for easier insertion; make certain that dentures are comfortably situated in patient's mouth before leaving the bedside	❏	❏	_____

	S	U	Comments
g. Before replacing dentures in patient's mouth or after storing dentures properly, gently brush patient's gums, tongue, and inside of cheeks and rinse thoroughly	❏	❏	_____
11. Dispose of gloves; clean and store supplies; perform hand hygiene	❏	❏	_____
12. Position patient for comfort, raise side rail, and lower bed	❏	❏	_____
13. Assess for patient comfort	❏	❏	_____
14. Document			
a. Procedure	❏	❏	_____
b. Pertinent observations	❏	❏	_____
c. Most facilities have flow sheets for documenting ADLs, but condition of oral cavity should be noted in nurse's notes	❏	❏	_____
d. Patient teaching	❏	❏	_____
15. Report bleeding or presence of lesions to nurse in charge or physician	❏	❏	_____

PERFORMANCE CHECKLIST 18-3

CARE OF THE HAIR, NAILS, AND FEET

	S	U	Comments
Prepare for procedure			
1. Refer to medical record, care plan, or Kardex	❏	❏	_____
2. Assemble supplies and complete necessary charges			
a. Bed shampoo	❏	❏	_____
b. Shaving	❏	❏	_____
c. Nail and foot care	❏	❏	_____
3. Introduce self	❏	❏	_____
4. Identify patient	❏	❏	_____
5. Explain procedure	❏	❏	_____
6. Perform hand hygiene and don clean gloves, as appropriate	❏	❏	_____
7. Assess patient			
a. Contraindications to shampooing, shaving, or nail care	❏	❏	_____
b. Restrictions to positioning	❏	❏	_____
c. Condition of scalp, hair, nails, or feet; color and temperature of toes, feet, and fingers	❏	❏	_____
d. Ability to care for own hair, nails, and feet	❏	❏	_____
e. Knowledge of foot and nail care practices	❏	❏	_____
8. Prepare patient for intervention			
a. Close door/pull privacy curtain	❏	❏	_____
b. Raise bed to a comfortable working height	❏	❏	_____
c. Arrange supplies at bedside or, if patient is able to perform procedure, have supplies available in the bathroom and offer assistance as needed	❏	❏	_____
9. Bed shampoo			
a. Position patient close to one side of bed; place shampoo board under patient's head and wash basin at end of spout; make sure spout extends over edge of mattress	❏	❏	_____

		S	U	Comments
b.	Position rolled-up bath towel under patient's neck	❑	❑	_____
c.	Brush and comb patient's hair; if hair is matted with blood, hydrogen peroxide is effective as a cleansing agent	❑	❑	_____
d.	Obtain water in pitcher at correct temperature	❑	❑	_____
e.	If patient is able, instruct patient to hold wash cloth over eyes; completely wet hair and apply small amount of shampoo	❑	❑	_____
f.	Massage scalp with fingertips, not nails; shampoo hairline, back of neck, and sides of hair	❑	❑	_____
g.	Rinse thoroughly and apply more shampoo, repeating steps e and f; rinse and repeat, rinsing until hair is free from shampoo	❑	❑	_____
h.	Wrap dry towel around patient's head; dry patient's face, neck, and shoulders; dry hair and scalp using second towel if necessary	❑	❑	_____
i.	Comb hair and/or dry with blow dryer	❑	❑	_____
j.	Complete styling hair and position patient for comfort	❑	❑	_____

10. Shaving the patient

		S	U	Comments
a.	Assist patient to sitting position	❑	❑	_____
b.	Observe face and neck	❑	❑	_____
c.	Use shaving cream or soap	❑	❑	_____
d.	Shave in direction hair grows; use short strokes; start with upper face and lips, and then extend to neck; if patient is able, it will help if he will hyperextend his head to help shave curved areas	❑	❑	_____
e.	Pull skin taut with nondominant hand below the area being shaved	❑	❑	_____
f.	Rinse razor after each stroke	❑	❑	_____
g.	Rinse and dry face	❑	❑	_____
h.	If patient desires, apply lotion or cologne	❑	❑	_____
i.	Dispose of blades in sharps container	❑	❑	_____

Student Name_____ Date_____ Instructor's name_____

	S	U	Comments

11. Hand and foot care

   a. Position patient in chair; place disposable mat under patient's feet ❑ ❑ _____

   b. Fill basin with water at correct temperature; place basin on disposable mat and assist patient to place feet into basin; allow to soak 10–20 minutes; rewarm water as necessary ❑ ❑ _____

   c. Place overbed table in low position in front of patient; fill emesis basin with water at 100°–110° F (43°–46° C); place basin on table and place patient's fingers in basin; allow fingernails to soak 10–20 minutes; rewarm water as necessary ❑ ❑ _____

   d. Using orangewood stick, gently clean under fingernails; with clippers, trim nails straight across and even with fingertips; with emery board, shape fingernails; push cuticles back gently with wash cloth or orangewood stick ❑ ❑ _____

   e. Don gloves and with wash cloth scrub areas of feet that are callused ❑ ❑ _____

   f. Trim and clean toenails following step d ❑ ❑ _____

   g. Apply lotion or cream to hands and feet; return patient to bed and position for comfort ❑ ❑ _____

   h. On completion of procedure, observe the nails and surrounding tissue for condition of skin and any remaining rough edges ❑ ❑ _____

   i. If the patient's nails are extremely hard or if the patient is unable to perform personal nail care, a podiatrist can provide nail care ❑ ❑ _____

12. Dispose of gloves in proper receptacle; clean and store supplies; place soiled laundry in hamper; perform hand hygiene ❑ ❑ _____

13. Assess for patient's comfort, lower bed level, raise side rails, and place call button within easy reach ❑ ❑ _____

14. Document

   a. Procedure ❑ ❑ _____

	S	U	Comments
b. Pertinent observations	❏	❏	_____
c. Most facilities have flow sheets for ADLs; shaving and nail and foot care are usually not recorded in nurse's notes; know agency policy	❏	❏	_____
d. Patient teaching	❏	❏	_____
15. Report abnormal findings	❏	❏	_____

Student Name_____ Date_____ Instructor's name_____

PERINEAL CARE: MALE AND FEMALE AND THE CATHETERIZED PATIENT

	S	U	Comments
Prepare for procedure			
1. Refer to medical record, care plan, or Kardex	❏	❏	_____
2. Assemble supplies and complete necessary charges			
a. Perineal care (uncatheterized patient)	❏	❏	_____
b. Perineal care (catheterized patient)	❏	❏	_____
3. Introduce self	❏	❏	_____
4. Identify patient	❏	❏	_____
5. Explain procedure	❏	❏	_____
6. Perform hand hygiene and don gloves to assess patient for			
a. Accumulated secretions	❏	❏	_____
b. Surgical incision	❏	❏	_____
c. Lesions	❏	❏	_____
d. Ability to perform self-care	❏	❏	_____
e. Extent of care required by patient	❏	❏	_____
f. Knowledge of importance of perineal care	❏	❏	_____
7. Remove gloves, discard appropriately	❏	❏	_____
8. Prepare patient for intervention			
a. Close door/pull privacy curtain	❏	❏	_____
b. Raise bed to comfortable working height and lower side rail	❏	❏	_____
c. Arrange supplies at bedside	❏	❏	_____
d. OB patients are allowed to perform this procedure by themselves while sitting on the stool by using a plastic squeeze bottle	❏	❏	_____

		S	U	Comments

e. Patients allowed tub/shower baths will do this by themselves; make certain supplies are close by

   (1) Assist patient to desired position in bed, supine for males or dorsal recumbent for females ❏ ❏ _____

   (2) Drape for procedure ❏ ❏ _____

   (3) When perineal care is given other than routinely during the bath, the nurse will need to fill the perineal bottle (peribottle) with cleansing solution and position the patient on the bedpan in bed ❏ ❏ _____

9. Perform hand hygiene and don clean gloves ❏ ❏ _____

10. Female perineal care

a. Raise side rail and fill basin two-thirds full of water at correct temperature ❏ ❏ _____

b. Position patient in bed with knees aligned and slightly abducted, with waterproof pad/towel under buttocks; drape for privacy ❏ ❏ _____

c. Using a disposable wash cloth wrapped around one hand, wash and dry patient's upper thighs ❏ ❏ _____

d. Wash both labia majora and labia minora; cleanse in direction anterior to posterior; use separate corner of wash cloth for each skin fold ❏ ❏ _____

e. Separate labia to expose the urinary meatus and vaginal orifice; wash downward toward rectum with smooth strokes; use separate corner of wash cloth for each smooth stroke ❏ ❏ _____

f. Cleanse, rinse, and dry thoroughly (if patient is on bedpan and peribottle is used, direct flow of cleansing solution down over perineal area and dry thoroughly) ❏ ❏ _____

g. Assist patient to side-lying position and cleanse rectal area with toilet tissue; wash area by cleansing from perineal area toward anus (several wash cloths may be needed). (Many facilitates have disposable wipes; if so, use them.) Wash, rinse, and dry thoroughly ❏ ❏ _____

Student Name_____ Date_____ Instructor's name_____

	S	U	Comments

11. Male perineal care

   a. Raise side rail, fill basin two-thirds full of water at the correct temperature, and position patient supine in bed ❏ ❏ _____

   b. Gently grasp shaft of penis; retract foreskin of uncircumcised patient ❏ ❏ _____

   c. Wash tip of penis with circular motion ❏ ❏ _____

   d. Cleanse from meatus outward; two wash cloths may be necessary; wash, rinse, and dry gently ❏ ❏ _____

   e. Replace foreskin, and wash shaft of penis with a firm but gentle downward stroke ❏ ❏ _____

   f. Rinse and dry thoroughly ❏ ❏ _____

   g. Cleanse scrotum gently; cleanse carefully in underlying skin folds; rinse and dry gently ❏ ❏ _____

   h. Assist patient to a side-lying position; cleanse anal area; follow step g of female perineal care ❏ ❏ _____

12. Catheter care

   a. Raise side rail and fill basin two-thirds full of water at the correct temperature ❏ ❏ _____

   b. Position and drape the female patient in bed, supine as described in step 11 ❏ ❏ _____

   c. Cleanse around urethral meatus and adjacent catheter; cleanse entire catheter with soap and water ❏ ❏ _____

   d. Repeat cleansing to remove all exudate from meatus and catheter ❏ ❏ _____

   e. If ointment is ordered, open package of sterile cotton-tipped applicators; do not touch cotton tip; apply ointment to applicator; do not touch wrapper to cotton tip ❏ ❏ _____

   f. Apply ointment to junction of catheter and urethral meatus ❏ ❏ _____

13. Remove gloves; clean and store equipment; dispose of contaminated supplies in proper receptacle; perform hand hygiene ❏ ❏ _____

14. Position patient for comfort ❏ ❏ _____

	S	U	Comments
15. Document			
a. Procedure	❑	❑	_____
b. Pertinent observations such as			
(1) Character and amount of discharge and odor if present	❑	❑	_____
(2) Condition of genitalia	❑	❑	_____
(3) Patient's ability to perform own care	❑	❑	_____
(4) Patient teaching	❑	❑	_____
16. Report abnormal findings to nurse in charge or physician	❑	❑	_____

PERFORMANCE CHECKLIST 18-5

Bedmaking

	S	U	Comments

Prepare for procedure

1. Refer to medical record, care plan, or Kardex ❑ ❑ _____

2. Assemble supplies and complete necessary charges ❑ ❑ _____

3. Introduce self ❑ ❑ _____

4. Identify patient ❑ ❑ _____

5. Explain procedure ❑ ❑ _____

6. Perform hand hygiene and don gloves as necessary ❑ ❑ _____

7. Prepare patient

   a. Close door/pull privacy curtain ❑ ❑ _____

   b. Raise bed to appropriate height and lower side rail on the side closest to the nurse ❑ ❑ _____

   c. Lower head of bed if patient can tolerate it ❑ ❑ _____

   d. Assess patient's tolerance of procedure; be alert for signs of discomfort and fatigue ❑ ❑ _____

8. Occupied bed

   a. Remove spread and blanket separately and, if soiled, place in laundry bag; if linens will be reused, fold neatly and place over back of chair ❑ ❑ _____

   b. Place bath blanket over patient on top of sheet ❑ ❑ _____

   c. Request patient to hold onto bath blanket and remove top linens ❑ ❑ _____

   d. Place soiled sheet in laundry bag ❑ ❑ _____

   e. With assistance from coworker, slide mattress to top of bed ❑ ❑ _____

   f. Position patient to far side of bed with the back toward nurse; adjust pillow for comfort; be sure side rail is up ❑ ❑ _____

		S	**U**	**Comments**
g.	Beginning at head and moving toward foot, loosen bottom linens; fan-fold linen draw sheet, protective draw sheet, and bottom sheet, tucking edges of linens under patient	❏	❏	_____
h.	Apply clean linens to bed by first placing mattress pad (if used); fold lengthwise, making sure crease is in center of bed; likewise, unfold bottom sheet and place over mattress pad; hem of bottom sheet (if flat is used) should be placed with rough edge down and just even with bottom edge of mattress	❏	❏	_____
i.	Miter corners (if flat sheet) at head of bed; continue to tuck in sheet along side toward front, keeping linens smooth	❏	❏	_____
j.	Reach under the patient to pull out protective draw sheet (if used), and smooth out over clean bottom sheet; tuck in; unfold linen draw sheet and place center fold along middle of bed, smooth out over protective draw sheet and tuck in; tuck in folded linens in center of bed so they are under patient's buttocks and torso	❏	❏	_____
k.	Keep palms down as linens are tucked under mattress	❏	❏	_____
l.	Raise side rail and assist patient to roll slowly toward nurse over folds of linen; go to opposite side of bed and lower side rail	❏	❏	_____
m.	Loosen edges of all soiled linens; remove by folding into a bundle and place in laundry bag	❏	❏	_____
n.	Spread clean linens, including protective draw sheet, out over mattress and smooth out wrinkles; assist patient to supine position and position pillow for comfort	❏	❏	_____
o.	Miter top corner of bottom sheet, pulling sheet taut; tuck bottom sheet under mattress all the way to foot of bed	❏	❏	_____
p.	Smooth out draw sheets; pulling sheet taut, tuck in protective draw sheet and then tuck in linen draw sheet	❏	❏	_____

	S	U	Comments
q. Place top sheet over bath blanket that is over patient; request patient to hold top sheet while nurse removes bath blanket; place blanket in laundry bag; if blanket is used, place over sheet and place spread over blanket; form cuff with top linens under patient's chin	❑	❑	_____
r. Tuck in all linens at foot of bed, making modified miter corner; raise side rail and make opposite side of bed; make toe pleat by placing fold either lengthwise down center of bed or across foot of bed	❑	❑	_____
s. Change pillow case; grasp closed end of pillow case, turning case inside out over hand; now grasp one end of pillow with hand in the case and smooth out wrinkles	❑	❑	_____

9. Unoccupied bed

	S	U	Comments
a. Starting at head of bed, loosen linens all the way to foot; go to opposite side of bed, loosen linens, roll all linens up in ball, and place in soiled laundry bag; perform hand hygiene after handling soiled linens	❑	❑	_____
b. If blanket and spread are to be reused, fold neatly and place over back of chair; remove soiled pillow case	❑	❑	_____
c. Slide mattress to head of bed	❑	❑	_____
d. If necessary, clean mattress with cloth moistened with antiseptic solution and dry thoroughly	❑	❑	_____
e. Begin to make bed standing on side where lines are placed; unfold bottom sheet, placing fold lengthwise down center of bed; make certain rough edge of hem lies down away from patient's heels and even with edge of mattress; smooth out sheet over top edge of mattress and miter corners; tuck remaining sheet under mattress all the way to foot	❑	❑	_____
f. Place draw sheet on bed so that center fold lies down middle of bed; if protective draw sheet is to be used, place it on first; smooth out over mattress and tuck in; keep palms down	❑	❑	_____

	S	U	Comments
g. Place top sheet over bed and smooth out; place blanket over top sheet; smooth out; place spread over blanket and smooth out; make cuff with top linens	❑	❑	_____
h. Allow for toe pleat; make modified mitered corner by not tucking tip of under mattress	❑	❑	_____
i. Move to opposite side of bed and complete making bed as described in steps 9e to 9h; pull linens tight and keep taut as linens are tucked in	❑	❑	_____
j. Put on clean pillow case (see step 8s); position pillow at head of bed; place call light within easy reach and lower bed level	❑	❑	_____
k. If patient is to return to bed, fan-fold top linens down to foot of bed; make sure cuff at top of linens is easily accessible to patient	❑	❑	_____
10. Arrange personal items on bed table or bedside stand and place within patient's easy reach	❑	❑	_____
11. Leave area neat and clean	❑	❑	_____
12. Place all soiled linens in proper receptacle; perform hand hygiene	❑	❑	_____
13. Assist patient to bed and position for comfort	❑	❑	_____
14. Documentation (Bedmaking does not need to be recorded. Record patient's vital signs, signs and symptoms only if there are changes.)	❑	❑	_____
15. Report any abnormal findings to nurse in charge or physician	❑	❑	_____

PERFORMANCE CHECKLIST 18-6

POSITIONING THE BEDPAN

	S	U	Comments
Prepare for procedure			
1. Refer to medical record, care plan, or Kardex	❏	❏	_____
2. Assemble supplies and complete necessary charges	❏	❏	_____
3. Introduce self	❏	❏	_____
4. Identify patient	❏	❏	_____
5. Explain procedure	❏	❏	_____
6. Perform hand hygiene and don clean gloves	❏	❏	_____
7. Assess patient's needs	❏	❏	_____
8. Prepare patient			
a. Close door/pull privacy curtain	❏	❏	_____
b. Arrange supplies close to the bedside	❏	❏	_____
c. Place protective pad under patient's buttocks	❏	❏	_____
9. Warm metal bedpan under running warm water	❏	❏	_____
10. Position patient in supine position with knees flexed and bottom of feet flat on bed surface; as patient raises hips, support patient's lower back with arm and position bedpan under patient; when patient has finished with elimination, remove bedpan in same manner	❏	❏	_____
11. For patient unable to assist self on bedpan			
a. Turn patient away toward opposite side rail, moving linens out of way	❏	❏	_____
b. Fit bedpan to patient's buttocks	❏	❏	_____
c. Assist patient to turn over onto bedpan while nurse secures bedpan	❏	❏	_____
d. Raise head of bed 30 degrees	❏	❏	_____
e. Place toilet tissue and call light within easy reach	❏	❏	_____

	S	U	Comments
12. For those patients who can be out of bed but are unable to ambulate far, there is the bedside commode; some are equipped with wheels that allow the patient to be moved to the bathroom	❏	❏	_____
13. When transferring a patient to the commode, assist the patient in the same manner as if assisting to a chair	❏	❏	_____
14. Document according to agency policy			
a. Amount	❏	❏	_____
b. Color	❏	❏	_____
c. Consistency	❏	❏	_____
d. Abnormal findings	❏	❏	_____
15. Report abnormal findings	❏	❏	_____

PERFORMANCE CHECKLIST 19-1

PREPARING PATIENT FOR DIAGNOSTIC EXAMINATION

	S	U	Comments
1. Refer to medical record, care plan, or Kardex	❑	❑	_____
2. Ensure that informed consent has been obtained when necessary (most invasive diagnostic tests require informed consent)	❑	❑	_____
3. Assemble equipment and supplies	❑	❑	_____
4. Introduce self	❑	❑	_____
5. Identify patient	❑	❑	_____
6. Explain procedure; assess patient's understanding of procedure and purpose; assess patient for allergy to dye (if dye is to be used)	❑	❑	_____
7. Perform hand hygiene and don clean gloves	❑	❑	_____
8. Prepare patient for procedure			
a. Transfer to examining room; maintain safety precautions	❑	❑	_____
b. Close door and pull curtains	❑	❑	_____
c. Raise bed or arrange examination table to convenient height	❑	❑	_____
d. Drape for procedure if necessary	❑	❑	_____
9. Assist physician with procedure	❑	❑	_____

Postprocedure

	S	U	Comments
10. Answer patient's questions	❑	❑	_____
11. Deliver specimen to laboratory promptly, label specimen according to agency policy: patient's name, birth date, age, room number, physician, date and time, type of specimen, and collector's initials; CDC and OSHA recommend inserting specimen (in container) into another plastic bag for transport to laboratory	❑	❑	_____

	S	U	Comments
12. Document procedure			
a. Type of procedure	❏	❏	_____
b. Time	❏	❏	_____
c. Specimen obtained	❏	❏	_____
d. Sent to laboratory with requisition	❏	❏	_____
e. Patient's response	❏	❏	_____
f. Patient teaching	❏	❏	_____

Student Name_____ Date_____ Instructor's name_____

COLLECTING A MIDSTREAM URINE SPECIMEN

	S	U	Comments
1. Refer to medical record, care plan, or Kardex	❏	❏	_____
2. Assemble supplies	❏	❏	_____
3. Introduce self	❏	❏	_____
4. Identify patient	❏	❏	_____
5. Explain procedure to patient; make certain patient understands how to perform procedure	❏	❏	_____
6. Prepare patient for procedure	❏	❏	_____
a. Close door/pull privacy curtain	❏	❏	_____
b. Offer assistance if required	❏	❏	_____
7. Perform hand hygiene and don clean gloves	❏	❏	_____
8. If patient is able, allow patient to cleanse perineum from anterior to posterior with antiseptic solution. Separate the labia well on a female patient. Retract foreskin of an uncircumcised male. Use each cotton ball that is saturated with antiseptic solution one time only. If patient is unable to cleanse area, the nurse will don gloves and assist with procedure	❏	❏	_____
9. Request that patient (1) begin to void into urine receptacle about 30 mL, then place the sterile specimen container so that sides of the labia of the female do not touch; (2) without stopping flow, void a small amount into specimen cup; and (3) without stopping flow, finish voiding into toilet	❏	❏	_____
10. Secure lid on container	❏	❏	_____
11. Cleanse and return toilet seat collector; empty and flush bedpan/urinal	❏	❏	_____
12. Label specimen appropriately; enclose in plastic bag for transport	❏	❏	_____
13. Remove gloves, discard in proper receptacle, and perform hand hygiene	❏	❏	_____

	S	U	Comments
14. Ensure that specimen is taken to laboratory with proper requisition slip (many facilities mandate within 1 hour)	❏	❏	_____
15. Document procedure per protocol	❏	❏	_____

Student Name_____ Date_____ Instructor's name_____

Collecting a Sterile Urine Specimen Via Catheter Port

	S	U	Comments
1. Refer to medical record, care plan, or Kardex	❑	❑	_____
2. Assemble supplies	❑	❑	_____
3. Introduce self	❑	❑	_____
4. Identify patient	❑	❑	_____
5. Explain procedure to patient	❑	❑	_____
6. Perform hand hygiene and don clean gloves	❑	❑	_____
7. Catheter port collection			
a. Clamp just below catheter port for about 30 minutes	❑	❑	_____
b. Return in 30 minutes; don clean gloves; clean port with alcohol prep	❑	❑	_____
c. Insert *needleless* adapter into port at 30-degree angle, and withdraw 5–10 mL of urine for a specimen	❑	❑	_____
d. Place urine in sterile specimen cup	❑	❑	_____
e. Unclamp catheter	❑	❑	_____
f. Label specimen, enclose in plastic bag, and send to laboratory with requisition	❑	❑	_____
8. Remove gloves and perform hand hygiene	❑	❑	_____
9. Document procedure and observations	❑	❑	_____

Student Name_____ Date_____ Instructor's name_____

COLLECTING A 24-HOUR URINE SPECIMEN

		S	U	Comments
1.	Refer to medical record, care plan, or Kardex	❑	❑	_____
2.	Assemble supplies and equipment	❑	❑	_____
3.	Introduce self	❑	❑	_____
4.	Identify patient	❑	❑	_____
5.	Explain procedure			
	a. Instruct patient about the importance of collecting all urine for a period of 24 hours	❑	❑	_____
	b. Instruct patient not to place toilet tissue or fecal material in urine	❑	❑	_____
6.	Post signs in all appropriate places	❑	❑	_____
7.	Perform hand hygiene and don gloves	❑	❑	_____
8.	Have patient void when the 24-hour specimen collection is to begin; discard this voiding	❑	❑	_____
9.	Place labeled container on ice if required	❑	❑	_____
10.	Save all urine for the 24-hour period; place each voided specimen into the larger container with preservative; all urine must be saved or results will be altered	❑	❑	_____
11.	Instruct patient to void a few minutes before end of 24 hours; this urine is part of the 24-hour specimen	❑	❑	_____
12.	Send specimen to lab promptly; be certain label is complete with all pertinent information. If more than one container is necessary, make certain all are labeled and numbered	❑	❑	_____
13.	Remove gloves, perform hand hygiene	❑	❑	_____
14.	Document procedure and observations	❑	❑	_____
15.	Do patient teaching	❑	❑	_____

Student Name_____ Date_____ Instructor's name_____

MEASURING BLOOD GLUCOSE LEVELS

	S	U	Comments
1. Refer to medical record, care plan, or Kardex	❏	❏	_____
2. Assemble supplies	❏	❏	_____
3. Introduce self	❏	❏	_____
4. Identify patient	❏	❏	_____
5. Explain procedure to patient	❏	❏	_____
6. Perform hand hygiene and don clean gloves	❏	❏	_____
7. Remove cap from lancet using sterile technique	❏	❏	_____
8. Place lancet into automatic lancing device according to instructions in operating manual	❏	❏	_____
9. Select site on side of any fingertip (heel used for infant)	❏	❏	_____
10. Wipe selected site with alcohol swab, and discard	❏	❏	_____
11. Ask patient to hold arm at side for 30 seconds	❏	❏	_____
12. Gently squeeze fingertip with thumb of same hand	❏	❏	_____
13. Hold lancing device	❏	❏	_____
14. Place trigger platform of lancing device on side of finger, and press	❏	❏	_____
15. Squeeze finger in downward motion (wipe off first drop of blood)	❏	❏	_____
16. While holding strip level, touch drop of blood to test pad (prevent skin from touching test pad)	❏	❏	_____
17. Begin recommended timing. After 60 seconds, blot blood off test strip, place reagent strip into appropriate site on meter, and wait for numeric readout	❏	❏	_____

	S	U	Comments
18. Remove lancet from device, and discard	❏	❏	_____
19. Remove gloves and discard; perform hand hygiene	❏	❏	_____
20. Document procedure and observations	❏	❏	_____
21. Do patient teaching	❏	❏	_____

Student Name_____ Date_____ Instructor's name_____

COLLECTING A STOOL SPECIMEN

	S	**U**	**Comments**
1. Refer to medical record, care plan, or Kardex	❑	❑	_____
2. Assemble supplies	❑	❑	_____
3. Introduce self	❑	❑	_____
4. Identify patient	❑	❑	_____
5. Explain procedure to patient; make certain patient understands what is expected	❑	❑	_____
6. Perform hand hygiene and don gloves	❑	❑	_____
7. Assist to bathroom when necessary	❑	❑	_____
8. Request that patient defecate into commode, specimen device, or bedpan, and prevent urine from entering specimen	❑	❑	_____
9. Transfer stool to specimen cup with use of a tongue blade and close lid securely	❑	❑	_____
10. Remove gloves and perform hand hygiene	❑	❑	_____
11. Attach requisition slip, enclose in plastic bag, and send specimen to laboratory; specimens for ova and parasites must be taken to the laboratory stat; other stool specimens may be kept at room temperature	❑	❑	_____
12. Assist patient to bed	❑	❑	_____
13. Document procedure and observations	❑	❑	_____
14. Do patient teaching	❑	❑	_____

Student Name_____ Date_____ Instructor's name_____

DETERMINING THE PRESENCE OF OCCULT BLOOD IN STOOL

	S	U	Comments
1. Refer to medical record, care plan, or Kardex	❏	❏	_____
2. Assemble supplies	❏	❏	_____
3. Introduce self	❏	❏	_____
4. Identify patient	❏	❏	_____
5. Explain procedure	❏	❏	_____
6. Perform hand hygiene, and don gloves	❏	❏	_____
7. Collect stool specimen appropriately	❏	❏	_____
8. Follow steps on Hemoccult slide test			
a. Open flap	❏	❏	_____
b. Smear very small amount of stool with tongue blade in first box (A)	❏	❏	_____
c. Smear very small amount of stool with tongue blade from another part of stool specimen, and transfer to box (B)	❏	❏	_____
d. Close card, label (label before collecting specimen), and place in plastic bag	❏	❏	_____
e. Send specimen to laboratory with requisition slip	❏	❏	_____
9. Remove gloves and perform hand hygiene	❏	❏	_____
10. Document procedure and observations	❏	❏	_____
11. Do patient teaching	❏	❏	_____

Collecting Gastric Secretions or Emesis Specimen

	S	U	Comments
1. Refer to medical record, care plan, or Kardex	❑	❑	_____
2. Assemble supplies	❑	❑	_____
3. Introduce self	❑	❑	_____
4. Identify patient	❑	❑	_____
5. Explain procedure	❑	❑	_____
6. Perform hand hygiene and don gloves	❑	❑	_____
7. To obtain specimen of gastric contents using NG or nasoenteral tube, position patient in high-Fowler's in bed or chair	❑	❑	_____
8. Verify NG tube placement	❑	❑	_____
9. Collect gastric contents via NG tube or nasoenteral tube			
a. Disconnect tube from suction or gravity drainage	❑	❑	_____
b. Attach bulb- or cone-tipped syringe	❑	❑	_____
c. Aspirate 5 to 10 mL	❑	❑	_____
d. To obtain sample of emesis, use a 3-mL syringe or wooden applicator	❑	❑	_____
e. Using applicator or syringe, apply 1 drop of gastric sample to Gastroccult blood test slide	❑	❑	_____
f. Apply 2 drops of commercial developer solution over sample and 1 drop between positive and negative performance monitors	❑	❑	_____
g. After 60 seconds, compare color of gastric sample with that of performance monitors	❑	❑	_____
h. Verify that performance monitor turns blue in 30 seconds	❑	❑	_____
10. Close card and label	❑	❑	_____

	S	U	Comments
11. Enclose specimen in plastic bag and send to laboratory with requisition slip	❏	❏	_____
12. Reconnect NG tube to drainage system, suction, or clamp as ordered	❏	❏	_____
13. Dispose of equipment, remove gloves, and perform hand hygiene	❏	❏	_____
14. Document procedure and observations	❏	❏	_____
15. Do patient teaching (patients are usually informed of test results)	❏	❏	_____

PERFORMANCE CHECKLIST 19-9

COLLECTING A SPUTUM SPECIMEN BY SUCTION

	S	U	Comments
1. Refer to medical record, care plan, or Kardex	❑	❑	_____
2. Assemble supplies	❑	❑	_____
3. Introduce self	❑	❑	_____
4. Identify patient	❑	❑	_____
5. Explain procedure; encourage patient to breathe normally to prevent hyperventilation	❑	❑	_____
6. Arrange equipment and prepare necessary charges	❑	❑	_____
7. Perform hand hygiene	❑	❑	_____
8. Assess patient			
a. Determine when patient last ate a meal	❑	❑	_____
b. Respiratory status: rate, depth, pattern, lung sounds, and color	❑	❑	_____
c. Anxiety level	❑	❑	_____
9. Position patient for procedure			
a. Close door/pull curtains	❑	❑	_____
b. The higher semi-Fowler's position is recommended	❑	❑	_____
c. Prepare suction machine or device and make certain it is functioning properly	❑	❑	_____
d. Drape patient as necessary	❑	❑	_____
e. Adjust bed to appropriate height and lower side rail	❑	❑	_____
10. Connect suction tube to adapter on sputum trap	❑	❑	_____
11. Apply sterile glove to dominant hand	❑	❑	_____
12. Preoxygenate the patient for 1 minute with 100% oxygen, if available	❑	❑	_____
13. Using sterile gloved hand, connect sterile suction catheter tubing on sputum trap	❑	❑	_____

	S	U	Comments
14. Gently insert tip of suction catheter prelubricated with sterile water through nasopharynx, endotracheal tube, or tracheostomy without applying suction	❏	❏	_____
15. Warn patient to expect to cough and gently and quickly advance catheter into trachea	❏	❏	_____
16. As patient coughs, apply suction for 5 to 10 seconds, collection 2 to 10 mL of sputum	❏	❏	_____
17. Release suction and remove catheter, then turn off suction	❏	❏	_____
18. Detach catheter from specimen trap, and dispose of catheter into appropriate receptacle; connect rubber tubing on sputum trap to plastic adapter	❏	❏	_____
19. If any sputum is present on outside of container, wash it off with disinfectant	❏	❏	_____
20. Offer patient tissues after suctioning; dispose of tissues in emesis basin or trash container; remove and dispose of gloves	❏	❏	_____
21. Securely attach properly completed identification label and laboratory requisition to side of specimen container (not the lid)	❏	❏	_____
22. Enclose specimen in a plastic bag; send specimen immediately to laboratory	❏	❏	_____
23. Offer patient mouth care and assist to a comfortable position and place needed items within easy reach	❏	❏	_____
24. Raise side rail and lower bed to lowest position	❏	❏	_____
25. Store, remove, or dispose of supplies and equipment as appropriate	❏	❏	_____
26. Document procedure			
a. Method used to obtain specimen	❏	❏	_____
b. Date and time collected	❏	❏	_____
c. Type of test ordered and how specimen was transported to the laboratory	❏	❏	_____
d. Characteristics of sputum specimen	❏	❏	_____
e. Patient's oxygenation and respiratory status	❏	❏	_____

Student Name_____ Date_____ Instructor's name_____

COLLECTING A SPUTUM SPECIMEN BY EXPECTORATION

	S	U	Comments
1. Refer to medical record, care plan, or Kardex	❑	❑	_____
2. Assemble supplies	❑	❑	_____
3. Introduce self	❑	❑	_____
4. Identify patient	❑	❑	_____
5. Explain procedure to patient	❑	❑	_____
6. Perform hand hygiene and don gloves	❑	❑	_____
7. Position patient in Fowler's position	❑	❑	_____
8. Instruct patient to take three breaths, and force cough into sterile container	❑	❑	_____
9. Label specimen container (if any sputum is present on outside of container, wash it off with disinfectant)	❑	❑	_____
10. Attach laboratory requisition, place in plastic bag, and send specimen to laboratory; specimen should be analyzed promptly for accurate results	❑	❑	_____
11. Remove gloves and perform hand hygiene	❑	❑	_____
12. Document procedure and observations	❑	❑	_____
13. Do patient teaching	❑	❑	_____

Student Name_____ Date_____ Instructor's name_____

Obtaining a Throat Specimen

	S	U	Comments
1. Refer to medical record, care plan, or Kardex	❏	❏	_____
2. Assemble supplies	❏	❏	_____
3. Introduce self	❏	❏	_____
4. Identify patient	❏	❏	_____
5. Explain procedure	❏	❏	_____
6. Perform hand hygiene and don gloves	❏	❏	_____
7. Instruct patient to tilt head backward; for patients in bed, place pillow behind shoulders	❏	❏	_____
8. Ask patient to open mouth and say "ah"	❏	❏	_____
9. Have swab stick ready for use (you may want to loosen top so swab can be removed easily)	❏	❏	_____
10. If pharynx is not visualized, depress tongue with tongue blade and note inflamed areas of pharynx of tonsils; depress anterior third tongue only (illuminate with penlight as needed)	❏	❏	_____
11. Insert swab without touching lips, teeth, tongue, or cheeks	❏	❏	_____
12. Gently but quickly swab tonsillar area side to side, making contact with inflamed or purulent sites	❏	❏	_____
13. Carefully withdraw swab without striking oral structures; immediately place swab in culture tube, using a 2 x 2 gauze; cover end of tube and crush ampule at bottom of tube; push tip of swab into liquid medium	❏	❏	_____
14. Securely attach properly completed label and requisition slip to side of specimen container (not the lid)	❏	❏	_____
15. Enclose in a plastic bag	❏	❏	_____

	S	U	Comments
16. Send specimen immediately to laboratory or refrigerate	❏	❏	_____
17. Discard gloves and perform hand hygiene	❏	❏	_____
18. Document procedure	❏	❏	_____

PERFORMANCE CHECKLIST 19-12

OBTAINING A NOSE CULTURE

	S	**U**	**Comments**
1. Refer to medical record, care plan, or Kardex	❏	❏	_____
2. Assemble supplies	❏	❏	_____
3. Introduce self	❏	❏	_____
4. Identify patient	❏	❏	_____
5. Explain procedure	❏	❏	_____
6. Perform hand hygiene and don gloves	❏	❏	_____
7. Ask patient to blow nose, and then check nostrils for patency with penlight; select nostril with greatest patency	❏	❏	_____
8. Ask patient to tilt head back; patients in bed should have a pillow behind the shoulders	❏	❏	_____
9. Gently insert nasal speculum in one nostril (optional); carefully pass swab into nostril until it reaches that portion of mucosa that is inflamed or containing exudate; rotate swab quickly (NOTE: If nasopharyngeal culture is to be obtained, use a special swab on a flexible wire that can be flexed downward to reach nasopharynx)	❏	❏	_____
10. With dominant hand, remove swab without touching sides of speculum or nasal canal	❏	❏	_____
11. With nondominant hand, carefully remove nasal speculum (if used) and place in basin; offer patient facial tissue	❏	❏	_____
12. Immediately place swab in culture tube	❏	❏	_____
13. Cover end of tube with 2 x 2 gauze, then crush ampule at bottom of tube to release culture medium; push tip of swab into liquid medium	❏	❏	_____
14. Place top on tube securely	❏	❏	_____
15. Discard supplies into trash	❏	❏	_____

	S	U	Comments
16. Send to laboratory with completed requisition and attached label (not attached to the lid); enclose in a plastic bag	❏	❏	_____
17. Remove and discard gloves, perform hand hygiene	❏	❏	_____
18. Document procedure	❏	❏	_____

PERFORMANCE CHECKLIST 19-13

PERFORMING THE VENIPUNCTURE

	S	U	Comments
1. Refer to medical record, care plan, or Kardex	❑	❑	_____
2. Assemble supplies	❑	❑	_____
3. Introduce self	❑	❑	_____
4. Identify patient	❑	❑	_____
5. Explain procedure	❑	❑	_____
6. Arrange equipment and complete necessary charges	❑	❑	_____
7. Perform hand hygiene and don clean gloves	❑	❑	_____
8. Assess patient	❑	❑	_____
9. Prepare patient for procedure			
a. Provide privacy; close door/pull curtain	❑	❑	_____
b. Position supine or semi-Fowler's with arm extended to form straight line from shoulders to waist	❑	❑	_____
c. Place small pillow or towel under upper arm	❑	❑	_____
d. Adjust bed to appropriate height and lower nearest side rail	❑	❑	_____
e. Drape patient	❑	❑	_____
10. Apply tourniquet 3–4 inches above puncture site	❑	❑	_____
11. Palpate distal pulse. If pulse is not palpable, reapply tourniquet more loosely	❑	❑	_____
12. Keep tourniquet on patient no longer than 1–2 minutes. If tourniquet is left on too long, remove and assess other extremity or wait 60 seconds before reapplying	❑	❑	_____
13. Request patient to open and close fist several times, finally leaving fist clenched; avoid vigorous opening and closing of fist, which may cause erroneous laboratory results	❑	❑	_____
14. Quickly assess extremity for best venipuncture site, looking for straight, prominent vein without edema or hematoma	❑	❑	_____

	S	U	Comments
15. Palpate selected vein with fingers; note if vein is firm and rebounds when palpated or if vein feels rigid and cordlike and rolls when palpated	❏	❏	_____
16. Select venipuncture site	❏	❏	_____
17. Obtain blood samples	❏	❏	_____

    a. Syringe method

	S	U	Comments
(1) Make certain syringe with appropriate needle is securely attached	❏	❏	_____
(2) Cleanse venipuncture site with alcohol swab, moving in circular motion from site for approximately 2 inches (5 cm) and allow to dry	❏	❏	_____
(3) Remove needle cover and inform patient a "stick" will be felt	❏	❏	_____
(4) Place thumb and forefinger of nondominant hand 1 inch below site and pull skin taut. Stretch skin down until vein is stabilized	❏	❏	_____
(5) Hold syringe and needle at 15- to 30-degree angle from patient's arm with bevel up	❏	❏	_____
(6) Slowly insert needle into vein	❏	❏	_____
(7) Hold syringe securely and pull back gently on plunger	❏	❏	_____
(8) Look for blood return	❏	❏	_____
(9) Obtain desired amount of blood, keeping needle stabilized	❏	❏	_____
(10) After obtaining specimen, release tourniquet	❏	❏	_____
(11) Apply a gauze pad or alcohol swab over needle site without applying pressure, quickly but carefully withdraw needle from vein, and apply pressure to puncture site	❏	❏	_____
(12) Carefully transfer blood from syringe into vacuum tube	❏	❏	_____
(13) Discard needle without recapping in proper receptacle	❏	❏	_____
(14) Remove and discard gloves; perform hand hygiene	❏	❏	_____

	S	U	Comments
b. Vacuum tube method			
(1) Attach double-ended needle to vacuum tube	❏	❏	_____
(2) Have proper blood specimen tube resting inside vacuum tube without puncturing rubber stopper	❏	❏	_____
(3) Cleanse venipuncture site properly with alcohol swab	❏	❏	_____
(4) Remove needle cover and inform patient "stick" will be felt	❏	❏	_____
(5) Place thumb and forefinger of nondominant hand 1 inch below site and pull taut. Stretch skin down until vein is stabilized	❏	❏	_____
(6) Hold vacuum tube at a 15- to 30-degree angle from arm with bevel up	❏	❏	_____
(7) Slowly insert needle into vein	❏	❏	_____
(8) Grasp vacuum tube securely and advance specimen tube into needle of holder	❏	❏	_____
(9) Note flow of blood into tube	❏	❏	_____
(10) After specimen tube is filled, grasp vacuum tube firmly and remove tube. Insert additional specimen tubes as needed	❏	❏	_____
(11) After last tube is filled, release tourniquet	❏	❏	_____
(12) Apply 2 x 2 gauze pad over needle site without applying pressure and quickly but carefully withdraw needle from vein, applying pressure over puncture site	❏	❏	_____
(13) Remove and discard gloves; perform hand hygiene	❏	❏	_____
18. For blood obtained by syringe, transfer specimen to tubes			
a. Using one-handed technique, insert needle through stopper of blood tube and allow vacuum to fill tube; do not force blood into tube	❏	❏	_____
b. Alternative method is to remove needle from syringe and stopper to each test tube; gently inject required amount of blood into each tube; reapply stopper	❏	❏	_____

	S	U	Comments
19. For blood obtained for culture			
a. Cleanse venipuncture site with providone-iodine or appropriate antiseptic; allow to dry	❏	❏	_____
b. Clean bottle tops of vacuum tubes or culture bottles with appropriate antiseptic (check agency policy)	❏	❏	_____
c. Collect 10 to 15 mL of venous blood by venipuncture from each venipuncture site	❏	❏	_____
d. Discard needle on syringe; replace with new sterile needle before injecting blood sample into culture bottles	❏	❏	_____
e. If both aerobic and anaerobic cultures are needed, inoculate anaerobic first	❏	❏	_____
f. Mix medium gently after inoculation	❏	❏	_____
g. After venipuncture, apply 2 x 2 gauze pad over puncture site without applying pressure, and quickly but carefully withdraw needle from vein	❏	❏	_____
20. For blood tubes containing additives, gently rotate back and forth 8–10 times	❏	❏	_____
21. Inspect puncture site for bleeding and apply adhesive tape with gauze	❏	❏	_____
22. Check tubes for any sign of external contamination with blood; decontaminate with alcohol, if necessary; remove and discard gloves; perform hand hygiene	❏	❏	_____
23. Securely attach properly completed ID label to each tube, affix proper requisition, and transfer to laboratory promptly	❏	❏	_____
24. Remove and appropriately discard gloves; perform hand hygiene	❏	❏	_____
25. Assist patient to a comfortable position and place needed items within easy reach	❏	❏	_____
26. Raise side rail and lower bed to lowest position	❏	❏	_____
27. Store, remove, and dispose of supplies and equipment as is appropriate	❏	❏	_____
28. Document procedure	❏	❏	_____

PERFORMANCE CHECKLIST 19-14

PERFORMING AN ELECTROCARDIOGRAM (ECG)

	S	U	Comments
1. Refer to medical record, care plan, or Kardex	❏	❏	_____
2. Assemble supplies	❏	❏	_____
3. Introduce self	❏	❏	_____
4. Identify patient	❏	❏	_____
5. Explain procedure	❏	❏	_____
6. Arrange equipment and complete necessary charges	❏	❏	_____
7. Perform hand hygiene and don clean gloves	❏	❏	_____
8. Assess patient for			
a. Chest pain	❏	❏	_____
b. Dyspnea	❏	❏	_____
c. Heart rate and rhythm	❏	❏	_____
d. Blood pressure, pulse, respirations	❏	❏	_____
9. Prepare patient for procedure			
a. Close door/pull curtain	❏	❏	_____
b. Position patient supine and provide for comfort	❏	❏	_____
c. Drape patient	❏	❏	_____
d. Adjust bed to proper height and lower nearest side rail	❏	❏	_____
10. Perform ECG			
a. Cleanse and wipe skin area with alcohol	❏	❏	_____
b. Apply electrode paste and attach leads. For 12-lead ECG			
(1) Chest (precordial leads)			
• V_1—Fourth intercostal space (ICS) at right sternal border	❏	❏	_____

	S	**U**	**Comments**
• V_2—Fourth ICS at left sternal border	❏	❏	_____
• V_3—Midway between V_2 and V_4	❏	❏	_____
• V_4—Fifth ICS at midclavicular line	❏	❏	_____
• V_5—Left anterior axillary line at level of V_4 horizontally	❏	❏	_____
• V_6—Left midaxillary line at level of V_4 horizontally	❏	❏	_____
(2) Extremities—one at lower portion of each extremity			
• aVR—Right wrist	❏	❏	_____
• aVL—Left wrist	❏	❏	_____
• AVF—Left ankle	❏	❏	_____
c. Obtain tracing	❏	❏	_____
d. Disconnect leads, wipe excess paste from chest	❏	❏	_____
e. Remove gloves, dispose of appropriately and perform hand hygiene	❏	❏	_____
f. Deliver EGG tracing promptly to laboratory or nursing unit	❏	❏	_____
11. Assist patient to position of comfort and place needed items within easy reach	❏	❏	_____
12. Raise side rail and lower bed to lowest position	❏	❏	_____
13. Store supplies and equipment as is appropriate	❏	❏	_____
14. Document procedure	❏	❏	_____

PERFORMANCE CHECKLIST 20-1

EYE IRRIGATION

	S	U	Comments
Prepare for procedure			
1. Refer to medical record, care plan, or Kardex	❑	❑	_____
2. Introduce self	❑	❑	_____
3. Identify patient	❑	❑	_____
4. Explain procedure and reason it is to be done	❑	❑	_____
5. Assess need for and provide patient teaching during procedure	❑	❑	_____
6. Assemble equipment and complete necessary charges	❑	❑	_____
7. Perform hand hygiene	❑	❑	_____
8. Assess patient	❑	❑	_____
9. Prepare patient for intervention			
a. Close door/pull privacy curtain	❑	❑	_____
b. Raise bed to comfortable working height; lower side rail on side nearest the nurse	❑	❑	_____
c. Position and drape patient as necessary	❑	❑	_____
During the skill			
10. Promote patient involvement as possible	❑	❑	_____
11. Assess patient's tolerance	❑	❑	_____
12. Assess condition of both eyes	❑	❑	_____
13. Place patient lying toward side to be irrigated	❑	❑	_____
14. Place towel under patient's head	❑	❑	_____
15. Use a sterile plastic squeeze bottle unless very large amounts of solution are needed (sometimes a medicine dropper is sufficient)	❑	❑	_____
16. Don gloves	❑	❑	_____
17. Place an emesis basin at side of face	❑	❑	_____

	S	U	Comments
18. Using the thumb and index finger of the nondominant hand, separate the patient's eyelids	❏	❏	_____
19. Gently direct the irrigating solution along the conjunctiva from the inner to the outer canthus	❏	❏	_____
20. Avoid directing a forceful stream onto the eyeball	❏	❏	_____
21. Avoid touching any parts of the eye with irrigation equipment	❏	❏	_____
22. A piece of gauze may be wrapped around the gloved index finger to raise upper lid	❏	❏	_____
23. Gently dry the eyelids	❏	❏	_____
24. Remove gloves and perform hand hygiene	❏	❏	_____

Postprocedure

	S	U	Comments
25. Assist patient to a position of comfort and place needed items within easy reach; be certain patient has a means to call for assistance and knows how to use it	❏	❏	_____
26. Raise side rails and lower bed to lowest position	❏	❏	_____
27. Store or remove and dispose of soiled supplies and equipment appropriately	❏	❏	_____
28. Remove gloves and all protective barriers; dispose of soiled supplies and equipment appropriately	❏	❏	_____
29. Perform hand hygiene after patient contact and after wearing gloves	❏	❏	_____
30. Document and do patient teaching	❏	❏	_____
31. Report any unexpected outcomes	❏	❏	_____

PERFORMANCE CHECKLIST 20-2

WARM, MOIST EYE COMPRESSES

	S	U	Comments
Prepare for procedure			
1. Refer to medical record, care plan, or Kardex	❏	❏	_____
2. Introduce self	❏	❏	_____
3. Identify patient	❏	❏	_____
4. Explain procedure and reason it is to be done	❏	❏	_____
5. Assess need for and provide patient teaching during procedure	❏	❏	_____
6. Assemble equipment and complete necessary charges	❏	❏	_____
7. Perform hand hygiene	❏	❏	_____
8. Assess patient	❏	❏	_____
9. Prepare patient for intervention			
a. Close door/pull privacy curtain	❏	❏	_____
b. Raise bed to comfortable working height; lower side rail on side nearest the nurse	❏	❏	_____
c. Position and drape patient as necessary	❏	❏	_____
During the skill			
10. Promote patient involvement as possible	❏	❏	_____
11. Assess patient's tolerance	❏	❏	_____
12. Don clean gloves	❏	❏	_____
13. Assess condition of both eyes	❏	❏	_____
14. Assist patient to a comfortable position; when applying warm compresses, have the patient sit if possible; support the head with a pillow and turn the head slightly to the unaffected side	❏	❏	_____
15. Place the towel/waterproof pad under the patient's head	❏	❏	_____
16. Use sterile technique when infection or ulceration is present; clean technique may be used for allergic reactions	❏	❏	_____

	S	U	Comments
17. Change gloves, dispose of in proper receptacle, and perform hand hygiene before treating each eye	❏	❏	_____
18. Temperature of compresses should not exceed 120° F (49° C); to heat solution, place the uncapped bottle of solution in a basin of hot water; pour the warmed solution into a sterile bowl, filling it halfway; place sterile gauze pads in the bowl	❏	❏	_____
19. Take two 4 x 4 gauze pads from the basin; squeeze out excess moisture	❏	❏	_____
20. Instruct the patient to close his or her eyes; gently apply the pads—one on top of the other—to the affected eye	❏	❏	_____
21. Do not exert pressure on eyelids	❏	❏	_____
22. Change compress every few minutes, as necessary, for the prescribed length of time	❏	❏	_____
23. If sterility is not necessary, moist heat may be applied by means of a clean wash cloth	❏	❏	_____
24. After removing each compress, assess the periorbital skin for signs that the compress solution is too hot	❏	❏	_____
25. Cleanse patient's eye and dry with the remaining gauze pads	❏	❏	_____
26. If ordered, apply ophthalmic ointment or eye patch	❏	❏	_____

Postprocedure

	S	U	Comments
27. Assist patient to a position of comfort and place needed items within easy reach; be certain patient has a means to call for assistance and knows how to use it	❏	❏	_____
28. Raise side rails and lower bed to lowest position	❏	❏	_____
29. Remove gloves and all protective barriers; dispose of soiled supplies and equipment appropriately	❏	❏	_____
30. Perform hand hygiene after patient contact and after wearing gloves	❏	❏	_____
31. Document and do patient teaching	❏	❏	_____
32. Report any unexpected outcomes	❏	❏	_____

PERFORMANCE CHECKLIST 20-3

EAR IRRIGATION

	S	U	Comments
Prepare for procedure			
1. Refer to medical record, care plan, or Kardex	❏	❏	_____
2. Introduce self	❏	❏	_____
3. Identify patient	❏	❏	_____
4. Explain procedure and reason it is to be done	❏	❏	_____
5. Assess need for and provide patient teaching during procedure	❏	❏	_____
6. Assemble equipment and complete necessary charges	❏	❏	_____
7. Perform hand hygiene	❏	❏	_____
8. Assess patient	❏	❏	_____
9. Prepare patient for intervention			
a. Close door/pull privacy curtain	❏	❏	_____
b. Raise bed to comfortable working height; lower side rail on side nearest the nurse	❏	❏	_____
c. Position and drape patient as necessary	❏	❏	_____
During the skill			
10. Promote patient involvement as possible	❏	❏	_____
11. Assess patient's tolerance	❏	❏	_____
12. Advise patient of sensations that might be experienced: vertigo, fullness, and warmth	❏	❏	_____
13. Don gloves as necessary	❏	❏	_____
14. Assess condition of external ear structures and canal for erythema, edema, and exudate	❏	❏	_____
15. Assist patient to either a side-lying or sitting position with head tilted toward affected ear and position emesis basin under ear	❏	❏	_____
16. Place towel under patient's shoulder just under ear and emesis basin	❏	❏	_____

	S	U	Comments
17. Inspect auditory canal for any accumulation of cerumen or debris. Remove what you can see with the naked eye or the otoscope using cotton or the applicator and solution (do not force cerumen into the canal)	❏	❏	_____
18. Assess irrigation solution for proper temperature; test temperature of solution by sprinkling a few drops of solution on inner wrist; fill bulb syringe with appropriate volume	❏	❏	_____
19. Straighten auditory canal for introduction of solution correctly according to age	❏	❏	_____
20. With tip of syringe just above canal, irrigate gently by creating steady flow of solution against roof of canal; do not occlude canal with tip of syringe	❏	❏	_____
21. Continue irrigation until all debris has been removed or all solution has been used; reassess auditory canal with otoscope	❏	❏	_____
22. Assess patient for vertigo or nausea; onset of symptoms may require temporary cessation of procedure	❏	❏	_____
23. Dry off auricle and apply cotton ball loosely to auditory meatus	❏	❏	_____
24. Position patient on side of affected ear for 10 minutes	❏	❏	_____
25. Return to patient to assess character and amount of drainage and determine patient's level of comfort	❏	❏	_____

Postprocedure

	S	U	Comments
26. Assist patient to a position of comfort and place needed items within easy reach; be certain patient has a means to call for assistance and knows how to use it	❏	❏	_____
27. Raise side rails and lower bed to lowest position	❏	❏	_____
28. Remove gloves and all protective barriers; dispose of soiled supplies and equipment appropriately	❏	❏	_____
29. Perform hand hygiene after patient contact and after wearing gloves	❏	❏	_____
30. Document and do patient teaching	❏	❏	_____
31. Report any unexpected outcomes	❏	❏	_____

PERFORMANCE CHECKLIST 20-4

Performing a Nasal Irrigation

	S	U	Comments
Prepare for procedure			
1. Refer to medical record, care plan or Kardex	❏	❏	_____
2. Introduce self	❏	❏	_____
3. Identify patient	❏	❏	_____
4. Explain procedure and reason it is to be done	❏	❏	_____
5. Assess need for and provide patient teaching during procedure	❏	❏	_____
6. Obtain equipment, assemble, and complete necessary charges	❏	❏	_____
7. Perform hand hygiene; don clean gloves	❏	❏	_____
8. Assess patient for comfort level and any nasal secretions	❏	❏	_____
9. Prepare patient			
a. Close door/pull privacy curtain	❏	❏	_____
b. Position patient sitting upright comfortably near equipment leaning over the basin or sink	❏	❏	_____
10. Prepare equipment			
a. Mix solution as needed	❏	❏	_____
b. Warm solution	❏	❏	_____
c. Fill irrigating device	❏	❏	_____
d. Place basin as collecting receptacle	❏	❏	_____
During the skill			
11. Instruct patient to keep mouth open and breathe rhythmically during procedure	❏	❏	_____
12. Teach patient neither to speak nor swallow during procedure	❏	❏	_____

	S	U	Comments
13. Remove irrigating device tip from nose if patient reports the need to cough or sneeze	❏	❏	_____
14. If using commercial kit, follow directions on package	❏	❏	_____
15. Don clean gloves and perform procedure			
a. Electrical irrigating device			
(1) Insert tip about 1/2 to 1 inch into patient's nostril	❏	❏	_____
(2) Begin with a low pressure setting	❏	❏	_____
(3) Irrigate both nostrils	❏	❏	_____
b. Bulb syringe			
(1) Fill bulb with warm saline solution	❏	❏	_____
(2) Insert tip 1/2 inch into patient's nostril	❏	❏	_____
(3) Squeeze bulb until a gentle stream of warm solution washes through the nose	❏	❏	_____
(4) Avoid forceful squeezing	❏	❏	_____
(5) Irrigate both nostrils until returns are clear	❏	❏	_____
16. Assess returns and report any abnormalities			
a. Color	❏	❏	_____
b. Viscosity	❏	❏	_____
c. Volume	❏	❏	_____
d. Blood	❏	❏	_____
e. Necrotic material	❏	❏	_____

Postprocedure

	S	U	Comments
17. Request patient to wait a few minutes before blowing nose	❏	❏	_____
18. Instruct patient to gently blow both nostrils at the same time	❏	❏	_____
19. Clean and store equipment	❏	❏	_____

Student Name_____ Date_____ Instructor's name_____

	S	U	Comments
20. Remove gloves and all protective barriers; dispose of soiled supplies and equipment appropriately	❑	❑	_____
21. Assist patient to cleanse and dry self	❑	❑	_____
22. Assist patient to a position of comfort and place needed items within easy reach; be certain patient has a means to call for assistance and knows how to use it	❑	❑	_____
23. If in bed, raise side rail and lower bed to lowest position	❑	❑	_____
24. Perform hand hygiene after patient contact and after wearing gloves	❑	❑	_____
25. Document	❑	❑	_____
26. Observe and assess patient for any adverse reactions	❑	❑	_____
27. Do patient teaching	❑	❑	_____

PERFORMANCE CHECKLIST 20-5

APPLYING A HOT, MOIST COMPRESS TO AN OPEN WOUND

	S	U	Comments
Prepare for procedure			
1. Refer to medical record, care plan, or Kardex	❏	❏	_____
2. Introduce self	❏	❏	_____
3. Identify patient	❏	❏	_____
4. Explain procedure and reason it is to be done	❏	❏	_____
5. Assess need for and provide patient teaching during procedure	❏	❏	_____
6. Assemble equipment and complete necessary charges	❏	❏	_____
7. Perform hand hygiene; don clean gloves	❏	❏	_____
8. Assess patient	❏	❏	_____
9. Prepare patient for intervention			
a. Close door/pull privacy curtain	❏	❏	_____
b. Raise bed to comfortable working height; lower side rail on side nearest the nurse	❏	❏	_____
c. Position and drape patient as necessary	❏	❏	_____
During the skill			
10. Promote patient involvement as possible	❏	❏	_____
11. Assess patient's tolerance	❏	❏	_____
12. Describe sensations to be felt; explain precautions to prevent burning	❏	❏	_____
13. Assess condition of exposed skin and wound on which compress is to be applied	❏	❏	_____
14. Place waterproof pad under area to be treated	❏	❏	_____
15. Assemble equipment; pour warmed solution into sterile container	❏	❏	_____

	S	U	Comments
16. Open sterile packages and drop gauze into container to immerse in solution; set Aquathermia pad (if used) to correct temperature and assess fluid level of unit	❏	❏	_____
17. Don disposable gloves; remove any existing dressings covering wound; dispose of gloves and dressings in proper receptacle	❏	❏	_____
18. Apply sterile gloves	❏	❏	_____
19. Apply sterile petroleum jelly (optional) with cotton swab to skin surrounding wound; do not apply jelly on impaired skin	❏	❏	_____
20. Pick up one layer of immersed gauze and squeeze out excess water	❏	❏	_____
21. Apply gauze lightly to open wound; observe response and ask whether patient feels discomfort; in a few seconds, lift edge of gauze to assess for erythema	❏	❏	_____
22. If patient tolerates compress, pack gauze snugly against wound; be certain all wound surfaces are covered by hot compress	❏	❏	_____
23. Wrap or cover moist compress with dry bath towel; if necessary, pin or tie in place	❏	❏	_____
24. Change hot compress frequently as ordered	❏	❏	_____
25. Apply Aquathermia or waterproof heating pad over compress (optional); keep it in place for desired duration of application	❏	❏	_____
26. Assess patient periodically for discomfort or burning sensation; observe area of skin not covered by compress	❏	❏	_____
27. Remove pad, towel, and compress; again assess wound and condition of skin	❏	❏	_____
28. Apply dry, sterile dressing as ordered	❏	❏	_____
29. Ask patient if any unusual burning sensation is noticed that was not felt before	❏	❏	_____

Student Name_____ Date_____ Instructor's name_____

	S	U	Comments

Postprocedure

30. Assist patient to a position of comfort and place needed items within easy reach; be certain patient has a means to call for assistance and knows how to use it ❏ ❏ _____

31. Raise side rails and lower bed to lowest position ❏ ❏ _____

32. Remove gloves and all protective barriers; dispose of soiled supplies and equipment appropriately ❏ ❏ _____

33. Perform hand hygiene after patient contact and after wearing gloves ❏ ❏ _____

34. Document and do patient teaching ❏ ❏ _____

35. Report an unexpected outcomes ❏ ❏ _____

Student Name_____ Date_____ Instructor's name_____

INITIATING INTRAVENOUS THERAPY

	S	U	Comments
Prepare for procedure			
1. Refer to medical record, care plan, or Kardex	❑	❑	_____
2. Introduce self	❑	❑	_____
3. Identify patient	❑	❑	_____
4. Explain procedure and reason it is to be done	❑	❑	_____
5. Assess need for and provide patient teaching during procedure	❑	❑	_____
6. Assemble equipment and IV solution to be infused	❑	❑	_____
7. Perform hand hygiene; don clean gloves	❑	❑	_____
8. Assess patient	❑	❑	_____
9. Prepare patient for intervention			
a. Close door/pull privacy curtain	❑	❑	_____
b. Raise bed to comfortable working height; lower side rail on side nearest the nurse	❑	❑	_____
c. Position and drape patient as necessary	❑	❑	_____
During the skill			
10. Promote patient involvement as possible	❑	❑	_____
11. Assess patient's tolerance	❑	❑	_____
12. Identify venipuncture sites	❑	❑	_____
13. Apply tourniquet	❑	❑	_____
14. Select venipuncture site	❑	❑	_____
15. Cleanse site with alcohol swab, or other special agent such as Betadine, using friction	❑	❑	_____
16. Stretch skin taut and stabilize vein with nondominant hand	❑	❑	_____
17. Holding angiocatheter bevel up, pierce skin above and slightly to side of vein at 45-degree angle	❑	❑	_____

	S	U	Comments
18. When using a needleless over-the-needle catheter safety device (ONC)			
a. Insert ONC with bevel up at 10- to 30-degree angle, slightly distal to actual site of venipuncture in direction of vein	❑	❑	_____
b. Look for blood return in flash back chamber on ONC; advance catheter off stylet into vein until head rests at venipuncture site; do not reinsert stylet once it is loosened; advance safety device by using push-off tab to thread catheter	❑	❑	_____
c. Stabilize catheter; apply gentle but firm pressure above insertion site; release tourniquet and retract stylet from ONC; do not recap stylet; for safety device slide, catheter off stylet while guiding protective guard over stylet	❑	❑	_____
19. Lower angle to 10 degrees and enter vein wall; slight resistance and "pop" accompany entry into vein	❑	❑	_____
20. Follow vein lumen with tip of needle to ensure placement within vein, watching for blood return through angiocatheter backflow chamber	❑	❑	_____
21. Release tourniquet	❑	❑	_____
22. Holding guide needle in place, gently thread plastic catheter off needle and into vein	❑	❑	_____
23. Applying gentle pressure over catheter in vein, remove guide needle, and attach sterile connection end of primed tubing into catheter hub	❑	❑	_____
24. Stabilizing insertion site, slowly open flow valve to begin intravenous infusion	❑	❑	_____
25. Following agency policy, secure and dress site with tape, medications, and dressings	❑	❑	_____
26. Label site and tubing according to agency policy	❑	❑	_____
27. Adjust fluid flow rate according to accurate drop-rate calculations or set infusion rate on infusion pump	❑	❑	_____
28. If infusion pump is used, set milliliters to be infused (volume to be infused)	❑	❑	_____

	S	U	Comments

Postprocedure

29. Assist patient to a position of comfort and place needed items within easy reach; be certain patient has a means to call for assistance and knows how to use it ❑ ❑ _____

30. Raise side rails and lower bed to lowest position ❑ ❑ _____

31. Remove gloves and all protective barriers; dispose of soiled supplies and equipment appropriately ❑ ❑ _____

32. Perform hand hygiene after patient contact and after wearing gloves ❑ ❑ _____

33. Document and do patient teaching ❑ ❑ _____

34. Report any unexpected outcomes ❑ ❑ _____

PERFORMANCE CHECKLIST 20-7A
MAINTAINING AN INTRAVENOUS SITE:

CHANGING A PERIPHERAL IV DRESSING

	S	U	Comments
Prepare for procedure			
1. Refer to medical record, care plan, or Kardex	❏	❏	_____
2. Introduce self	❏	❏	_____
3. Identify patient	❏	❏	_____
4. Explain procedure and reason it is to be done	❏	❏	_____
5. Assess need for dressing change and provide patient teaching	❏	❏	_____
6. Assemble equipment and complete necessary charges	❏	❏	_____
7. Perform hand hygiene; don clean gloves	❏	❏	_____
8. Assess patient	❏	❏	_____
9. Prepare patient for intervention			
a. Close door/pull privacy curtain	❏	❏	_____
b. Raise bed to comfortable working height; lower side rail on side nearest the nurse	❏	❏	_____
c. Position and drape patient as necessary	❏	❏	_____
During the skill			
10. Promote patient involvement as possible	❏	❏	_____
11. Assess patient's tolerance	❏	❏	_____
12. Prepare equipment	❏	❏	_____
13. Assess IV site			
a. When was dressing last changed	❏	❏	_____
b. Assess present dressing	❏	❏	_____
c. Observe present IV system for proper functioning or complications	❏	❏	_____
d. Palpate catheter site through intact dressing	❏	❏	_____

	S	U	Comments
e. Inspect exposed catheter site	❏	❏	_____
f. Monitor body temperature	❏	❏	_____
g. Determine patient's understanding of need for procedure	❏	❏	_____
14. Remove any overlying tape, transparent membrane dressing, gauze dressing and tape; leave tape securing catheter to skin	❏	❏	_____
15. Observe insertion site	❏	❏	_____
16. If IV is infusing properly, remove tape securing catheter; stabilize catheter with one finger; remove adhesive residue if necessary	❏	❏	_____
17. Cleanse peripheral insertion site properly; allow to dry; apply skin protectant solution if necessary	❏	❏	_____
18. Transparent dressing			
a. Place transparent dressing over venipuncture site correctly	❏	❏	_____
b. Taking a 1-inch piece of tape, place correctly over transparent dressing	❏	❏	_____
19. Gauze dressing			
a. Apply single 4-inch strip of sterile nonallergic tape under catheter hub correctly	❏	❏	_____
b. Place gauze over venipuncture site and catheter hub properly; secure edges	❏	❏	_____
20. Secure dressing and tubing to arm at insertion site; place gauze under catheter tubing correctly; curl a loop of tubing as directed in skill; secure tubing in two places (Transparent dressings are also currently used.)	❏	❏	_____

Postprocedure

	S	U	Comments
21. Label dressing completely and accurately	❏	❏	_____
22. Secure arm or hand to board as necessary	❏	❏	_____

	S	U	Comments

23. Assist patient to a position of comfort and place needed items within easy reach; be certain patient has a means to call for assistance and knows how to use it ❏ ❏ _____

24. Raise side rails and lower bed to lowest position ❏ ❏ _____

25. Remove gloves and all protective barriers; dispose of soiled supplies and equipment appropriately ❏ ❏ _____

26. Perform hand hygiene after patient contact and after wearing gloves ❏ ❏ _____

27. Document ❏ ❏ _____

28. Report any unexpected outcomes ❏ ❏ _____

PERFORMANCE CHECKLIST 20-7B
MAINTAINING AN INTRAVENOUS SITE:

CHANGING INFUSION TUBING

	S	U	Comments
Prepare for procedure			
1. Refer to medical record, care plan, or Kardex	❏	❏	_____
2. Introduce self	❏	❏	_____
3. Identify patient	❏	❏	_____
4. Explain procedure and reason it is to be done	❏	❏	_____
5. Assess need for tubing change and provide patient teaching	❏	❏	_____
6. Assemble equipment and complete necessary charges	❏	❏	_____
7. Perform hand hygiene; don clean gloves	❏	❏	_____
8. Assess patient's IV setup	❏	❏	_____
9. Prepare patient for intervention			
a. Close door/pull privacy curtain	❏	❏	_____
b. Raise bed to comfortable working height; lower side rail on side nearest the nurse	❏	❏	_____
c. Position and drape patient as necessary	❏	❏	_____
During the skill			
10. Promote patient involvement as possible	❏	❏	_____
11. Assess patient's tolerance	❏	❏	_____
12. Prepare equipment	❏	❏	_____
13. Assess			
a. New infusion set necessary	❏	❏	_____
b. Observe tubing	❏	❏	_____
c. Determine patient's need for continued IV infusion	❏	❏	_____

	S	U	Comments
14. Open new infusion set, connect add-on pieces (keeping sterile where necessary); secure all junctions correctly; avoid use of tape	❏	❏	_____
15. If necessary, remove IV dressing as catheter hub needs to be visible; maintain catheter securely to skin; if necessary, place small piece of sterile tape across hub	❏	❏	_____
16. For existing continuous infusion			
a. Close roller clamp on new tubing	❏	❏	_____
b. Slow rate of flow on existing IV properly	❏	❏	_____
c. Compress and fill drip chamber of old tubing	❏	❏	_____
17. a. Remove IV container from pole	❏	❏	_____
b. Invert container	❏	❏	_____
c. Remove old tubing from solution container	❏	❏	_____
d. Hold container 36 inches above IV site	❏	❏	_____
18. Place insertion spike of new tubing into old fluid container opening; hang container on IV pole and adjust correctly	❏	❏	_____
19. a. Slowly open roller clamp	❏	❏	_____
b. Remove protector cap from adapter	❏	❏	_____
c. Flush new tubing with solution	❏	❏	_____
d. Stop infusion and replace cap	❏	❏	_____
20. Turn roller clamp on old tubing off	❏	❏	_____
21. a. Stabilize hub of catheter and apply pressure appropriately	❏	❏	_____
b. Disconnect old tubing and insert adapter of new tubing correctly	❏	❏	_____
22. a. Open roller clamp and adjust correctly	❏	❏	_____
b. Regulate per physician's order	❏	❏	_____
c. Monitor hourly rate	❏	❏	_____
23. Provide reference (label) to determine next time for tubing change	❏	❏	_____
24. If necessary, apply new dressing to insertion site	❏	❏	_____

	S	U	Comments
25. Secure tubing to patient's arm	❑	❑	_____

Postprocedure

	S	U	Comments
26. Assist patient to a position of comfort and place needed items within easy reach; be certain patient has a means to call for assistance and knows how to use it	❑	❑	_____
27. Raise side rails and lower bed to lowest position	❑	❑	_____
28. Remove gloves and all protective barriers; dispose of soiled supplies and equipment appropriately	❑	❑	_____
29. Perform hand hygiene after patient contact and after wearing gloves	❑	❑	_____
30. Document	❑	❑	_____
31. Report any unexpected outcomes	❑	❑	_____

Student Name_____ Date_____ Instructor's name_____

CHANGING FLUID CONTAINER

	S	U	Comments
Prepare for procedure			
1. Refer to medical record, care plan, or Kardex	❏	❏	_____
2. Introduce self	❏	❏	_____
3. Identify patient	❏	❏	_____
4. Explain procedure and reason it is to be done	❏	❏	_____
5. Assess need for container change and provide patient teaching	❏	❏	_____
6. Assemble equipment and complete necessary charges	❏	❏	_____
7. Perform hand hygiene; don clean gloves	❏	❏	_____
8. Prepare patient for intervention			
a. Close door/pull privacy curtain	❏	❏	_____
b. Raise bed to comfortable working height; lower side rail on side nearest the nurse	❏	❏	_____
c. Position and drape patient as necessary	❏	❏	_____
During the skill			
9. Promote patient involvement as possible	❏	❏	_____
10. Assess patient's tolerance	❏	❏	_____
11. Prepare equipment	❏	❏	_____
12. Determine compatibility of all IV fluids and additives	❏	❏	_____
13. Assess patency of current IV site	❏	❏	_____
14. a. Prepare next solution at least 1 hour before needed	❏	❏	_____
b. Order up from pharmacy if necessary	❏	❏	_____
c. Check that solution is correct and properly labeled	❏	❏	_____

	S	U	Comments
d. Check solution expiration date	❏	❏	_____
e. Observe for precipitate or discoloration	❏	❏	_____
15. Change solution when fluid is in neck of container or when new type of solution has been ordered	❏	❏	_____
16. Stop flow rate correctly and remove old IV fluid container from IV pole	❏	❏	_____
17. a. Quickly remove spike from old container	❏	❏	_____
b. Remove protective cover from new fluid container	❏	❏	_____
c. Insert spike into new bag or bottle using sterile technique	❏	❏	_____
18. Hang new bag or bottle of solution on pole	❏	❏	_____
19. Check tubing for air; remove bubbles appropriately	❏	❏	_____
20. Make certain drip chamber is 1/3 to 1/2 full	❏	❏	_____
21. Regulate flow to prescribed rate	❏	❏	_____
22. Place time label on side of container with appropriate information	❏	❏	_____

Postprocedure

	S	U	Comments
23. Assist patient to a position of comfort and place needed items within easy reach; be certain patient has a means to call for assistance and knows how to use it	❏	❏	_____
24. Raise side rails and lower bed to lowest position	❏	❏	_____
25. Remove gloves and all protective barriers; dispose of soiled supplies and equipment appropriately	❏	❏	_____
26. Perform hand hygiene after patient contact and after wearing gloves	❏	❏	_____
27. Document correctly; do patient teaching	❏	❏	_____
28. Report any unexpected outcomes	❏	❏	_____

PERFORMANCE CHECKLIST 20-7D
MAINTAINING AN INTRAVENOUS SITE:

Discontinuing IV Medications

	S	U	Comments
Prepare for procedure			
1. Refer to medical record, care plan, or Kardex	❏	❏	_____
2. Introduce self	❏	❏	_____
3. Identify patient	❏	❏	_____
4. Explain procedure and reason it is to be done	❏	❏	_____
5. Assess need for discontinuation and provide patient teaching	❏	❏	_____
6. Assemble equipment and complete necessary charges	❏	❏	_____
7. Perform hand hygiene; don clean gloves	❏	❏	_____
8. Prepare patient for intervention			
a. Close door/pull privacy curtain	❏	❏	_____
b. Raise bed to comfortable working height; lower side rail on side nearest the nurse	❏	❏	_____
c. Position and drape patient as necessary	❏	❏	_____
During the skill			
9. Promote patient involvement as possible	❏	❏	_____
10. Assess patient's tolerance	❏	❏	_____
11. Prepare equipment	❏	❏	_____
12. a. Observe for complete infusion of all medication	❏	❏	_____
b. Review orders for any necessary blood samples	❏	❏	_____
c. Continue to monitor patient's response to medication	❏	❏	_____
13. Move roller clamp on infusion tubing to off	❏	❏	_____

	S	U	Comments
14. Remove any clasping devices and discontinue medication delivery tubing from injection port	❏	❏	_____
15. Remove needle or needleless adapter; discard appropriately; replace with sterile cap or cover as indicated	❏	❏	_____
16. Swab injection port or adapter on main IV tubing	❏	❏	_____
17. a. If medication is piggybacked into a continuous infusion, flush line appropriately but gently	❏	❏	_____
b. Regulate fluid flow as ordered	❏	❏	_____
18. If using a saline/heparin lock, flush catheter appropriately but gently; if necessary, attach sterile injection port cover	❏	❏	_____
19. Prepare patient for blood samples if necessary after medication infusion	❏	❏	_____

Postprocedure

	S	U	Comments
20. Assist patient to a position of comfort and place needed items within easy reach; be certain patient has a means to call for assistance and knows how to use it	❏	❏	_____
21. Raise side rails and lower bed to lowest position	❏	❏	_____
22. Remove gloves and all protective barriers; dispose of soiled supplies and equipment appropriately	❏	❏	_____
23. Perform hand hygiene after patient contact and after wearing gloves	❏	❏	_____
24. Document correctly; do patient teaching	❏	❏	_____
25. Report any unexpected outcomes	❏	❏	_____

Student Name_____ Date_____ Instructor's name_____

PERFORMANCE CHECKLIST 20-7E
MAINTAINING AN INTRAVENOUS SITE:

Discontinuing Peripheral IV Access

	S	U	Comments

Prepare for procedure

1. Refer to medical record, care plan, or Kardex ❑ ❑ _____

2. Introduce self ❑ ❑ _____

3. Identify patient ❑ ❑ _____

4. Explain procedure and reason it is to be done ❑ ❑ _____

5. Assess need for discontinuation and provide patient teaching ❑ ❑ _____

6. Assemble equipment and complete necessary charges ❑ ❑ _____

7. Perform hand hygiene; don clean gloves ❑ ❑ _____

8. Prepare patient for intervention

   a. Close door/pull privacy curtain ❑ ❑ _____

   b. Raise bed to comfortable working height; lower side rail on side nearest the nurse ❑ ❑ _____

   c. Position and drape patient as necessary ❑ ❑ _____

During the skill

9. Promote patient involvement as possible ❑ ❑ _____

10. Assess patient's tolerance ❑ ❑ _____

11. Prepare equipment ❑ ❑ _____

12. a. Observe existing IV site for signs and symptoms of infection ❑ ❑ _____

   b. Determine patient's understanding of procedure ❑ ❑ _____

13. Turn IV tubing roller clamp to "off" position; remove tape securing tubing ❑ ❑ _____

14. Remove IV site dressing and tape; stabilize catheter ❑ ❑ _____

	S	U	Comments
15. Hold dry gauze or alcohol swab over site; apply light pressure; withdraw catheter appropriately	❏	❏	_____
16. Apply pressure to site for 2 to 3 minutes using a dry, sterile gauze pad; secure with tape	❏	❏	_____
17. Inspect the removed catheter for intactness, noting tip integrity and length	❏	❏	_____
18. Instruct patient to report any abnormal signs and symptoms	❏	❏	_____

Postprocedure

	S	U	Comments
19. Assist patient to a position of comfort and place needed items within easy reach; be certain patient has a means to call for assistance and knows how to use it	❏	❏	_____
20. Raise side rails and lower bed to lowest position	❏	❏	_____
21. Remove gloves and all protective barriers; dispose of soiled supplies and equipment appropriately	❏	❏	_____
22. Perform hand hygiene after patient contact and after wearing gloves	❏	❏	_____
23. Document correctly; do patient teaching	❏	❏	_____
24. Report any unexpected outcomes	❏	❏	_____

PERFORMANCE CHECKLIST 20-8

Oxygen Administration

	S	U	Comments
Prepare for procedure			
1. Refer to medical record, care plan, or Kardex	❏	❏	_____
2. Introduce self	❏	❏	_____
3. Identify patient	❏	❏	_____
4. Explain procedure and reason it is to be done	❏	❏	_____
5. Assess need for (perform oximetry to obtain oxygen saturation) and provide patient teaching during procedure	❏	❏	_____
6. Assemble equipment and complete necessary charges	❏	❏	_____
7. Perform hand hygiene; don clean gloves	❏	❏	_____
8. Assess patient	❏	❏	_____
9. Prepare patient for intervention			
a. Close door/pull privacy curtain	❏	❏	_____
b. Raise bed to comfortable working height; lower side rail on side nearest the nurse	❏	❏	_____
c. Position and drape patient as necessary	❏	❏	_____
During the skill			
10. Promote patient involvement as possible	❏	❏	_____
11. Assess patient's tolerance	❏	❏	_____
12. Explain necessary precautions during oxygen therapy	❏	❏	_____
13. Place patient in Fowler's or semi-Fowler's position	❏	❏	_____
14. Assess patient's airway	❏	❏	_____
15. Consider laboratory reports	❏	❏	_____
16. Suction any secretions obstructing the airway and reassess lung sounds with stethoscope	❏	❏	_____

	S	U	Comments
17. Fill humidifier container to designated level, if used: use sterile, distilled water or as prescribed	❏	❏	_____
18. Attach flowmeter to humidifier and insert in proper oxygen source	❏	❏	_____
19. Administer oxygen therapy	❏	❏	_____

Nasal cannula

	S	U	Comments
a. Attach nasal cannula to oxygen tubing, then attach to flowmeter	❏	❏	_____
b. Place prongs in cup of water; adjust flow meter to 6–10 L to flush tubing and prongs with oxygen; wipe off water	❏	❏	_____
c. Adjust flow rate to the prescribed amount	❏	❏	_____
d. Place a nasal prong into each naris of the patient; adjust liter flow per physician's order or to maintain oxygen saturation at 91% or greater	❏	❏	_____
e. Adjust straps of the cannula over the ears and tighten under the chin	❏	❏	_____
f. Place padding between strap and ears	❏	❏	_____
g. Provide slack in tubing and secure to patient's garment	❏	❏	_____
h. Maintain regular assessment			
(1) Assess cannula frequently for possible obstruction	❏	❏	_____
(2) Observe external nasal area, nares, and superior surface of both ears for skin impairment every 6–8 hours	❏	❏	_____
(3) Assess nares and prongs and cleanse with cotton-tipped applicator as needed; apply water-soluble lubricant to nares to prevent from drying	❏	❏	_____
(4) Refer to physician's orders for any prescribed changes in flow rate	❏	❏	_____
(5) Auscultate lung sounds	❏	❏	_____
(6) Monitor oxygen saturation	❏	❏	_____

	S	U	Comments

(7) Maintain solution in humidifier container at appropriate level at all times   ❏ ❏ _____

Face masks

i. Adjust flow rate of oxygen per physician's order; monitor oxygen saturation   ❏ ❏ _____

j. Allow patient to hold mask and place your hand over patient's hand   ❏ ❏ _____

k. Place mask over bridge of nose, then cover mouth   ❏ ❏ _____

l. Adjust straps around patient's head and over ears; place cotton ball or gauze over ears under elastic straps   ❏ ❏ _____

m. Observe reservoir bag if one is attached to mask   ❏ ❏ _____

    (1) Partial-rebreather mask: reservoir should fill on exhalation and almost collapse on inhalation   ❏ ❏ _____

    (2) Nonrebreathing mask: reservoir should fill on exhalation and should never totally collapse on inhalation   ❏ ❏ _____

n. Maintain regular assessments

    (1) Remove mask and clean and dry skin regularly   ❏ ❏ _____

    (2) Refer to physician's orders for prescribed flow rate and any changes to maintain oxygen saturation of 91% or greater   ❏ ❏ _____

    (3) Maintain solution in humidifier container, if used, at appropriate level at all times   ❏ ❏ _____

Postprocedure

20. Assist patient to a position of comfort and place needed items within easy reach; be certain patient has a means to call for assistance and knows how to use it   ❏ ❏ _____

	S	U	Comments
21. Raise side rails and lower bed to lowest position	❏	❏	_____
22. Remove gloves and all protective barriers; dispose of soiled supplies and equipment appropriately	❏	❏	_____
23. Perform hand hygiene after patient contact and after wearing gloves	❏	❏	_____
24. Document, including oxygen saturation levels, and do patient teaching	❏	❏	_____
25. Report any unexpected outcomes	❏	❏	_____

PERFORMANCE CHECKLIST 20-9

TRACHEOSTOMY CARE AND SUCTIONING

	S	U	Comments
Prepare for procedure			
1. Refer to medical record, care plan, or Kardex	❏	❏	_____
2. Introduce self	❏	❏	_____
3. Identify patient	❏	❏	_____
4. Explain procedure and reason it is to be done	❏	❏	_____
5. Assess need for and provide patient teaching during procedure	❏	❏	_____
6. Assemble equipment and complete necessary charges	❏	❏	_____
7. Perform hand hygiene; don clean gloves	❏	❏	_____
8. Assess patient	❏	❏	_____
9. Prepare patient for intervention			
a. Close door/pull privacy curtain	❏	❏	_____
b. Raise bed to comfortable working height; lower side rail on side nearest the nurse	❏	❏	_____
c. Position and drape patient as necessary	❏	❏	_____
During the skill			
10. Promote patient involvement as possible	❏	❏	_____
11. Assess patient's tolerance	❏	❏	_____
12. Assess patient's tracheostomy	❏	❏	_____
13. Position patient in semi-Fowler's position	❏	❏	_____
14. Provide paper and pencil for patient	❏	❏	_____
15. Position self at head of bed facing patient	❏	❏	_____
16. Auscultate lungs; monitor oxygen saturation	❏	❏	_____
17. Place towel or prepackaged drape under tracheostomy and across chest	❏	❏	_____

	S	U	Comments
18. Prepare equipment and supplies on overbed table			
a. Open suction catheter, leaving it in its wrapper, and attach it to suction machine	❏	❏	_____
b. Pour cleansing solution (hydrogen peroxide) in one basin and rinsing solution (normal saline) in another basin	❏	❏	_____
c. Turn on suction machine (120 mm Hg in adults); apply sterile glove; keep dominant hand sterile	❏	❏	_____
d. Apply another sterile glove, still keeping dominant hand sterile	❏	❏	_____
19. Unlock and remove inner cannula; place in cleansing solution; place fingers on tabs of outer cannula	❏	❏	_____
20. Suction inner aspect of outer cannula			
a. Aspirate sterile rinsing solution through catheter	❏	❏	_____
b. Ask patient to take several deep breaths or if patient is receiving oxygen, remove oxygen immediately before suctioning	❏	❏	_____
c. Remove thumb from suction control or pinch catheter with gloved thumb and index finger; insert catheter 5–6 inches	❏	❏	_____
d. Apply intermittent suction	❏	❏	_____
e. Suction for a maximum of 10 seconds	❏	❏	_____
f. Allow patient to rest between each episode of suctioning	❏	❏	_____
g. Rinse catheter with sterile normal saline and repeat suctioning if needed	❏	❏	_____
h. Turn off suction and dispose of catheter appropriately	❏	❏	_____
21. Apply second sterile glove, if one-glove technique is used, or apply new pair of sterile gloves; clean inner cannula			

	S	U	Comments
a. Use pipe cleaners and brush to clean inside and outside of inner cannula with hydrogen peroxide solution	❏	❏	_____
b. Place inner cannula in sterile normal saline solution, rinse thoroughly	❏	❏	_____
c. Inspect inner and outer areas of inner cannula; remove excess liquid	❏	❏	_____
d. Insert inner cannula and lock in place	❏	❏	_____
22. Clean skin around tracheostomy and tabs of outer cannula; use wipes that are free of lint around the tracheostomy opening	❏	❏	_____
23. Thoroughly rinse cleansing solution from skin; place dry, sterile dressing around tracheostomy face plate	❏	❏	_____
24. Change cotton tapes			
a. Untie one side of cotton tape from outer cannula and replace with clean one	❏	❏	_____
b. Bring clean tape under back of neck	❏	❏	_____
c. Untie other side from outer cannula and replace with clean tape	❏	❏	_____
d. Tie ends of two clean cotton tapes together and position knot appropriately	❏	❏	_____
25. Auscultate lung sounds; monitor oxygen saturation	❏	❏	_____
26. Provide mouth care	❏	❏	_____
27. Remove gloves and all protective barriers and/or remove and dispose of soiled supplies and equipment appropriately	❏	❏	_____
28. Perform hand hygiene after patient contact and after wearing gloves	❏	❏	_____

	S	U	Comments

Postprocedure

29. Assist patient to a position of comfort and place needed items within easy reach; be certain patient has a means to call for assistance and knows how to use it ❑ ❑ _____

30. Raise side rails and lower bed to lowest position ❑ ❑ _____

31. Place call light, paper, and pencil within easy reach ❑ ❑ _____

32. Reassess patient's tracheostomy ❑ ❑ _____

33. Document and do patient teaching ❑ ❑ _____

34. Report any unexpected outcomes ❑ ❑ _____

Student Name_____ Date_____ Instructor's name_____

CARE OF THE PATIENT WITH A CUFFED TRACHEOSTOMY TUBE

	S	U	Comments
Prepare for procedure			
1. Refer to medical record, care plan, or Kardex	❏	❏	_____
2. Introduce self	❏	❏	_____
3. Identify patient	❏	❏	_____
4. Explain procedure and reason it is to be done	❏	❏	_____
5. Assess need for and provide patient teaching during procedure	❏	❏	_____
6. Assemble equipment and complete necessary charges	❏	❏	_____
7. Perform hand hygiene; don clean gloves	❏	❏	_____
8. Assess patient	❏	❏	_____
9. Prepare patient for intervention			
a. Close door/pull privacy curtain	❏	❏	_____
b. Raise bed to comfortable working height; lower side rail on side nearest the nurse	❏	❏	_____
c. Position and drape patient as necessary	❏	❏	_____
During the skill			
10. Promote patient involvement as possible	❏	❏	_____
11. Assess patient's tolerance; monitor oxygen saturation	❏	❏	_____
12. Suction patient as in Skill 20-8 steps 12 through 20h; connect syringe to pilot balloon valve	❏	❏	_____
13. Position stethoscope in sternal notch or above tracheostomy tube and listen for minimal amount of air leak at end of inspiration	❏	❏	_____
14. Remove all air from cuff if no air leak is auscultated	❏	❏	_____

	S	U	Comments
15. While listening with stethoscope, slowly inflate cuff with 0.5–1 mL of air at a time; when no air leak is heard, stop injecting air and slowly withdraw up to 0.5 mL of air until air leak is auscultated with stethoscope	❏	❏	_____
16. If excessive air leak is heard, slowly add air as in step 15	❏	❏	_____
17. Remove stethoscope and cleanse diaphragm with alcohol swab	❏	❏	_____
18. Do not leave syringe attached to pilot balloon valve; remove syringe and either discard in proper container or store per agency's policy	❏	❏	_____

Postprocedure

	S	U	Comments
19. Assist patient to a position of comfort and place needed items within easy reach; be certain patient has a means to call for assistance and knows how to use it	❏	❏	_____
20. Raise side rails and lower bed to lowest position	❏	❏	_____
21. Remove gloves and all protective barriers; dispose of soiled supplies and equipment appropriately	❏	❏	_____
22. Perform hand hygiene after patient contact and after wearing gloves	❏	❏	_____
23. Document and do patient teaching	❏	❏	_____
24. Report any unexpected outcomes	❏	❏	_____

PERFORMANCE CHECKLIST 20-11

CLEARING THE AIRWAY

	S	U	Comments
Prepare for procedure			
1. Refer to medical record, care plan, or Kardex	❏	❏	_____
2. Introduce self	❏	❏	_____
3. Identify patient	❏	❏	_____
4. Explain procedure and reason it is to be done	❏	❏	_____
5. Assess need for and provide patient teaching during procedure	❏	❏	_____
6. Assemble equipment and complete necessary charges	❏	❏	_____
7. Perform hand hygiene; don clean gloves	❏	❏	_____
8. Assess patient	❏	❏	_____
9. Prepare patient for intervention			
a. Close door/pull privacy curtain	❏	❏	_____
b. Raise bed to comfortable working height; lower side rail on side nearest the nurse	❏	❏	_____
c. Position and drape patient as necessary	❏	❏	_____
During the skill			
10. Promote patient involvement as possible	❏	❏	_____
11. Assess patient's tolerance; monitor oxygen saturation	❏	❏	_____
12. Position patient			
a. If patient is alert and conscious, place in semi-Fowler's position with head to one side	❏	❏	_____
b. If patient is unconscious, place in side-lying position facing nurse	❏	❏	_____
(1) Place towel lengthwise under patient's chin and over pillow	❏	❏	_____

	S	U	Comments
13. Pour sterile normal saline solution into sterile container	❏	❏	_____
14. Turn on suction machine, and select appropriate suction pressure, usually 120 mm Hg for adults	❏	❏	_____
15. Select appropriate catheter size	❏	❏	_____
16. Aspirate solution through catheter	❏	❏	_____
17. Remove thumb from Y-connector opening or pinch catheter with thumb and index finger; if using suction catheter with vent, remove thumb from vent opening	❏	❏	_____
18. Insert catheter	❏	❏	_____

Oropharyngeal suctioning

	S	U	Comments
a. Gently insert Yankauer into one side of mouth	❏	❏	_____
b. Glide Yankauer toward oropharynx without suction	❏	❏	_____
c. Apply suction and move Yankauer tonsillar tip catheter around mouth until secretions are cleared	❏	❏	_____
d. Encourage patient to cough	❏	❏	_____
e. Rinse Yankauer; turn off suction	❏	❏	_____
f. Repeat procedure as necessary	❏	❏	_____

Nasopharyngeal suctioning

	S	U	Comments
g. Holding catheter, assess for correct length of insertion	❏	❏	_____
h. Lubricate catheter with water-soluble lubricant	❏	❏	_____
i. Hold catheter to observe its natural curvature and gently insert catheter into one side of nasal passage	❏	❏	_____

Nasotracheal suctioning

	S	U	Comments
j. Holding catheter, measure for correct length	❏	❏	_____

	S	U	Comments
k. Lubricate catheter with water-soluble lubricant	❑	❑	_____
l. Ask patient if either side of nose is obstructed; use unobstructed side; hold catheter to observe its natural curvature and gently insert catheter into one side of nasal passage	❑	❑	_____
m. Stimulate coughing reflex, or ask patient to cough to guide catheter into trachea; if no cough reflex is present or if patient cannot assist, insert catheter when patient inhales	❑	❑	_____
19. Apply intermittent suction	❑	❑	_____
20. Observe patient closely and limit suction for the appropriate time	❑	❑	_____
21. Repeat suctioning if needed	❑	❑	_____
22. Allow 1 to 2 minutes rest between suctioning if procedure must be repeated; if oxygen is administered by nasal cannula, mask, or other means, reapply oxygen during rest period	❑	❑	_____
23. If patient is alert and can cooperate, request patient to breathe deeply and cough	❑	❑	_____
24. When suctioning is complete, suction between cheeks and gum line and under tongue; suction mouth last	❑	❑	_____
25. Place catheter in solution and supply suction	❑	❑	_____
26. Discard catheter	❑	❑	_____
27. Place sterile, unopened catheter at patient's bedside	❑	❑	_____
28. Provide mouth care	❑	❑	_____
29. Assess patient's breathing patterns	❑	❑	_____
30. Monitor oxygen saturation	❑	❑	_____

Postprocedure

| 31. Assist patient to a position of comfort and place needed items within easy reach; be certain patient has a means to call for assistance and knows how to use it | ❑ | ❑ | _____ |

	S	U	Comments
32. Raise side rails and lower bed to lowest position	❏	❏	_____
33. Remove gloves and all protective barriers; dispose of soiled supplies and equipment appropriately	❏	❏	_____
34. Perform hand hygiene after patient contact and after wearing gloves	❏	❏	_____
35. Document and do patient teaching	❏	❏	_____
36. Report any unexpected outcomes	❏	❏	_____

PERFORMANCE CHECKLIST 20-12

Catheterization: Male and Female

	S	U	Comments
Prepare for procedure			
1. Refer to medical record, care plan, or Kardex	❏	❏	_____
2. Introduce self	❏	❏	_____
3. Identify patient	❏	❏	_____
4. Explain procedure and reason it is to be done	❏	❏	_____
5. Assess need for and provide patient teaching during procedure	❏	❏	_____
6. Assemble equipment and complete necessary charges	❏	❏	_____
7. Perform hand hygiene; don clean gloves	❏	❏	_____
8. Assess patient	❏	❏	_____
9. Prepare patient for intervention			
a. Close door/pull privacy curtain	❏	❏	_____
b. Raise bed to comfortable working height; lower side rail on side nearest the nurse	❏	❏	_____
c. Position and drape patient as necessary	❏	❏	_____
During the skill			
10. Promote patient involvement as possible	❏	❏	_____
11. Assess patient's tolerance	❏	❏	_____
12. Arrange for extra nursing personnel to assist	❏	❏	_____
13. Position patient			
a. Male: Supine position with thighs slightly abducted	❏	❏	_____
b. Female: Dorsal recumbent position with knees flexed, soles of feet flat on bed, and feet about 2 feet apart	❏	❏	_____
14. Drape patient with bath blanket	❏	❏	_____

	S	U	Comments
15. Place waterproof, absorbent pad under patient's buttocks	❏	❏	_____
16. Arrange supplies and equipment on bedside table; provide a good light	❏	❏	_____
17. Don clean gloves and wash perineal area	❏	❏	_____
18. Remove disposable gloves and place in proper receptacle	❏	❏	_____
19. Facing patient, stand on left side of bed if right-handed (on right side if left-handed)	❏	❏	_____
20. Open packaging using sterile technique; don sterile gloves	❏	❏	_____
21. If indwelling catheter is used, test balloon appropriately	❏	❏	_____
22. Add antiseptic to cotton balls; open lubricant container; lubricate catheter the appropriate length	❏	❏	_____
23. Wrap edges of sterile drape around gloved hands and request patient to raise hips, then slide drape under patient's buttocks	❏	❏	_____
24. Cleanse perineal area using forceps to hold cotton balls soaked in antiseptic solution			
a. Male: If male is not circumcised, retract foreskin with nondominant hand; if erection does occur, discontinue procedure momentarily			
(1) Grasp penis at shaft below glans with one hand; continue to hold throughout insertion of catheter	❏	❏	_____
(2) With other hand, use forceps to hold cotton balls soaked in antiseptic solution	❏	❏	_____
(3) Cleanse meatus in circular motion	❏	❏	_____
(4) Repeat cleansing two more times using sterile cotton balls each time	❏	❏	_____
b. Female			
(1) Have assistant hold pen light or flashlight to provide adequate lighting	❏	❏	_____

	S	U	Comments
(2) Spread labia minora with thumb and index finger of nondominant hand and be prepared to hold throughout the insertion of the catheter	❏	❏	_____
(3) With other hand, use forceps to hold cotton balls soaked in antiseptic solution	❏	❏	_____
(4) Cleanse area from clitoris toward anus, using a different sterile cotton ball each time—first to the right of the meatus, then to the left of the meatus, then down the center over meatus	❏	❏	_____
25. Pick up catheter with free sterile, gloved hand near the tip; hold remaining part of catheter coiled in hands; place distal end in basin	❏	❏	_____
26. Insert catheter gently, 15–18 cm (6–7 inches) for male or 5–10 cm (2–4 inches) for female	❏	❏	_____
27. Collect urine specimen, if needed	❏	❏	_____
28. Type of catheter			
a. Indwelling catheter			
(1) Inflate balloon with required amount of normal saline or sterile water	❏	❏	_____
(2) Pull gently to feel resistance	❏	❏	_____
(3) Attach drainage bag below the level of bladder (most catheters are presealed to the collecting tube of the drainage system)	❏	❏	_____
(4) Attach collection bag to side of bed	❏	❏	_____
(5) Secure catheter to patient			
• Male: Tape catheter to top of thigh appropriately	❏	❏	_____
• Female: Tape catheter to inner thigh appropriately	❏	❏	_____
(6) Clip drainage tubing to bed linen appropriately	❏	❏	_____

	S	U	Comments
b. Straight catheter			
(1) Hold coiled catheter in hand with opening draining into sterile basin or into presealed plastic drainage bag	❑	❑	_____
(2) Empty bladder	❑	❑	_____
(3) Withdraw catheter slowly	❑	❑	_____
29. Dry perineal area	❑	❑	_____

Postprocedure

	S	U	Comments
30. Assist patient to a position of comfort and place needed items within easy reach; be certain patient has a means to call for assistance and knows how to use it	❑	❑	_____
31. Raise side rails and lower bed to lowest position	❑	❑	_____
32. Assess flow of urine and drainage tubing setup	❑	❑	_____
33. Remove gloves and all protective barriers; dispose of soiled supplies and equipment appropriately	❑	❑	_____
34. Perform hand hygiene after patient contact and after wearing gloves	❑	❑	_____
35. Document type of catheter used, amount and color of urine, and do patient teaching	❑	❑	_____
36. Report any unexpected outcomes	❑	❑	_____
37. Label urine specimen appropriately	❑	❑	_____
38. Transport to laboratory immediately	❑	❑	_____

PERFORMING ROUTINE CATHETER CARE

	S	U	Comments
Prepare for procedure			
1. Refer to medical record, care plan, or Kardex	❏	❏	_____
2. Introduce self	❏	❏	_____
3. Identify patient	❏	❏	_____
4. Explain procedure and reason it is to be done	❏	❏	_____
5. Assess need for and provide patient teaching during procedure	❏	❏	_____
6. Assemble equipment and complete necessary charges	❏	❏	_____
7. Perform hand hygiene; don clean gloves	❏	❏	_____
8. Assess patient	❏	❏	_____
9. Prepare patient for intervention			
a. Close door/pull privacy curtain	❏	❏	_____
b. Raise bed to comfortable working height; lower side rail on side nearest the nurse	❏	❏	_____
c. Position and drape patient as necessary	❏	❏	_____
During the skill			
10. Promote patient involvement as possible	❏	❏	_____
11. Assess patient's tolerance	❏	❏	_____
12. Position patient			
a. Male: In bed in supine position	❏	❏	_____
b. Female: In bed in dorsal recumbent position	❏	❏	_____
13. Place waterproof disposable pad under patient's buttocks and to the side from which catheter care will be given	❏	❏	_____
14. Drape patient with bath blanket, exposing only perineal area	❏	❏	_____

	S	U	Comments
15. If using sterile catheter care kit			
a. Open supplies using sterile technique and arrange on bedside table	❏	❏	_____
b. Don sterile gloves	❏	❏	_____
c. Place cotton balls in sterile basin and saturate with sterile solution	❏	❏	_____
d. With one hand expose urethral meatus			
(1) **Male**: retract foreskin, then hold penis erect	❏	❏	_____
(2) **Female**: gently retract labia minora away from urinary meatus and hold in position	❏	❏	_____
e. Wash the area at the meatus and around the catheter with cotton balls saturated with sterile solution			
(1) **Male**			
• With one cotton ball, cleanse around meatus and catheter in a circular motion	❏	❏	_____
• Repeat twice more, using different cotton balls each time	❏	❏	_____
(2) **Female**			
• With one cotton ball, swab to one side of labia minora from anterior to posterior	❏	❏	_____
• Repeat with second cotton ball on opposite side	❏	❏	_____
• Repeat with third cotton ball down middle over meatus and around catheter	❏	❏	_____
f. Discard soiled cotton balls in other basin in kit	❏	❏	_____
g. With forceps, pick up cotton ball soaked in antiseptic solution or mild soap and water and cleanse around catheter from urethral opening	❏	❏	_____
16. If using a collection of sterile supplies			
a. Open separate sterile packages observing sterile technique	❏	❏	_____

		S	U	Comments
b.	Don clean gloves	❑	❑	_____
c.	Arrange refuse bag	❑	❑	_____
d.	Cleanse the perineal area with mild soap and warm water; pat dry			
	(1) Male: retract foreskin then hold the penis erect	❑	❑	_____
	(2) Female: gently retract labia away from urinary meatus and hold in position	❑	❑	_____
e.	Apply in appropriate amount of sterile antiinfective ointment (if used) on sterile cotton-tipped applicator and gently apply around catheter at site of insertion (this is seldom used now)	❑	❑	_____
f.	Release labia of female patient; replace foreskin of male patient	❑	❑	_____
17.	Observe meatus, catheter, and surrounding tissue to assess normal or abnormal condition; determine presence or absence of inflammation, edema, malodorous exudate, color of tissue, and burning sensation	❑	❑	_____
18.	Dispose of equipment and linen; remove gloves and all protective barriers; dispose of soiled supplies and equipment appropriately	❑	❑	_____
19.	Retape catheter to thigh	❑	❑	_____

Postprocedure

		S	U	Comments
20.	Assist patient to a position of comfort and place needed items within easy reach; be certain patient has a means to call for assistance and knows how to use it	❑	❑	_____
21.	Raise side rails and lower bed to lowest position	❑	❑	_____
22.	Perform hand hygiene after patient contact and after wearing gloves	❑	❑	_____
23.	Document and do patient teaching	❑	❑	_____
24.	Report any unexpected outcomes	❑	❑	_____

PERFORMANCE CHECKLIST 20-14

Catheter Irrigation: Open, Intermittent, Continuous, and Bladder Instillation

	S	U	Comments
Prepare for procedure			
1. Refer to medical record, care plan, or Kardex	❑	❑	_____
2. Introduce self	❑	❑	_____
3. Identify patient	❑	❑	_____
4. Explain procedure and reason it is to be done	❑	❑	_____
5. Assess need for and provide patient teaching	❑	❑	_____
6. Assemble equipment and complete necessary charges	❑	❑	_____
7. Perform hand hygiene; don clean gloves	❑	❑	_____
8. Assess patient	❑	❑	_____
9. Prepare patient for intervention			
a. Close door/pull privacy curtain	❑	❑	_____
b. Raise bed to comfortable working height; lower side rail on side nearest the nurse	❑	❑	_____
c. Position and drape patient as necessary	❑	❑	_____
During the skill			
10. Promote patient involvement as possible	❑	❑	_____
11. Assess patient	❑	❑	_____
12. Position patient			
a. **Male:** Supine in bed	❑	❑	_____
b. **Female:** Dorsal recumbent in bed	❑	❑	_____
13. Place waterproof absorbent pad under patient's buttocks and to the side from which bladder irrigation will be done	❑	❑	_____
14. Arrange supplies and equipment at bedside on overbed table	❑	❑	_____

	S	U	Comments

15. Open method

   a. Pour sterile irrigating solution (normal saline unless otherwise specified) into sterile graduated container and recap solution bottle; irrigating solution should be at room temperature   ❏ ❏ _____

   b. Don sterile gloves   ❏ ❏ _____

   c. Place sterile basin between patient's legs, close to perineal area   ❏ ❏ _____

   d. Disconnect catheter from drainage system and plug drainage tubing with sterile plug   ❏ ❏ _____

   e. Draw 30 mL of sterile solution into syringe   ❏ ❏ _____

   f. Cleanse catheter end with antiseptic swab   ❏ ❏ _____

   g. Place tip of syringe into end of catheter and gently insert solution   ❏ ❏ _____

   h. Withdraw syringe and allow solution to drain into basin by gravity   ❏ ❏ _____

   i. If solution does not return, turn patient on side facing nurse   ❏ ❏ _____

   j. Repeat injection of solution until amount ordered is injected and returned   ❏ ❏ _____

   k. Remove plug from drainage tubing, and connect tubing to catheter   ❏ ❏ _____

   l. Measure solution (to determine amount returned and amount of urine expelled)   ❏ ❏ _____

16. Closed intermittent method (repeat steps 1 to 14)

   a. Pour sterile irrigating solution (normal saline unless otherwise specified) into graduated container   ❏ ❏ _____

   b. Draw up sterile solution into syringe   ❏ ❏ _____

   c. Clamp catheter below injection port   ❏ ❏ _____

   d. Cleanse port with antiseptic   ❏ ❏ _____

   e. Insert needle of syringe into port   ❏ ❏ _____

   f. Inject solution into catheter slowly   ❏ ❏ _____

17. Closed continuous method or continuous bladder irrigation (CBI)

		S	U	Comments
a.	Set up irrigating solution (normal saline unless otherwise specified) by attaching tubing to irrigation bag	❏	❏	_____
b.	Clamp off tubing so no solution flows through	❏	❏	_____
c.	Suspend bag on IV pole	❏	❏	_____
d.	Open clamp and allow solution to flow through tubing	❏	❏	_____
e.	Cleanse irrigating lumen on end of triple lumen catheter	❏	❏	_____
f.	Connect irrigating solution tubing to catheter lumen	❏	❏	_____
g.	Restore flow as ordered; run drip rate to keep drainage system clear	❏	❏	_____
h.	Deduct solution from urine in drainage bag when emptying to compute true urine	❏	❏	_____

18. Bladder instillation

		S	U	Comments
a.	Disconnect catheter from tubing—stabilize tubing to prevent touching the floor (triple lumen catheter does not require disconnection from drainage tubing)	❏	❏	_____
b.	Cleanse end of catheter with antiseptic swab	❏	❏	_____
c.	Draw medication or solution ordered into syringe	❏	❏	_____
d.	Place tip of syringe into end of catheter and slowly inject medication or solution ordered	❏	❏	_____
e.	Clamp off end of catheter for period of time necessary; then reconnect catheter and tubing, making certain the system is tightly connected	❏	❏	_____
f.	Measure solution	❏	❏	_____

	S	U	Comments

Postprocedure

19. Assist patient to a position of comfort and place needed items within easy reach; be certain patient has a means to call for assistance and knows how to use it ❏ ❏ _____

20. Raise side rails and lower bed to lowest position ❏ ❏ _____

21. Remove gloves and all protective barriers; dispose of soiled supplies and equipment appropriately ❏ ❏ _____

22. Perform hand hygiene after patient contact and after wearing gloves ❏ ❏ _____

23. Document and do patient teaching ❏ ❏ _____

24. Report any unexpected outcomes ❏ ❏ _____

PERFORMANCE CHECKLIST 20-15

REMOVING AN INDWELLING CATHETER

	S	U	Comments
Prepare for procedure			
1. Refer to medical record, care plan, or Kardex	❑	❑	_____
2. Introduce self	❑	❑	_____
3. Identify patient	❑	❑	_____
4. Explain procedure and reason it is to be done	❑	❑	_____
5. Assess need for procedure and provide patient teaching	❑	❑	_____
6. Assemble equipment and complete necessary charges	❑	❑	_____
7. Perform hand hygiene; don clean gloves	❑	❑	_____
8. Assess patient	❑	❑	_____
9. Prepare patient for intervention			
a. Close door/pull privacy curtain	❑	❑	_____
b. Raise bed to comfortable working height; lower side rail on side nearest the nurse	❑	❑	_____
c. Position and drape patient as necessary	❑	❑	_____
During the skill			
10. Position patient supine	❑	❑	_____
11. a. Females: place waterproof pad under catheter; abduct legs and place drape between thighs	❑	❑	_____
b. Males: lay drape on thighs	❑	❑	_____
12. Insert hub of syringe into inflation valve (balloon port) and aspirate until tubing collapses	❑	❑	_____
13. Remove catheter steadily and smoothly; do not use force	❑	❑	_____
14. Wrap catheter in waterproof pad	❑	❑	_____

	S	U	Comments
15. Unhook collection bag and drainage tubing from bed	❏	❏	_____
16. Measure urine and empty drainage bag	❏	❏	_____
17. Record output	❏	❏	_____
18. Cleanse perineum; dry thoroughly	❏	❏	_____
19. Do patient teaching	❏	❏	_____
20. Place urine hat on toilet seat	❏	❏	_____

Postprocedure

	S	U	Comments
21. Assist patient to a position of comfort and place needed items within easy reach; be certain patient has a means to call for assistance and knows how to use it	❏	❏	_____
22. Raise side rails and lower bed to lowest position	❏	❏	_____
23. Remove gloves and all protective barriers; dispose of soiled supplies and equipment appropriately	❏	❏	_____
24. Perform hand hygiene after patient contact and after wearing gloves	❏	❏	_____
25. Document and finish patient teaching	❏	❏	_____
26. Report any unexpected outcomes	❏	❏	_____

PERFORMANCE CHECKLIST 20-16

Performing a Vaginal Irrigation or Douche

	S	U	Comments
Prepare for procedure			
1. Refer to medical record, care plan, or Kardex	❏	❏	_____
2. Introduce self	❏	❏	_____
3. Identify patient	❏	❏	_____
4. Explain procedure and reason it is to be done	❏	❏	_____
5. Assess need for and provide patient teaching during procedure	❏	❏	_____
6. Assemble equipment and complete necessary charges	❏	❏	_____
7. Perform hand hygiene; don clean gloves	❏	❏	_____
8. Assess patient	❏	❏	_____
9. Prepare patient for intervention			
a. Close door/pull privacy curtain	❏	❏	_____
b. Raise bed to comfortable working height; lower side rail on side nearest the nurse	❏	❏	_____
c. Position and drape patient as necessary	❏	❏	_____
During the skill			
10. Promote patient involvement as possible	❏	❏	_____
11. Assess patient's tolerance	❏	❏	_____
12. Prepare equipment			
a. Solution should be at body temperature	❏	❏	_____
b. Allow some solution to drain down the tubing out through the nozzle into bedpan	❏	❏	_____
13. Gently retract labial folds and direct nozzle toward the sacrum, following the floor of the vagina	❏	❏	_____
14. Raise the container approximately 30–50 cm (12–20 in) above level of vagina	❏	❏	_____

	S	U	Comments
15. Insert nozzle appropriately through vaginal meatus	❏	❏	_____
16. Allow solution to flow while inserting and rotating nozzle	❏	❏	_____
17. Instruct patient to tighten perineal muscles as if to suppress urination and then relax; repeat four to five times during procedure	❏	❏	_____
18. Administer all of the solution while rotating nozzle gently during instillation	❏	❏	_____
19. Withdraw nozzle and assist patient to a comfortable position while she remains on the bedpan	❏	❏	_____
20. Allow patient to remain on bedpan a short time (10 minutes), then don clean gloves; remove bedpan, assessing results; dispose of remaining solution in proper manner	❏	❏	_____
21. Cleanse and dry patient or allow her to cleanse and dry herself	❏	❏	_____

Postprocedure

	S	U	Comments
22. Assist patient to a position of comfort and place needed items within easy reach; be certain patient has a means to call for assistance and knows how to use it	❏	❏	_____
23. Raise side rails and lower bed to lowest position	❏	❏	_____
24. Remove gloves and all protective barriers; dispose of soiled supplies and equipment appropriately	❏	❏	_____
25. Perform hand hygiene after patient contact and after wearing gloves	❏	❏	_____
26. Document and do patient teaching	❏	❏	_____
27. Report any unexpected outcomes	❏	❏	_____

PERFORMANCE CHECKLIST 20-17

Inserting a Nasogastric Tube

	S	U	Comments
Prepare for procedure			
1. Refer to medical record, care plan, or Kardex	❏	❏	_____
2. Introduce self	❏	❏	_____
3. Identify patient	❏	❏	_____
4. Explain procedure and reason it is to be done	❏	❏	_____
5. Assess need for and provide patient teaching during procedure	❏	❏	_____
6. Assemble equipment and complete necessary charges	❏	❏	_____
7. Perform hand hygiene; don clean gloves	❏	❏	_____
8. Assess patient	❏	❏	_____
9. Prepare patient for intervention			
a. Close door/pull privacy curtain	❏	❏	_____
b. Raise bed to comfortable working height; lower side rail on side nearest the nurse	❏	❏	_____
c. Position and drape patient as necessary	❏	❏	_____
During the skill			
10. Promote patient involvement as possible	❏	❏	_____
11. Assess patient's tolerance	❏	❏	_____
12. Assess patient for condition of nares and oral cavity	❏	❏	_____
13. Assess patient's oral cavity	❏	❏	_____
14. Position patient in high Fowler's position with pillow behind head and shoulders	❏	❏	_____
15. Stand at right side of bed if right-handed and left side if left-handed	❏	❏	_____
16. Place bath towel over patient's chest; give tissues to patient	❏	❏	_____

	S	U	Comments
17. Instruct patient to relax and breathe normally while occluding one naris; repeat this action for other naris	❏	❏	_____
18. Measure distance to insert tube correctly (measure distance from tip of nose to earlobe to xiphoid process)	❏	❏	_____
19. Mark length of tube to be inserted with piece of tape or note distance from next tube marking	❏	❏	_____
20. Curve end of tube tightly around index finger; release	❏	❏	_____
21. Lubricate end of tube generously with water-soluble lubricating jelly	❏	❏	_____
22. Initially instruct patient to extend neck back against pillow; insert tube slowly through naris with curved end pointing downward	❏	❏	_____
23. Continue to pass tube along floor of nasal passage, aiming down toward ear; when resistance is felt, apply gentle downward pressure to advance tube (do not force past resistance)	❏	❏	_____
24. If resistance continues, withdraw tube, allow patient to rest, relubricate tube, and insert into other naris	❏	❏	_____
25. Continue insertion of tube until just past nasopharynx by gently rotating tube toward opposite naris			
a. Stop tube advancement, allow patient to relax, and provide tissues	❏	❏	_____
b. Explain that the next step requires swallowing	❏	❏	_____
26. With tube just above oropharynx, instruct patient to flex head forward and dry swallow or suck in air through straw; advance with each swallow; if patient has trouble swallowing and is allowed fluids, offer glass of water; advance tube with each swallow of water; while advancing the tube in an unconscious patient (or in a patient who cannot swallow), stroke the patient's neck	❏	❏	_____
27. If patient begins to cough, gag, or choke, stop tube advancement; instruct patient to breathe easily and take sips of water	❏	❏	_____

	S	U	Comments
28. If patient continues to cough, pull tube back slightly	❏	❏	_____
29. If patient continues to gag, assess back of oral pharynx using flashlight and tongue blade	❏	❏	_____
30. After patient relaxes, continue to advance tube desired distance	❏	❏	_____
31. Ask patient to talk	❏	❏	_____
32. Assess posterior pharynx for presence of coiled tube	❏	❏	_____
33. Attach cone-tipped syringe to end of tube; aspirate gently back on syringe to obtain gastric contents	❏	❏	_____
34. Measure pH of aspirate with color-coded pH paper	❏	❏	_____
35. If tube is not in the stomach, advance another 2.5–5 cm (1–2 in) and repeat step 33	❏	❏	_____
36. After tube is properly inserted, clamp end or connect it to suction	❏	❏	_____
37. Cleanse nose with alcohol and Skin Prep for better adherence of nasal guard	❏	❏	_____
38. Secure tube to nose with a nasal guard; avoid putting pressure on nares	❏	❏	_____
39. Fasten end of tube to gown by looping rubber band around tube in slip knot; pin rubber band to gown	❏	❏	_____
40. Unless physician orders otherwise, head of bed should be elevated 30 degrees	❏	❏	_____

Postprocedure

	S	U	Comments
41. Assist patient to a position of comfort and place needed items within easy reach; be certain patient has a means to call for assistance and knows how to use it	❏	❏	_____
42. Raise side rails and lower bed to lowest position	❏	❏	_____
43. Remove gloves and all protective barriers; dispose of soiled supplies and equipment appropriately	❏	❏	_____

	S	U	Comments
44. Perform hand hygiene after patient contact and after wearing gloves	❏	❏	_____
45. Document and do patient teaching	❏	❏	_____
46. Report any unexpected outcomes	❏	❏	_____

PERFORMANCE CHECKLIST 20-18

NASOGASTRIC TUBE IRRIGATION

	S	U	Comments
Prepare for procedure			
1. Refer to medical record, care plan, or Kardex	❑	❑	_____
2. Introduce self	❑	❑	_____
3. Identify patient	❑	❑	_____
4. Explain procedure and reason it is to be done	❑	❑	_____
5. Assess need for and provide patient teaching during procedure	❑	❑	_____
6. Assemble equipment and complete necessary charges	❑	❑	_____
7. Perform hand hygiene; don clean gloves	❑	❑	_____
8. Assess patient	❑	❑	_____
9. Prepare patient for intervention			
a. Close door/pull privacy curtain	❑	❑	_____
b. Raise bed to comfortable working height; lower side rail on side nearest the nurse	❑	❑	_____
c. Position and drape patient as necessary	❑	❑	_____
During the skill			
10. Promote patient involvement as possible	❑	❑	_____
11. Assess patient's tolerance	❑	❑	_____
12. Place patient in semi-Fowler's position	❑	❑	_____
13. Verify that tube is in right place by attaching syringe to end of tube and aspirating for stomach content	❑	❑	_____
14. Assess abdomen	❑	❑	_____
15. Pour normal saline into container; draw up 30 mL (or amount ordered) into piston syringe	❑	❑	_____

	S	U	Comments
16. Clamp connection tubing distal to connection site for drainage or suction apparatus; disconnect tubing and lay end on a towel or waterproof pad	❏	❏	_____
17. Insert tip of irrigating syringe into end of NG tube; hold syringe with tip pointed toward the floor and instill 30 mL or ordered amount saline slowly and evenly **(do not force solution)**	❏	❏	_____
18. If resistance is met, assess tubing for kinks, change patient's position, and repeat attempt; if resistance continues, confer with RN or physician	❏	❏	_____
19. Withdraw fluid into syringe and measure; continue irrigating with ordered amount of saline until purpose of irrigation has been accomplished	❏	❏	_____
20. Reconnect NG tube to suction, introduce 30 mL of air into blue air vent lumen to clear air vent tubing; do not put liquid irrigant into blue airway lumen; secure airway lumen above level of stomach	❏	❏	_____
21. Note amount of saline instilled and withdrawn; subtract amount instilled from amount withdrawn and record difference as output	❏	❏	_____

Postprocedure

	S	U	Comments
22. Assist patient to a position of comfort and place needed items within easy reach; be certain patient has a means to call for assistance and knows how to use it	❏	❏	_____
23. Raise side rails and lower bed to lowest position	❏	❏	_____
24. Remove gloves and all protective barriers; dispose of soiled supplies and equipment appropriately	❏	❏	_____
25. Perform hand hygiene after patient contact and after wearing gloves	❏	❏	_____
26. Document and do patient teaching	❏	❏	_____
27. Report any unexpected outcomes	❏	❏	_____

Student Name_____ Date_____ Instructor's name_____

GASTRIC AND INTESTINAL SUCTIONING CARE

	S	U	Comments
Prepare for procedure			
1. Refer to medical record, care plan, or Kardex	❑	❑	_____
2. Introduce self	❑	❑	_____
3. Identify patient	❑	❑	_____
4. Explain procedure and reason it is to be done	❑	❑	_____
5. Assess need for and provide patient teaching during procedure	❑	❑	_____
6. Assemble equipment and complete necessary charges	❑	❑	_____
7. Perform hand hygiene; don clean gloves	❑	❑	_____
8. Assess patient	❑	❑	_____
9. Prepare patient for intervention			
a. Close door/pull privacy curtain	❑	❑	_____
b. Raise bed to comfortable working height; lower side rail on side nearest the nurse	❑	❑	_____
c. Position and drape patient as necessary	❑	❑	_____
During the skill			
10. Promote patient involvement as possible	❑	❑	_____
11. Assess patient's tolerance	❑	❑	_____
12. Assess suction apparatus	❑	❑	_____
a. For suction machine (Gomco)			
(1) Make certain machine is plugged in securely	❑	❑	_____
(2) Make certain light is blinking on and off	❑	❑	_____
(3) Make certain tubing connections are secure	❑	❑	_____
(4) Make certain setting is correct	❑	❑	_____

	S	U	Comments
b. For wall suction			
(1) Make certain pressure gauge connections are tight	❏	❏	_____
(2) Make certain pressure indicated on gauge is as ordered or according to agency policy, 80–100 mm Hg; pressure above 120 mm Hg results in gastric bleeding	❏	❏	_____
(3) Suction is set on intermittent or continuous as ordered	❏	❏	_____
13. Assess patient			
a. Oral/nasal cavities	❏	❏	_____
b. Abdomen for bowel sounds and extent of distention (be certain to turn off wall suctioning during assessment to prevent hearing Salem sump sounds)	❏	❏	_____
c. NPO status	❏	❏	_____
d. Lips and oral mucosa	❏	❏	_____
14. Ensure that tubing is not kinked and that patient is not lying on tubing	❏	❏	_____
15. Pin NG tube to patient's gown with enough slack to allow movement	❏	❏	_____
16. Verify that drainage is moving through tubing to drainage collection bottle	❏	❏	_____
17. For Salem sump tube see that vent is pointing upward; listen at opening of blue air vent; if no hissing sounds are heard, instruct patient to cough or reposition to the right or left Sims' or supine position; it may be necessary to momentarily disconnect the NG tube from the suction tubing; be certain to reconnect immediately	❏	❏	_____
18. Measure amount of drainage in bottle, noting color; empty when becoming full and at end of each shift	❏	❏	_____

Student Name_____ Date_____ Instructor's name_____

	S	U	**Comments**

Postprocedure

19. Assist patient to a position of comfort and place needed items within easy reach; be certain patient has a means to call for assistance and knows how to use it ❏ ❏ _____

20. Raise side rails and lower bed to lowest position ❏ ❏ _____

21. Remove gloves and all protective barriers; dispose of soiled supplies and equipment appropriately ❏ ❏ _____

22. Perform hand hygiene after patient contact and after wearing gloves ❏ ❏ _____

23. Document and do patient teaching ❏ ❏ _____

24. Report any unexpected outcomes ❏ ❏ _____

PERFORMANCE CHECKLIST 20-20

Nasogastric Tube Removal

	S	U	Comments
Prepare for procedure			
1. Refer to medical record, care plan, or Kardex	❑	❑	_____
2. Introduce self	❑	❑	_____
3. Identify patient	❑	❑	_____
4. Explain procedure and reason it is to be done	❑	❑	_____
5. Assess need for and provide patient teaching during procedure	❑	❑	_____
6. Assemble equipment and complete necessary charges	❑	❑	_____
7. Perform hand hygiene; don clean gloves	❑	❑	_____
8. Assess patient	❑	❑	_____
9. Prepare patient for intervention			
a. Close door/pull privacy curtain	❑	❑	_____
b. Raise bed to comfortable working height; lower side rail on side nearest the nurse	❑	❑	_____
c. Position and drape patient as necessary	❑	❑	_____
During the skill			
10. Promote patient involvement as possible	❑	❑	_____
11. Assess patient's tolerance	❑	❑	_____
12. Reassure that removal is less distressing than insertion	❑	❑	_____
13. Assess			
a. Patient's abdomen for bowel sounds (turn off wall suction during assessment to prevent misinterpreting Salem sump sounds for peristalsis)	❑	❑	_____
b. Patient's nasal and oral cavity	❑	❑	_____

	S	U	Comments
14. If tube is attached to suction, turn off suction machine and disconnect tubing, remove nose guard, and unfasten pin from gown	❏	❏	_____
15. Place towel or waterproof pad across patient's chest	❏	❏	_____
16. Instruct patient to take deep breath and hold it; pinch tube with fingers or clamp; quickly and smoothly remove tube while patient is holding breath	❏	❏	_____
17. Provide patient with tissues to cleanse nasal passage	❏	❏	_____
18. Place tubing in plastic bag or towel	❏	❏	_____
19. Cleanse nose with alcohol to remove residue from nasal guard placement	❏	❏	_____
20. Provide oral and nasal care; make patient comfortable	❏	❏	_____
21. Dispose of tube and equipment; measure drainage; note color and write down for documentation	❏	❏	_____
22. Inspect condition of nares and oral cavity	❏	❏	_____

Postprocedure

	S	U	Comments
23. Assist patient to a position of comfort and place needed items within easy reach; be certain patient has a means to call for assistance and knows how to use it	❏	❏	_____
24. Raise side rails and lower bed to lowest position	❏	❏	_____
25. Palpate abdomen periodically, noting any distention, pain, and rigidity; auscultate abdomen for bowel sounds	❏	❏	_____
26. Remove gloves and all protective barriers; dispose of soiled supplies and equipment appropriately	❏	❏	_____
27. Perform hand hygiene after patient contact and after wearing gloves	❏	❏	_____
28. Document and do patient teaching	❏	❏	_____
29. Report any unexpected outcomes	❏	❏	_____

PERFORMANCE CHECKLIST 20-21

INSERTING A RECTAL TUBE

	S	U	Comments
Prepare for procedure			
1. Refer to medical record, care plan, or Kardex	❏	❏	_____
2. Introduce self	❏	❏	_____
3. Identify patient	❏	❏	_____
4. Explain procedure and reason it is to be done	❏	❏	_____
5. Assess need for and provide patient teaching	❏	❏	_____
6. Assemble equipment and complete necessary charges	❏	❏	_____
7. Perform hand hygiene; don clean gloves	❏	❏	_____
8. Assess patient	❏	❏	_____
9. Prepare patient for intervention			
a. Close door/pull privacy curtain	❏	❏	_____
b. Raise bed to comfortable working height; lower side rail on side nearest the nurse	❏	❏	_____
c. Position and drape patient as necessary	❏	❏	_____
During the skill			
10. Promote patient involvement as possible	❏	❏	_____
11. Assess bowel sounds	❏	❏	_____
12. Request patient to assume Sims' position	❏	❏	_____
13. Arrange gown and top sheet to prevent soiling	❏	❏	_____
14. Place waterproof pad under buttocks	❏	❏	_____
15. Don gloves	❏	❏	_____
16. Lubricate tube well	❏	❏	_____
17. Expose anus	❏	❏	_____
18. Insert tube appropriately	❏	❏	_____

	S	U	Comments
19. Insert drainage end into receptacle or use commercially prepared set	❏	❏	_____
20. Instruct patient to lie quietly	❏	❏	_____
21. Leave tube in place the allotted time	❏	❏	_____
22. Notify physician as necessary	❏	❏	_____
23. Remove tube and assist patient to bedpan/ toilet or commode	❏	❏	_____
24. Assess for bowel movement	❏	❏	_____
25. Provide for hygiene	❏	❏	_____
26. Assess for bowel sounds	❏	❏	_____

Postprocedure

	S	U	Comments
27. Assist patient to a position of comfort and place needed items within easy reach; be certain patient has a means to call for assistance and knows how to use it	❏	❏	_____
28. Raise side rails and lower bed to lowest position	❏	❏	_____
29. Remove gloves and all protective barriers; dispose of soiled supplies and equipment appropriately	❏	❏	_____
30. Perform hand hygiene after patient contact and after wearing gloves	❏	❏	_____
31. Document and do patient teaching	❏	❏	_____
32. Report any unexpected outcomes	❏	❏	_____

PERFORMANCE CHECKLIST 20-22

ADMINISTERING AN ENEMA

	S	U	Comments
Prepare for procedure			
1. Refer to medical record, care plan, or Kardex	❏	❏	_____
2. Introduce self	❏	❏	_____
3. Identify patient	❏	❏	_____
4. Explain procedure and reason it is to be done	❏	❏	_____
5. Assess need for and provide patient teaching during procedure	❏	❏	_____
6. Assemble equipment and complete necessary charges	❏	❏	_____
7. Perform hand hygiene; don clean gloves	❏	❏	_____
8. Assess patient	❏	❏	_____
9. Prepare patient for intervention			
a. Close door/pull privacy curtain	❏	❏	_____
b. Raise bed to comfortable working height; lower side rail on side nearest the nurse	❏	❏	_____
c. Position and drape patient as necessary	❏	❏	_____
During the skill			
10. Promote patient involvement as possible	❏	❏	_____
11. Assess patient's tolerance	❏	❏	_____
12. Prepare solution	❏	❏	_____
13. Arrange equipment at bedside	❏	❏	_____
14. Assist patient to Sims' position; when giving an enema to a patient who is unable to contract the external sphincter, position the patient on the bedpan	❏	❏	_____
15. Place waterproof pad under patient	❏	❏	_____
16. Place bath blanket over patient and fan-fold linen to foot of bed; adjust patient's gown	❏	❏	_____
17. Clamp tubing 28 cm (7 in) from end; fill container with correctly warmed solution (usually 1000 mL at 105° F for adults) and any additives; allow solution to fill tubing to prevent air in colon	❏	❏	_____

	S	U	Comments

18. Lubricate tubing; spread patient's buttocks to expose anus; while rotating tube, gently insert it 7–10 cm (3–4 in); instruct patient to breathe out slowly through mouth (for commercially prepared enemas, remove cover from tip of enema device; add additional lubricant and insert entire tip into anus, squeeze container until it is empty; continue to squeeze container and remove and discard device appropriately) ❏ ❏ _____

19. Elevate container 30–45 cm (12–18 in) above level of anus ❏ ❏ _____

20. Release clamp; allow more solution to flow slowly while holding clamp ❏ ❏ _____

21. Lower container or clamp tubing if patient complains of cramping; encourage slow, deep breathing (when severe cramping, bleeding, or sudden abdominal pain occurs that is unrelieved by temporarily stopping or slowing flow of solution, stop enema and notify physician) ❏ ❏ _____

22. Clamp and remove tube when all of the solution has been administered; encourage patient to retain solution at least 5 minutes ❏ ❏ _____

23. When patient can no longer retain solution, assist to bedpan, bedside commode, or bathroom ❏ ❏ _____

24. Instruct patient to call for nurse to inspect results before flushing stool; observe characteristics of feces/solution ❏ ❏ _____

25. Provide for patient hygiene ❏ ❏ _____

Postprocedure

26. Assist patient to a position of comfort and place needed items within easy reach; be certain patient has a means to call for assistance and knows how to use it ❏ ❏ _____

27. Raise side rails and lower bed to lowest position ❏ ❏ _____

28. Remove gloves and all protective barriers; dispose of soiled supplies and equipment appropriately ❏ ❏ _____

Student Name_____ Date_____ Instructor's name_____

	S	U	Comments
29. Perform hand hygiene after patient contact and after wearing gloves; provide for patient hygiene and assist patient to the bed or to the chair	❏	❏	_____
30. Document and do patient teaching	❏	❏	_____
31. Report any unexpected outcomes	❏	❏	_____

DIGITAL EXAMINATION WITH REMOVAL OF FECAL IMPACTION

	S	U	Comments
Prepare for procedure			
1. Refer to medical record, care plan, or Kardex	❑	❑	_____
2. Introduce self	❑	❑	_____
3. Identify patient	❑	❑	_____
4. Explain procedure and reason it is to be done	❑	❑	_____
5. Assess need for and provide patient teaching during procedure	❑	❑	_____
6. Assemble equipment and complete necessary charges	❑	❑	_____
7. Perform hand hygiene; don clean gloves	❑	❑	_____
8. Assess patient	❑	❑	_____
9. Prepare patient for intervention			
a. Close door/pull privacy curtain	❑	❑	_____
b. Raise bed to comfortable working height; lower side rail on side nearest the nurse	❑	❑	_____
c. Position and drape patient as necessary	❑	❑	_____
During the skill			
10. Promote patient involvement as possible	❑	❑	_____
11. Assess patient's tolerance	❑	❑	_____
12. Assist patient to assume the Sims' position and place waterproof pad under patient's buttocks	❑	❑	_____
13. Place the bedpan on the bed close to the patient's buttocks	❑	❑	_____
14. Don gloves; lubricate forefinger well with petroleum or water-soluble lubricant; use the index finger of your dominant hand	❑	❑	_____

	S	U	Comments
15. Insert finger gently; slowly but gently move finger into and around the fecal mass; as pieces of the mass are broken off, remove them to bedpan	❏	❏	_____
16. Instruct patient to take slow, deep breaths	❏	❏	_____
17. Continue procedure until impaction is removed	❏	❏	_____
18. Stop procedure for a few minutes if patient complains of severe discomfort; give patient opportunity to rest; be alert for complications such as adverse vagal response	❏	❏	_____
19. After removal is complete, wash and dry perineal area	❏	❏	_____
20. Assist the patient to toilet or position on the bedpan if urge to defecate develops	❏	❏	_____

Postprocedure

	S	U	Comments
21. Assist patient to a position of comfort and place needed items within easy reach; be certain patient has a means to call for assistance and knows how to use it	❏	❏	_____
22. Raise side rails and lower bed to lowest position	❏	❏	_____
23. Remove gloves and all protective barriers; dispose of soiled supplies and equipment appropriately	❏	❏	_____
24. Perform hand hygiene after patient contact and after wearing gloves	❏	❏	_____
25. Document and do patient teaching	❏	❏	_____
26. Report any unexpected outcomes	❏	❏	_____

PERFORMANCE CHECKLIST 20-24

Performing Colostomy, Ileostomy, and Urostomy Care

	S	U	Comments
Prepare for procedure			
1. Refer to medical record, care plan, or Kardex	❏	❏	_____
2. Introduce self	❏	❏	_____
3. Identify patient	❏	❏	_____
4. Explain procedure and reason it is to be done	❏	❏	_____
5. Assess need for and provide patient teaching during procedure	❏	❏	_____
6. Assemble equipment and complete necessary charges	❏	❏	_____
7. Perform hand hygiene; don clean gloves	❏	❏	_____
8. Assess patient	❏	❏	_____
9. Prepare patient for intervention			
a. Close door/pull privacy curtain	❏	❏	_____
b. Raise bed to comfortable working height; lower side rail on side nearest the nurse	❏	❏	_____
c. Position and drape patient as necessary	❏	❏	_____
During the skill			
10. Promote patient involvement as possible	❏	❏	_____
11. Assess patient's tolerance	❏	❏	_____
12. Arrange supplies/equipment at bedside or in bathroom	❏	❏	_____
13. Position patient supine and make comfortable	❏	❏	_____
14. Unfasten and remove belt, if worn; carefully remove wafer seal from skin	❏	❏	_____
15. Place reusable pouch in bedpan or disposable pouch in plastic bag. Place bag away from patient to prevent unpleasant odors	❏	❏	_____
16. Cleanse skin with warm water; pat dry	❏	❏	_____

	S	U	Comments
17. Measure stoma using measuring device	❏	❏	_____
18. Place toilet tissue or disposable wash cloth over stoma; use gauze for ileostomy; if using Skin Prep, apply to skin and allow to dry	❏	❏	_____
19. Apply protective skin barrier about 1/16 inch from stoma; assess stoma to determine color and viability	❏	❏	_____
20. Apply protective wafer with flange, cutting an opening in the center of wafer to 1/16 inch larger than stoma	❏	❏	_____
21. Gently attach pouch to flange by compressing the two together (a device is available called Autolok which snaps into place with a smooth lock, thus eliminating the need to compress the flange to the pouch)	❏	❏	_____
22. Remove tissue or gauze from stoma and backing from protectant; center opening over stoma and press against skin for 1–2 minutes	❏	❏	_____
23. Fold bottom edges of pouch over one time to fit clamp	❏	❏	_____
24. Secure clamp	❏	❏	_____
25. If belt is used, attach properly	❏	❏	_____
26. Assist patient to comfortable position in bed or chair; remove equipment from bedside	❏	❏	_____
27. Empty, wash, and dry reusable pouch	❏	❏	_____

Urostomy care

	S	U	Comments
28. Follow steps 1 to 13 of ostomy care procedure	❏	❏	_____
29. Empty urine into graduated pitcher; write down amount and characteristics of urine for later documentation (mucus will be present in urine from shedding of mucus by mucous membrane of intestine as urine passes over the intestinal conduit)	❏	❏	_____
30. Carefully remove water seal from skin and place pouch in plastic bag	❏	❏	_____
31. Cleanse skin with warm water and pat dry	❏	❏	_____
32. Measure stoma using measuring device	❏	❏	_____

	S	U	Comments
33. Place gauze over stoma	❏	❏	_____
34. If using Skin Prep, apply to skin and allow to dry; apply protective stoma paste about 1/16 inch from the stoma	❏	❏	_____
35. Apply protective wafer with flange, cutting an opening in the center of wafer 1/16 inch larger than stoma; assess stoma to determine color and viability	❏	❏	_____

Postprocedure

	S	U	Comments
36. Assist patient to a position of comfort and place needed items within easy reach; be certain patient has a means to call for assistance and knows how to use it	❏	❏	_____
37. Raise side rails and lower bed to lowest position	❏	❏	_____
38. Remove gloves and all protective barriers; dispose of soiled supplies and equipment appropriately	❏	❏	_____
39. Perform hand hygiene after patient contact and after wearing gloves	❏	❏	_____
40. Document and do patient teaching	❏	❏	_____
41. Report any unexpected outcomes	❏	❏	_____

PERFORMANCE CHECKLIST 20-25

PERFORMING A COLOSTOMY IRRIGATION

	S	U	Comments
Prepare for procedure			
1. Refer to medical record, care plan, or Kardex	❑	❑	_____
2. Introduce self	❑	❑	_____
3. Identify patient	❑	❑	_____
4. Explain procedure and reason it is to be done	❑	❑	_____
5. Assess need for and provide patient teaching during procedure	❑	❑	_____
6. Assemble equipment and complete necessary charges	❑	❑	_____
7. Perform hand hygiene; don clean gloves	❑	❑	_____
8. Assess patient	❑	❑	_____
9. Prepare patient for intervention			
a. Close door/pull privacy curtain	❑	❑	_____
b. Raise bed to comfortable working height; lower side rail on side nearest the nurse	❑	❑	_____
c. Position and drape patient as necessary	❑	❑	_____
During the skill			
10. Promote patient involvement as possible	❑	❑	_____
11. Assess patient's tolerance	❑	❑	_____
12. Position patient			
a. Bathroom: instruct patient to sit on toilet or on a chair in front of the toilet	❑	❑	_____
b. Bed: have patient lie comfortably with head of bed slightly elevated	❑	❑	_____

	S	U	Comments
13. Remove pouch, cleanse skin, and place irrigation sleeve over stoma; attach belt if using; place end of sleeve in toilet	❏	❏	_____
14. Close clamp on irrigating tubing; fill irrigating container with 1000 mL tepid water (or as otherwise ordered); container may be hung on a hook at patient's shoulder level	❏	❏	_____
15. Allow a small amount of water to flow through tubing	❏	❏	_____
16. Attach cone to tubing; lubricate cone; gently insert cone into stoma through top of sleeve	❏	❏	_____
17. While holding cone in place, allow solution to flow slowly into colon (500–1000 mL over 15 minutes)	❏	❏	_____
18. After all solution is instilled, remove cone and close top of sleeve	❏	❏	_____
19. Instruct patient to sit about 15–20 minutes while returns flow into toilet	❏	❏	_____
20. Drain sleeve; remove and rinse it	❏	❏	_____
21. Observe patient and results of irrigation; flush toilet	❏	❏	_____
22. Perform colostomy care	❏	❏	_____

Postprocedure

	S	U	Comments
23. Assist patient to a position of comfort and place needed items within easy reach; be certain patient has a means to call for assistance and knows how to use it	❏	❏	_____
24. Raise side rails and lower bed to lowest position	❏	❏	_____
25. Remove gloves and all protective barriers; dispose of soiled supplies and equipment appropriately	❏	❏	_____
26. Perform hand hygiene after patient contact and after wearing gloves	❏	❏	_____
27. Document and do patient teaching	❏	❏	_____
28. Report any unexpected outcomes	❏	❏	_____

Student Name_____ Date_____ Instructor's name_____

PERFORMANCE CHECKLIST 21-1

ADMINISTERING NASOGASTRIC TUBE FEEDINGS

	S	U	Comments
1. Refer to medical record, care plan, or Kardex for special interventions; physician's order will state formula, rate, route, and frequency of feeding	❏	❏	_____
2. Introduce self	❏	❏	_____
3. Identify patient	❏	❏	_____
4. Explain procedure	❏	❏	_____
5. Assess need for patient teaching	❏	❏	_____
6. Assemble equipment and complete necessary charges; organize procedure	❏	❏	_____
7. Perform hand hygiene; don clean gloves	❏	❏	_____
8. Assess patient, auscultate for active bowel sounds to assess abdomen for distention or tenderness	❏	❏	_____
9. Prepare patient for intervention			
a. Close door/pull privacy curtain	❏	❏	_____
b. Raise bed to a comfortable working height	❏	❏	_____
c. Elevate level of bed to Fowler's, at least 30 degrees, or reverse Trendelenburg if spinal injury present	❏	❏	_____
10. Check for placement of feeding tube			
a. Aspirate gastric or intestinal contents with appropriate cone-tipped syringe inserted into end of tube	❏	❏	_____
b. Place drop of GI contents on pH test paper (gastric content should have a pH of 0–4, tracheobronchial and pleural secretions should have a pH > 6 and intestinal contents usually have a pH of 7 or greater)	❏	❏	_____
c. Inspect oral cavity for tube kinking or curling in back of pharynx	❏	❏	_____
d. If unable to aspirate, consider tube is occluded or kinked, and attempt to flush with 30 mL of warm water	❏	❏	_____

Copyright © 2011, 2006, 2003, 1999, 1995, 1991 by Mosby, Inc., an affiliate of Elsevier Inc. All rights reserved.

	S	U	Comments
11. Readminister residual volume to patient slowly	❑	❑	_____
a. If residual amounts are greater than last infusion or 150 mL, hold feeding for one hour and reassess residual	❑	❑	_____
12. Prepare formula for administration	❑	❑	_____
13. Bolus or intermittent feedings			
a. Administer tube feeding with 60 mL bulb or plunger syringe	❑	❑	_____
b. Remove cap or plug from end of feeding tube and pinch closed	❑	❑	_____
c. Attach syringe by removing bulb or plunger and inserting tip into end of tube; elevate to no more than 18 inches above insertion site	❑	❑	_____
d. Fill syringe with formula, release tube, and allow syringe to empty gradually, refilling until prescribed ordered amount has been administered	❑	❑	_____
e. Flush tube with 30–60 mL tap water	❑	❑	_____
f. Recap/plug tube	❑	❑	_____
14. Continuous drip method			
a. Administer tube feeding with gavage bag	❑	❑	_____
b. Prepare administration set: clamp tubing, prepare gavage bag with prescribed type and amount of formula, unclamp and prime tubing to remove air, then reclamp tubing	❑	❑	_____
c. Label bag with tube feeding type, strength, and amount. Include date, time, and initials	❑	❑	_____
d. Pinch end of feeding tube. Remove plug/cap and securely attach gavage tubing to end of feeding tube	❑	❑	_____
e. Set rate by adjusting roller clamp on tubing	❑	❑	_____
f. Flush tube with 30–60 mL tap water	❑	❑	_____
g. Recap/plug tube	❑	❑	_____
15. Feeding via infusion pump			
a. Administer tube feeding as a continuous drip via infusion pump	❑	❑	_____

	S	U	Comments

b. Prepare administration set. Clamp tubing, spike bag, unclamp and prime tubing. Reclamp tubing ❏ ❏ _____

c. Label bag with tube feeding type, strength, and amount. Include date, time, and initials ❏ ❏ _____

d. Hang tube feeding set on IV pole with infusion pump. Connect tubing to pump and set rate ❏ ❏ _____

e. Pinch end of feeding tube. Remove plug/cap. Connect infusion tubing to patient feeding tube ❏ ❏ _____

f. Open roller clamp on infusion tubing ❏ ❏ _____

g. Check residual volumes every 4 hours ❏ ❏ _____

16. Fill a 60 mL syringe with ordered volume of water (30–50 mL). Inject into feeding tube to flush after bolus or as ordered with continuous drip ❏ ❏ _____

17. Flush tube with water every 4–8 hours, clamp it when no feedings are infusing ❏ ❏ _____

18. Rinse syringe or bag and tubing with warm water. Remove and discard gloves and wash hands ❏ ❏ _____

19. Ask if patient is comfortable while infusion is continuing; diarrhea should be reported to physician ❏ ❏ _____

20. Assist patient to a position of comfort and place needed items within reach ❏ ❏ _____

21. Raise side rails and lower bed to lowest position ❏ ❏ _____

22. Remove gloves, dispose of used supplies and perform hand hygiene ❏ ❏ _____

23. Document ❏ ❏ _____

24. Monitor weight and laboratory values daily ❏ ❏ _____

25. Observe and assess patient for any adverse reactions, such as shortness of breath, low oxygenation saturation, and presence of feeding from airway ❏ ❏ _____

Student Name_____ Date_____ Instructor's name_____

ADMINISTERING ENTERAL FEEDINGS VIA GASTROSTOMY OR JEJUNOSTOMY TUBE

	S	U	Comments

Observe all guidelines for nasal gastric tube feedings and follow steps 1 to 9 of Skill 21-1 and then continue with the steps below.

1. Verify tube placement—see Skill 21-1, step 10

   a. Gastrostomy tube: aspirate gastric secretions, check pH; return aspirated contents to stomach unless volume exceeds 150 mL ❑ ❑ _____

   b. Jejunostomy tube: aspirate intestinal secretions, check pH ❑ ❑ _____

2. Flush with 30 mL water ❑ ❑ _____

3. Initiate feedings. Usually gastrostomy and jejunostomy feedings are given continuously to ensure proper absorption. However, initial feedings may be given by bolus to assess patient's tolerance to formula

   a. Syringe feedings

      (1) Pinch proximal end of gastrostomy tube ❑ ❑ _____

      (2) Remove plunger and attach barrel of syringe to end of tube, then fill syringe with formula ❑ ❑ _____

      (3) Allow syringe to empty gradually. Refill until prescribed amount has been delivered to patient ❑ ❑ _____

      (4) Flush with ordered volume of water (30-50 mL) ❑ ❑ _____

   b. Continuous drip method

      (1) Fill feeding container with enough formula for 4 hours of feeding ❑ ❑ _____

      (2) Hang container on IV pole, and clear tubing of air ❑ ❑ _____

      (3) Thread tubing on pump according to manufacturer's directions ❑ ❑ _____

	S	U	Comments
(4) Connect tubing to end of feeding tube	❏	❏	_____
(5) Begin infusion at prescribed rate	❏	❏	_____
4. Assess skin around tube exit site; skin around tube should be cleansed daily with warm water and mild soap	❏	❏	_____
5. Dispose of supplies and perform hand hygiene	❏	❏	_____
6. Monitor finger-stick blood glucose every 6 hrs until maximum administration rate is reached and maintained for 24 hours	❏	❏	_____
7. Monitor intake and output	❏	❏	_____
8. Weigh patient daily	❏	❏	_____
9. Observe laboratory values	❏	❏	_____
10. Inspect enteral site for signs of pressure	❏	❏	_____
11. Document	❏	❏	_____
12. Observe for any adverse reactions	❏	❏	_____

PERFORMANCE CHECKLIST 21-3

ASSISTING PATIENTS WITH EATING

		S	U	Comments
1.	Complete or delay care that will interfere with eating	❏	❏	_____
2.	Provide period of rest or quiet before meals; offer patient a bedpan or urinal before mealtime	❏	❏	_____
3.	Provide patient with opportunity for hand-washing; offer mouth care before eating	❏	❏	_____
4.	Remove any soiled articles or clutter from room	❏	❏	_____
5.	Make patient comfortable for eating; use pain relief techniques if needed	❏	❏	_____
6.	Raise head of bed to sitting position if possible	❏	❏	_____
7.	Cover patient's upper chest with napkin or towel	❏	❏	_____
8.	Sit beside patient; avoid appearing hurried	❏	❏	_____
9.	Encourage patients to take part in their eating as much as possible and to extent that their condition permits	❏	❏	_____
10.	Provide flexible straw for patients who are unable to use a cup or glass (unless contraindicated)	❏	❏	_____
11.	Serve manageable amounts of food with each bite	❏	❏	_____
12.	For a stroke patient, direct food toward side of mouth that is not paralyzed	❏	❏	_____
13.	Serve food in order of patient's preference	❏	❏	_____
14.	Give patient time to chew thoroughly and swallow food	❏	❏	_____
15.	Modify utensils and texture of food if patient must remain flat while eating; use child's training cup or large syringe with flexible rubber tube; puree or grind foods if necessary	❏	❏	_____
16.	If you have begun to feed a patient, do not leave until he or she has finished eating; a meal should not be interrupted	❏	❏	_____

	S	U	Comments
17. Talk with patient about pleasant subjects; eating is a social occasion	❏	❏	_____
18. Use suggested actions that involve removing a tray (see Skill 21-4)	❏	❏	_____

PERFORMANCE CHECKLIST 21-4

SERVING AND REMOVING TRAYS

	S	U	Comments
1. Be available when trays arrive from dietary department	❑	❑	_____
2. Clear area where patient will eat	❑	❑	_____
3. Check general appearance of tray for spilled liquids, missing items, or ordered food that is missing	❑	❑	_____
4. Compare name on tray with name on patient's identification bracelet	❑	❑	_____
5. Ensure that patients who are undergoing special tests have food withheld or provided according to test directions	❑	❑	_____
6. Check to see that patient is not being served foods to which he or she is allergic, or that he or she cannot tolerate	❑	❑	_____
7. Place tray so that it faces patient; remove food covers	❑	❑	_____
8. Open milk cartons and cereal boxes, butter toast, cut up meat, and otherwise assist as necessary	❑	❑	_____
9. Serve trays that have been kept warm last to those patients who need help with eating	❑	❑	_____
10. Note kinds and amounts of food that patient is not eating	❑	❑	_____
11. Observe whether patient feels satisfied with amounts of food served; serving sizes need to match appetite	❑	❑	_____
12. Follow agency policies about serving food brought from home; ensure that food is covered, labeled, refrigerated, or stored properly	❑	❑	_____
13. Be considerate and visit with patients who are on special diets and may be denied food they like because of a health problem	❑	❑	_____
14. Encourage patients to eat, but do not scold those who feel they cannot	❑	❑	_____

	S	U	Comments
15. Remove trays as soon as possible, and restore cleanliness of the eating area	❏	❏	_____
16. Assist or offer patient an opportunity to brush and floss teeth	❏	❏	_____
17. Record how patient ate and enter amounts of fluid consumed if appropriate	❏	❏	_____
18. Always assess patient's appetite during first assessment of the day; ask how he or she ate breakfast, etc.	❏	❏	_____
19. Use fractions (such as 1/4, 1/3, 1/2) or percentages (such as 35%, 50%, 100%) when documenting food eaten, or follow agency policy	❏	❏	_____

Student Name_____ Date_____ Instructor's name_____

Measuring Intake and Output (I&O)

	S	U	Comments
1. Identify patient	❏	❏	_____
2. Explain procedure	❏	❏	_____
3. Instruct patient to inform staff of all oral intake; provide a marked I&O container	❏	❏	_____
4. Instruct patient not to empty any output collection receptacles and to notify the nurse after elimination	❏	❏	_____
5. Alert all staff and remind patient of need to measure I&O	❏	❏	_____
6. Measure and record all fluids taken orally or per feeding tube, and all fluids administered parenterally	❏	❏	_____
7. Perform hand hygiene and don gloves	❏	❏	_____
8. Measure and record output in urinary drainage system, diarrhea stools, nasogastric suction, emesis, ileostomy, and output in surgical wound receptacles such as Davol, Jackson-Pratt, and Hemovac	❏	❏	_____
9. Remove gloves and perform hand hygiene	❏	❏	_____
10. Compute and document I&O on patient's record	❏	❏	_____
11. Be vigilant to maintain accurate I&O when ordered	❏	❏	_____

Student Name_____ Date_____ Instructor's name_____

ADMINISTERING TABLETS, PILLS, AND CAPSULES

	S	U	Comments
1. Follow the six rights	❑	❑	_____
2. Perform the three label checks	❑	❑	_____
3. Follow standard precautions	❑	❑	_____
4. Perform hand hygiene	❑	❑	_____
5. Check for allergies	❑	❑	_____
6. If using unit dose package, place unopened package in medicine cup	❑	❑	_____
7. If using a multidose bottle, pour tablet (without touching it) into cap of bottle appropriately	❑	❑	_____
8. Pour tablet from cap into medicine cup	❑	❑	_____
9. If using medicine tray (for several patients), set it up from left to right, front to back with patient's name and room number	❑	❑	_____
10. If pouring from multidose bottle and patient is to receive several tablets, use separate cup for medications such as digitalis. If the patient's pulse is less than 60/BPM, withhold the medication and report this to the RN. Place digitalis in a separate cup marked with a red heart to allow for easy identification	❑	❑	_____
11. Do not use pills, tablets, or capsules that come from multidose bottles if they have been handled or dropped on the floor	❑	❑	_____
12. Take medication to patient's room	❑	❑	_____
13. Identify room, bed, patient, and patient's birthdate	❑	❑	_____
14. Check again for allergies	❑	❑	_____
15. Explain procedure to patient	❑	❑	_____

	S	U	Comments
16. Document administration of medication in Medex or computer with initials, date, and time	❑	❑	_____
17. Return to assess patient's response to medication	❑	❑	_____
18. Document assessment	❑	❑	_____

Student Name_____ Date_____ Instructor's name_____

ADMINISTERING LIQUID MEDICATIONS

	S	U	Comments
1. Follow the six rights	❏	❏	_____
2. Perform the three label checks	❏	❏	_____
3. Follow standard precautions	❏	❏	_____
4. Perform hand hygiene	❏	❏	_____
5. Check for allergies	❏	❏	_____
6. Remove liquid preparation from patient's drug box/bin (or from medication cabinet or refrigerator)	❏	❏	_____
7. Check dosage/mL and total volume of medication in container	❏	❏	_____
8. Calculate dosage; if the dosage ordered is different from the dosage/mL stated on the label, calculate correct dose; if ordered medication is labeled in a different measurement system, convert by using appropriate equivalent. Work problem on paper correctly	❏	❏	_____
9. Check calculations with another nurse	❏	❏	_____
10. Obtain graduated medicine cup or appropriate syringe	❏	❏	_____
11. Face label of bottle toward palm of hand to avoid soiling label; if label becomes soiled, return the bottle to the pharmacy; do not give medication if label is unreadable	❏	❏	_____
12. Place medicine cup on flat surface, or hold at eye level while pouring	❏	❏	_____
13. Place cap of bottle with inner rim up	❏	❏	_____
14. Read dosage amount at lower level of meniscus	❏	❏	_____
15. Transport medication to patient's room	❏	❏	_____
16. Identify room, bed, patient, and patient's birthdate	❏	❏	_____

	S	U	Comments
17. Check for allergies	❏	❏	_____
18. Explain procedure to patient	❏	❏	_____
19. Document administration of medication in Medex or computer with initials, date, and time	❏	❏	_____
20. Return to assess patient's response to medication	❏	❏	_____
21. Document assessment	❏	❏	_____

PERFORMANCE CHECKLIST 23-3

ADMINISTERING TUBAL MEDICATIONS

	S	U	Comments
1. Follow the six rights	❏	❏	_____
2. Perform the three label checks	❏	❏	_____
3. Follow standard precautions	❏	❏	_____
4. Perform hand hygiene	❏	❏	_____
5. Check for allergies	❏	❏	_____
6. Prepare medication using the same procedure as for liquid medications	❏	❏	_____
7. If tablet, crush pill, dissolve in 15-20 mL warm water. For capsules, open and dissolve powder in 15-30 mL warm water. For gelatin capsules, aspirate with syringe or capsule may be dissolved in warm water and remove gelatin outer layer	❏	❏	_____
8. Gather equipment: 10 mL syringe, towel, stethoscope, bulb or Asepto syringe, tap water	❏	❏	_____
9. Take equipment and medication to patient's room	❏	❏	_____
10. Identify room, bed, patient, and patient's birthdate	❏	❏	_____
11. Recheck for allergies	❏	❏	_____
12. Explain procedure; answer questions patient may have about the procedure	❏	❏	_____
13. Place patient in high Fowler's position	❏	❏	_____
14. Put towel over patient's chest	❏	❏	_____
15. Don disposable, unsterile gloves	❏	❏	_____
16. Check and recheck placement and patency of tube with the appropriate procedure			
a. Method A: Attach bulb or Asepto syringe to end of NG tube; pull plunger back or release suction of bulb syringe to aspirate stomach contents; if stomach contents are seen, instill 10 to 20 mL of water before medication administration to clear tube; proceed with medication	❏	❏	_____

	S	U	Comments
b. Method B: Place stethoscope over stomach; push 10 mL of air through NG tube with syringe	❏	❏	_____
c. Method C: Many authorities now recommend the litmus test instead of the auscultatory (air-instillation) method: measure pH of aspirate with color-coded pH paper with range of whole numbers from 1 to 11; gastric aspirates have decidedly acidic pH values (preferably 4 or less); proceed with medication	❏	❏	_____
17. Clamp tube with rubber-tipped hemostat or other clamping device	❏	❏	_____
18. Attach syringe to end of tube correctly (with plunger out of syringe)	❏	❏	_____
19. Pour medication into syringe	❏	❏	_____
20. Unclamp tubing to allow medication to slowly flow by gravity	❏	❏	_____
21. Follow medication with 30–50 mL of water	❏	❏	_____
22. Clamp tubing; secure tube after medication is given	❏	❏	_____
23. If NG tube is attached to suction, do not reconnect suction for 30 minutes	❏	❏	_____
24. Remove towel from patient	❏	❏	_____
25. Remove gloves and dispose of properly	❏	❏	_____
26. Leave patient in comfortable position	❏	❏	_____
27. Gather equipment; clean up patient and area appropriately	❏	❏	_____
28. Perform hand hygiene	❏	❏	_____
29. Document administration of NG medication in Medex or computer with initials, date, and time	❏	❏	_____
30. Return to assess patient's response to medication	❏	❏	_____
31. Document assessment	❏	❏	_____

Student Name_____ Date_____ Instructor's name_____

ADMINISTERING RECTAL SUPPOSITORIES

	S	U	Comments
1. Follow the six rights	❑	❑	_____
2. Perform the three label checks	❑	❑	_____
3. Follow standard precautions	❑	❑	_____
4. Perform hand hygiene	❑	❑	_____
5. Check for allergies	❑	❑	_____
6. Obtain water-soluble lubricant	❑	❑	_____
7. Obtain suppository from refrigerator or from patient's medication bin	❑	❑	_____
8. Place unopened suppository into medicine cup or souffle cup	❑	❑	_____
9. Take disposable, unsterile gloves or finger cot to patient's room	❑	❑	_____
10. Identify room, bed, patient, and patient's birthdate	❑	❑	_____
11. Explain procedure to patient	❑	❑	_____
12. Gain patient's cooperation	❑	❑	_____
13. Provide privacy	❑	❑	_____
14. Position patient appropriately in Sims' position (on left side with upper leg flexed at knee)	❑	❑	_____
15. Unwrap suppository	❑	❑	_____
16. Maintain privacy; expose buttocks	❑	❑	_____
17. Don gloves	❑	❑	_____
18. Apply lubricant, such as KY jelly, to tapered end of suppository	❑	❑	_____
19. Ask patient to take deep breath; insert beyond internal anal sphincter; insert suppository as patient exhales to relax anal sphincter	❑	❑	_____
20. Ask patient to retain suppository as long as possible; hold the buttocks together to help patient to retain suppository	❑	❑	_____

	S	U	Comments
21. Discard gloves correctly	❏	❏	_____
22. Help patient assume comfortable position	❏	❏	_____
23. Perform hand hygiene	❏	❏	_____
24. Document administration of suppository in Medex or computer with initials, date, and time	❏	❏	_____
25. Return to assess patient's response to medication	❏	❏	_____
26. Document assessment	❏	❏	_____

PERFORMANCE CHECKLIST 23-5

APPLYING TOPICAL AGENTS

	S	U	Comments
1. Follow the six rights	❑	❑	_____
2. Perform the three label checks	❑	❑	_____
3. Follow standard precautions	❑	❑	_____
4. Perform hand hygiene	❑	❑	_____
5. Check for allergies	❑	❑	_____
6. Transport medication to patient's room	❑	❑	_____
7. Identify room, bed, patient, and patient's birthdate	❑	❑	_____
8. Recheck for allergies	❑	❑	_____
9. Introduce self; explain procedure to patient	❑	❑	_____
10. Provide privacy; place patient in comfortable position that allows exposure to selected site	❑	❑	_____
11. Don gloves	❑	❑	_____
12. Cleanse site with appropriate materials, removing debris, encrustations, and previous medications	❑	❑	_____
13. Read prescription instructions carefully	❑	❑	_____
14. Prepare medicinal agent (ointments, creams, and lotions may have to be squeezed or removed with a tongue blade, depending on preparation)	❑	❑	_____
15. Apply paper applicator, disk, lotion, ointment, or cream	❑	❑	_____
16. Remove gloves	❑	❑	_____
17. Leave patient properly draped or clothed in comfortable position	❑	❑	_____
18. Answer patient's questions, and teach patient to perform self-applications if appropriate	❑	❑	_____
19. Clean work area	❑	❑	_____

	S	U	Comments
20. Perform hand hygiene	❏	❏	_____
21. Document administration of medication in Medex or computer with initials, date, and time	❏	❏	_____
22. Return to assess patient's response to medication	❏	❏	_____
23. Document assessment	❏	❏	_____

Student Name_____ Date_____ Instructor's name_____

PERFORMANCE CHECKLIST 23-6

ADMINISTERING EYEDROPS AND EYE OINTMENTS

	S	U	Comments
1. Follow the six rights	❑	❑	_____
2. Perform the three label checks	❑	❑	_____
3. Follow standard precautions	❑	❑	_____
4. Perform hand hygiene	❑	❑	_____
5. Check for allergies	❑	❑	_____
6. Transport medications to patient's room	❑	❑	_____
7. Identify medications as ophthalmic	❑	❑	_____
8. Identify room, bed, patient, and patient's birthdate	❑	❑	_____
9. Recheck for allergies	❑	❑	_____
10. Introduce self; explain procedure	❑	❑	_____
11. Provide privacy, position back of patient's head on pillow; direct patient's face upward toward ceiling. Review which eye or eyes to receive the medication; left eye, right eye, or both eyes	❑	❑	_____
12. Recheck for allergies	❑	❑	_____
13. Don gloves	❑	❑	_____
14. Remove exudate; clean eye as needed using sterile solution of saline; use cotton balls to wipe away exudate; use one cotton ball per stroke, wiping from inner canthus outward	❑	❑	_____
15. To apply drops, expose lower conjunctival sac by having patient look upward while gentle traction is applied to lower eyelid	❑	❑	_____
16. Put prescribed number of drops into conjunctival sac, not onto eyeball; conjunctival sac normally holds one or two drops	❑	❑	_____
17. Using a cotton ball or tissue, apply gentle pressure above bone at inner corner of eyelid for 1–2 minutes	❑	❑	_____
18. Apply sterile dressing if ordered	❑	❑	_____

	S	U	Comments
19. To apply ointment, expose lower conjunctival sac by having patient look upward while gentle traction is applied to lower eyelid	❏	❏	_____
20. Squeeze ointment into lower conjunctival sac	❏	❏	_____
21. Ask patient to close eye and to move it around in circular motion to spread medication	❏	❏	_____
22. Apply sterile dressing if ordered	❏	❏	_____
23. After applying drops or ointment to an eye, leave patient in comfortable position; clean up the work area	❏	❏	_____
24. Remove gloves and perform hand hygiene	❏	❏	_____
25. Answer patient's questions and if appropriate, teach patient to perform self-care	❏	❏	_____
26. Document administration of medications in Medex or computer with initials, date, and time	❏	❏	_____
27. Return to assess patient's response to medication	❏	❏	_____
28. Document assessment in nurse's notes	❏	❏	_____

PERFORMANCE CHECKLIST 23-7

ADMINISTERING EARDROPS

	S	U	Comments
1. Follow the six rights	❏	❏	_____
2. Perform the three label checks	❏	❏	_____
3. Follow standard precautions	❏	❏	_____
4. Perform hand hygiene	❏	❏	_____
5. Check for allergies	❏	❏	_____
6. Transport medication to patient's room	❏	❏	_____
7. Identify medications as otic	❏	❏	_____
8. Identify room, bed, patient, and patient's birthdate	❏	❏	_____
9. Recheck for allergies	❏	❏	_____
10. Introduce self; explain procedure	❏	❏	_____
11. Provide privacy; position patient with affected ear upward	❏	❏	_____
12. Don gloves	❏	❏	_____
13. Remove external exudate from ear; an order must be obtained before irrigating the ear	❏	❏	_____
14. Draw medication into dropper	❏	❏	_____
15. For adults and for children over 3 years old, turn head with affected side up; pull earlobe upward and back to straighten external auditory canal; give drops without touching ear with dropper	❏	❏	_____
16. For children under 3 years old, turn head with affected side up; pull earlobe downward and back; instill drops without touching ear with dropper	❏	❏	_____
17. Tell patient to remain in same position for a few minutes to allow medication to drain into ear by gravity	❏	❏	_____

	S	U	Comments
18. A cotton ball may be placed loosely into ear as needed	❏	❏	_____
19. Remove gloves	❏	❏	_____
20. Leave patient in comfortable position; clean work area	❏	❏	_____
21. Answer patient's questions and if appropriate, teach patient self-care	❏	❏	_____
22. Perform hand hygiene	❏	❏	_____
23. Document administration of medication in Medex or computer with initials, date, and time	❏	❏	_____
24. Return to assess patient's response to medication	❏	❏	_____
25. Document assessment in nurse's notes	❏	❏	_____

PERFORMANCE CHECKLIST 23-8

ADMINISTERING NOSE DROPS

	S	U	Comments
1. Follow the six rights	❏	❏	_____
2. Perform the three label checks	❏	❏	_____
3. Follow standard precautions	❏	❏	_____
4. Perform hand hygiene	❏	❏	_____
5. Check for allergies	❏	❏	_____
6. Transport medication to patient's room	❏	❏	_____
7. Identify room, bed, patient, and patient's birthdate	❏	❏	_____
8. Recheck for allergies	❏	❏	_____
9. Introduce self; explain procedure	❏	❏	_____
10. Provide privacy	❏	❏	_____
11. Don gloves	❏	❏	_____
12. Ask adult or older child to clear nose of accumulations by blowing gently into tissue	❏	❏	_____
13. Determine which nostril (or both) is to receive the medication	❏	❏	_____
14. Have patient lie down, hanging head backward over edge of bed or with pillow under shoulders to hyperextend the neck if patient can tolerate it	❏	❏	_____
15. After drawing medication into dropper, instill medication while holding dropper above nostril being treated	❏	❏	_____
16. If ordered, repeat procedure to instill drops in other nostril	❏	❏	_____
17. Tell patient to hold position for a few minutes to allow medication to remain in place	❏	❏	_____
18. Administer nosedrops to a younger child after positioning child on bed with head backward and downward, or to an infant while holding his head backward and downward	❏	❏	_____

	S	U	Comments
19. Administer drops in same way as to an adult	❏	❏	_____
20. Remove gloves	❏	❏	_____
21. Tell patient to refrain from blowing nose immediately after instillation	❏	❏	_____
22. Offer tissues for later use	❏	❏	_____
23. Leave patient in comfortable position; clean work area	❏	❏	_____
24. Answer patient's questions and if appropriate, teach patient self-care	❏	❏	_____
25. Perform hand hygiene	❏	❏	_____
26. Document administration of medication in Medex or computer with initials, date, and time	❏	❏	_____
27. Return to assess patient's response to medication	❏	❏	_____
28. Document assessment in nurse's notes	❏	❏	_____

Student Name_____ Date_____ Instructor's name_____

Administering Nasal Sprays

	S	U	Comments
1. Follow the six rights	❑	❑	_____
2. Perform the three label checks	❑	❑	_____
3. Follow standard precautions	❑	❑	_____
4. Perform hand hygiene	❑	❑	_____
5. Check for allergies	❑	❑	_____
6. Transport medication to patient's room	❑	❑	_____
7. Identify room, bed, patient, and patient's birthdate	❑	❑	_____
8. Recheck for allergies	❑	❑	_____
9. Introduce self; explain procedure	❑	❑	_____
10. Provide privacy; position patient upright	❑	❑	_____
11. Don gloves	❑	❑	_____
12. Determine which nostril (or both) is to receive medication	❑	❑	_____
13. Have patient gently blow nose to clear nasal passages of accumulations	❑	❑	_____
14. Compress one nostril	❑	❑	_____
15. Shake bottle while holding it upright	❑	❑	_____
16. Insert tip of spray bottle into patient's patent nostril	❑	❑	_____
17. Instruct patient to inhale; while he inhales, squeeze bottle	❑	❑	_____
18. If ordered, repeat procedure for other nostril	❑	❑	_____
19. Tell patient to refrain from blowing nose for a few minutes; offer tissues for later use	❑	❑	_____
20. Answer patient's questions and if appropriate, teach self-administration	❑	❑	_____
21. Remove gloves and perform hand hygiene	❑	❑	_____

	S	U	Comments
22. Document administration of medication in Medex or computer with initials, date, and time	❏	❏	_____
23. Return to assess patient's response to medication	❏	❏	_____
24. Document assessment in nurse's notes	❏	❏	_____

PERFORMANCE CHECKLIST 23-10

ADMINISTERING INHALANTS

		S	U	Comments
1.	Follow the six rights	❑	❑	_____
2.	Perform the three label checks	❑	❑	_____
3.	Follow standard precautions	❑	❑	_____
4.	Perform hand hygiene	❑	❑	_____
5.	Check for allergies	❑	❑	_____
6.	Transport medication to patient's room	❑	❑	_____
7.	Identify room, bed, patient, and patient's birthdate	❑	❑	_____
8.	Recheck for allergies	❑	❑	_____
9.	Introduce self; explain procedure	❑	❑	_____
10.	Provide privacy	❑	❑	_____
11.	Allow patient opportunity to manipulate inhaler, canister, and spacer device (aerochamber); explain and demonstrate how canister fits into inhaler	❑	❑	_____
12.	Explain what metered dose is and warn patient about overuse of inhaler, including drug side effects	❑	❑	_____
13.	Remove mouthpiece cover from inhaler; shake inhaler well	❑	❑	_____
14.	Without aerochamber (spacer): Open lips and place inhaler 1–2 cm (1/2 to 1 inch) from mouth with opening toward back of pharynx. Lips should not touch inhaler. Avoid rapid influx of inhaled medication and subsequent airway irritation	❑	❑	_____
15.	With aerochamber (spacer): Exhale fully, then grasp mouthpiece with teeth and lips while holding inhaler with thumb at the mouthpiece and fingers at the top	❑	❑	_____
16.	Press down on inhaler to release medication while inhaling slowly and deeply through mouth	❑	❑	_____

	S	U	Comments
17. Breathe in slowly for 2–3 seconds; hold breath for approximately 10 seconds	❑	❑	_____
18. Exhale through pursed lips	❑	❑	_____
19. Instruct patient to wait 2 to 5 minutes between puffs; more than one puff is usually prescribed	❑	❑	_____
20. If more than one type of inhaled medications are prescribed, wait 5–10 minutes between inhalations or as ordered by physician	❑	❑	_____
21. Explain that patient may feel gagging sensation in throat caused by droplets of medication on pharynx or tongue	❑	❑	_____
22. Instruct patient in removing medication canister and cleaning inhaler in warm water	❑	❑	_____
23. Teach patient to measure the amount of medication remaining in the canister by immersing it in a large bowl or pan of water	❑	❑	_____
24. Record administration in Medex or computer with initials, date, and time	❑	❑	_____
25. Return to assess patient's response to medication	❑	❑	_____
26. Document assessment in nurse's notes	❑	❑	_____

PERFORMANCE CHECKLIST 23-11

Administering Sublingual Medications

	S	U	Comments
1. Follow the six rights	❑	❑	_____
2. Perform the three label checks	❑	❑	_____
3. Follow standard precautions	❑	❑	_____
4. Perform hand hygiene	❑	❑	_____
5. Check for allergies	❑	❑	_____
6. Identify room, bed, patient, and patient's birthdate	❑	❑	_____
7. Recheck for allergies	❑	❑	_____
8. Wear gloves to place tablet under patient's tongue	❑	❑	_____
9. Do not follow with water	❑	❑	_____
10. Instruct patient not to swallow tablet	❑	❑	_____
11. Explain to patient how to place medication under tongue; instruct patient to let it dissolve	❑	❑	_____
12. Remove gloves and perform hand hygiene	❑	❑	_____
13. Document sublingual administration in Medex or computer with initials, date, and time	❑	❑	_____
14. Return to assess patient's response to medication	❑	❑	_____
15. Document assessment in nurse's notes	❑	❑	_____

Student Name_____ Date_____ Instructor's name_____

ADMINISTERING BUCCAL MEDICATIONS

	S	U	Comments
1. Follow the six rights	❏	❏	_____
2. Perform the three label checks	❏	❏	_____
3. Follow standard precautions	❏	❏	_____
4. Perform hand hygiene	❏	❏	_____
5. Check for allergies	❏	❏	_____
6. Identify room, bed, patient, and patient's birthdate	❏	❏	_____
7. Recheck for allergies	❏	❏	_____
8. Wear gloves to place tablet between patient's cheek and gum	❏	❏	_____
9. Do not follow with water	❏	❏	_____
10. Instruct patient not to swallow tablet; let it dissolve	❏	❏	_____
11. Explain to patient how to place medication between cheek and gum	❏	❏	_____
12. Remove gloves and perform hand hygiene	❏	❏	_____
13. Document buccal administration in Medex or computer with initials, date, and time	❏	❏	_____
14. Return to assess patient's response to medication	❏	❏	_____
15. Document assessment in nurse's notes	❏	❏	_____

Student Name_____ Date_____ Instructor's name_____

PERFORMANCE CHECKLIST 23-13A
PREPARING PARENTERAL MEDICATIONS:

WITHDRAWING MEDICATION FROM A VIAL

	S	U	Comments
1. Follow the six rights	❏	❏	_____
2. Perform the three label checks	❏	❏	_____
3. Follow standard precautions	❏	❏	_____
4. Check for allergies	❏	❏	_____
5. Perform hand hygiene before handling equipment; prepare medication in clean area; reduce distractions	❏	❏	_____
6. Keep sterile parts of syringe and needle sterile; use aseptic technique throughout preparation	❏	❏	_____
7. Compare drug and dosage ordered with drug and dosage on hand; check expiration date, dosage per milliliter, total volume of solution in vial; look for contaminants or defects in vial	❏	❏	_____
8. Calculate drug dosage and check calculations with another nurse	❏	❏	_____
9. Check compatibility chart or consult pharmacy if mixing two medications	❏	❏	_____
10. Remove metal cap from top of vial; wipe rubber diaphragm briskly with alcohol sponge	❏	❏	_____
11. Pull plunger of syringe back to aspirate air into syringe equal to amount of drug to be withdrawn	❏	❏	_____
12. Insert needle into inverted vial; inject air and withdraw volume of solution to be given; keep needle under solution to prevent aspiration of air into syringe	❏	❏	_____
13. Push plunger gently to disperse solution to tip of needle; remove air bubbles by gently tapping syringe	❏	❏	_____

Student Name_____ Date_____ Instructor's name_____

WITHDRAWING MEDICATION FROM AN AMPULE

	S	U	Comments
1. Follow the six rights	❏	❏	_____
2. Perform the three label checks	❏	❏	_____
3. Follow standard precautions	❏	❏	_____
4. Check for allergies	❏	❏	_____
5. Perform hand hygiene before handling equipment; prepare medication in clean area; reduce distractions	❏	❏	_____
6. Keep sterile parts of syringe and needle sterile; use aseptic technique throughout preparation	❏	❏	_____
7. Compare drug and dosage ordered with drug and dosage on hand; check expiration date, dosage per milliliter, total volume of solution in ampule; look for contaminants or defects in ampule	❏	❏	_____
8. Calculate drug dosage and check calculations with another nurse	❏	❏	_____
9. Check compatibility chart or consult pharmacy if mixing two medications	❏	❏	_____
10. Tap the top of ampule to move solution from top of ampule to bottom of ampule	❏	❏	_____
11. Cover neck of ampule with an alcohol sponge, break off top of ampule; deposit top of glass ampule in sharps container	❏	❏	_____
12. Use a filter needle to aspirate medication from ampule. Filter or aspiration needles catch particles of glass that may be in the solution from the broken ampule	❏	❏	_____
13. Insert filter needle into open neck of ampule, invert ampule to withdraw correct dose	❏	❏	_____
14. Replace filter needle with needle appropriate for purpose of solution and viscosity of solution	❏	❏	_____
15. Push plunger gently until the plunger measures the correct dose	❏	❏	_____

Student Name_____ Date_____ Instructor's name_____

Reconstituting a Powdered Dosage Form

	S	U	Comments
1. Follow the six rights	❑	❑	_____
2. Perform the three label checks	❑	❑	_____
3. Follow standard precautions	❑	❑	_____
4. Check for allergies	❑	❑	_____
5. Perform hand hygiene before handling equipment; prepare medication in clean area; reduce distractions	❑	❑	_____
6. Keep sterile parts of syringe and needle sterile; use aseptic technique throughout preparation	❑	❑	_____
7. Compare drug and dosage ordered with drug and dosage on hand; check expiration date, dosage per milliliter, total volume of solution in vial; look for contaminants or defects in vial	❑	❑	_____
8. Calculate drug dosage and check calculations with another nurse	❑	❑	_____
9. Check compatibility chart or consult pharmacy if mixing two medications	❑	❑	_____
10. Follow instructions on manufacturer's box and drug insert; the instructions will specify the type and amount of diluent to use (for example, add 10 mL bacteriostatic normal saline to prepare a ratio of 500 mg/mL)	❑	❑	_____
11. Remove the protective cap from diluent and cleanse with alcohol pad; withdraw diluent using sterile technique	❑	❑	_____
12. Withdraw needle from diluent vial	❑	❑	_____
13. Inject diluent into vial of powdered drug; remove syringe and needle; gently shake and tap vial to dissolve powder into solution	❑	❑	_____
14. If solution is multidose vial, label solution with			
a. Date and time mixed	❑	❑	_____

	S	**U**	**Comments**
b. Name of person who mixed drug and diluent	❏	❏	_____
c. Dosage per milliliter obtained (concentration)	❏	❏	_____
d. Amount and type of diluent used	❏	❏	_____
15. Withdraw correct dose; change needle with a new needle; select appropriate needle gauge and length for patient	❏	❏	_____

Student Name_____ Date_____ Instructor's name_____

PLACING TWO MEDICATIONS INTO ONE SYRINGE (INSULIN EXAMPLE USED)

	S	U	Comments
1. Follow the six rights	☐	☐	_____
2. Perform the three label checks	☐	☐	_____
3. Follow standard precautions	☐	☐	_____
4. Check for allergies	☐	☐	_____
5. Perform hand hygiene before handling equipment; prepare medication in clean area; reduce distractions	☐	☐	_____
6. Keep sterile parts of syringe and needle sterile; use aseptic technique throughout preparation	☐	☐	_____
7. Compare drug and dosage ordered with drug and dosage on hand; check expiration date, dosage per milliliter, total volume of solution in vial; look for contaminants	☐	☐	_____
8. Calculate drug dosage and check calculations with another nurse	☐	☐	_____
9. Check compatibility of two drugs with a compatibility chart or call pharmacy	☐	☐	_____
10. Check and compare label of each drug ordered with label of each drug on hand	☐	☐	_____
11. Compare each label with medication order	☐	☐	_____
12. Roll long- and intermediate-acting insulin between the palms; do not shake any insulin [note: do not mix long-acting glargine insulin (Lantus) with regular insulin; Lantus insulin is clear and does not need to be rolled to mix]	☐	☐	_____
13. Briskly wipe tops of both vials with separate alcohol swab	☐	☐	_____
14. Pull back plunger of syringe to amount equal to volume of longer-acting insulin to be given	☐	☐	_____
15. Insert needle and inject air into vial of longer-acting insulin	☐	☐	_____

	S	U	Comments
16. Withdraw needle from vial; do not remove insulin	❑	❑	_____
17. Pull back plunger of syringe to amount equal to volume of shorter-acting (regular) insulin to be given	❑	❑	_____
18. Insert needle through rubber stopper of second vial; inject air into vial	❑	❑	_____
19. Invert vial; withdraw volume of shorter-acting (regular) insulin first	❑	❑	_____
20. Check and verify dosage in syringe with second nurse against medication order	❑	❑	_____
21. Wipe rubber stopper of longer-acting insulin; insert needle of the syringe containing shorter-acting insulin and withdraw ordered dose of longer-acting insulin. Verify dosage with second nurse	❑	❑	_____
22. Remove needle/syringe from vial	❑	❑	_____
23. Check labels of both vials against medication order	❑	❑	_____
24. Pull plunger back far enough to allow space in barrel of syringe for insulin to be gently mixed; mix by tilting syringe back and forth; remove air	❑	❑	_____
25. Administer mixture of insulin within 5 minutes of preparation; regular insulin binds with NPH and the action of regular insulin is reduced	❑	❑	_____
26. Identify room, bed, patient, and patient's birthdate	❑	❑	_____
27. Don gloves	❑	❑	_____
28. Inject subcutaneously	❑	❑	_____
29. Record administration in Medex or computer with site, initials, date, and time including witness of second nurse	❑	❑	_____
30. Return to assess patient's response to medication	❑	❑	_____
31. Document assessment in nurse's notes	❑	❑	_____

Student Name_____ Date_____ Instructor's name_____

PERFORMANCE CHECKLIST 23-14

Giving an Intramuscular Injection

		S	U	Comments
1.	Follow the six rights	❏	❏	_____
2.	Perform the three label checks	❏	❏	_____
3.	Follow standard precautions	❏	❏	_____
4.	Perform hand hygiene	❏	❏	_____
5.	Check for allergies	❏	❏	_____
6.	Prepare medication according to standard procedure for injectables	❏	❏	_____
7.	Identify room, bed, patient, and patient's birthdate	❏	❏	_____
8.	Recheck for allergies	❏	❏	_____
9.	Don gloves	❏	❏	_____
10.	Explain procedure			
11.	Select and expose site (according to IM site selection procedure); provide privacy	❏	❏	_____
12.	Clean skin with alcohol swab (from center outward), spread skin tight with thumb and index finger, and let dry	❏	❏	_____
13.	Ask patient to take a deep breath and exhale slowly to relax muscle as needle is inserted (lessens pain from injection)	❏	❏	_____
14.	Insert needle at a 90-degree angle quickly in a dartlike motion; quickness reduces discomfort	❏	❏	_____
15.	Maintain needle in muscle; gently aspirate (pull back plunger) to be certain needle is in muscle and not in a vein or an artery	❏	❏	_____
16.	If blood is seen, needle is in a vein or artery; withdraw needle; discard solution; prepare new medication; select another site	❏	❏	_____
17.	Slowly inject medication into muscle to lessen discomfort	❏	❏	_____

	S	U	Comments
18. Withdraw needle quickly without bending or twisting it	❏	❏	_____
19. Use pressure and gauze (2 x 2) or Band-Aid to stop any bleeding	❏	❏	_____
20. Do not recap needle (if safety glide needle used, advance protective glide); dispose directly into sharps container	❏	❏	_____
21. Remove gloves and perform hand hygiene	❏	❏	_____
22. Document administration in Medex or computer including site used and amount and type of medication (for example, meperidine [Demerol] 50 mg given IM left ventrogluteal); record initials, date, and time. Remember, a quick, dartlike insertion followed by slow injection of the medication is much less painful to the patient	❏	❏	_____
23. Return to assess patient's response to medication	❏	❏	_____
24. Document assessment in nurse's notes	❏	❏	_____

PERFORMANCE CHECKLIST 23-15

Giving a Z-Track Injection

	S	U	Comments
1. Follow the six rights	❏	❏	_____
2. Perform the three label checks	❏	❏	_____
3. Follow standard precautions	❏	❏	_____
4. Perform hand hygiene	❏	❏	_____
5. Check for allergies	❏	❏	_____
6. Prepare medication according to standard procedure for injectables	❏	❏	_____
7. Use one needle to withdraw dose from container; use another needle (1½ to 2 inches) to inject medication so that no solution remains on the outside of needle shaft	❏	❏	_____
8. Draw up to 0.2 mL of air to create an air lock	❏	❏	_____
9. Identify room, bed, patient, and patient's birthdate	❏	❏	_____
10. Recheck for allergies	❏	❏	_____
11. Don gloves	❏	❏	_____
12. Expose and locate dorsogluteal or ventrogluteal site according to IM site selection procedure; provide privacy	❏	❏	_____
13. Clean site with an alcohol swab	❏	❏	_____
14. Ask the patient to take a deep breath and to slowly exhale (to relax the muscle); pull skin tightly in a lateral direction (move skin at least 1 to 1½ inch laterally) to one side; hold the skin taut with the nondominant hand	❏	❏	_____
15. Insert needle at a 90-degree angle; aspirate; if no blood is seen, inject medication and air slowly; wait 10 seconds to allow the medication to disperse slowly	❏	❏	_____

	S	U	Comments
16. Withdraw needle quickly; allow skin to return to its normal position, which leaves a zigzag path that seals the needle track wherever tissue planes slide across each other. The drug cannot escape from the muscle tissue	❏	❏	_____
17. Use a 2 x 2 gauze pad or Band-Aid as needed	❏	❏	_____
18. Do not massage site	❏	❏	_____
19. Do not recap needle (if safety glide needle used, advance protective glide); dispose directly into sharps container	❏	❏	_____
20. Remove gloves and perform hand hygiene	❏	❏	_____
21. Document administration in Medex or computer, including site used, Z-track method used, and amount and type of medication given; record initials, date, and time	❏	❏	_____
22. Return to assess patient's response to medication	❏	❏	_____
23. Document assessment in nurse's notes	❏	❏	_____

Student Name_____ Date_____ Instructor's name_____

GIVING AN INTRADERMAL INJECTION

	S	U	Comments
1. Follow the six rights	❑	❑	_____
2. Perform the three label checks	❑	❑	_____
3. Follow standard precautions	❑	❑	_____
4. Perform hand hygiene	❑	❑	_____
5. Check for allergies	❑	❑	_____
6. Prepare medication according to standard procedure for injectables	❑	❑	_____
7. Identify room, bed, patient, and patient's birthdate; explain procedure	❑	❑	_____
8. Recheck for allergies	❑	❑	_____
9. Don gloves	❑	❑	_____
10. Select and expose inner aspect of lower arm	❑	❑	_____
11. Clean site gently with alcohol swab from center outward; let dry	❑	❑	_____
12. Two injections are made if test is for sensitivity. One injection is a control using sterile water or bacteriostatic normal saline; the other is the substance that is to be tested	❑	❑	_____
13. Advance needle through epidermis to approximately 1/8 inch (3 mm) below skin surface using a 25-gauge needle at approximately a 15-degree angle with bevel up directly under skin to make a small bleb (wheal) with test solution; needle can be seen through skin. Do not inject into subcutaneous tissue. Inject control of normal saline into another site for comparison with test substance at designated time interval	❑	❑	_____
14. Do not massage site	❑	❑	_____
15. Draw a circle around skin test with a marker; label area with date, time, and name of test. Another method is to make a diagram in patient's chart to indicate location of site	❑	❑	_____

	S	U	Comments
16. Do not recap needle (if safety glide needle used, advance protective glide); dispose directly into sharps container	❏	❏	_____
17. Remove gloves and perform hand hygiene	❏	❏	_____
18. Chart site; intradermal; record initials, date, and time	❏	❏	_____
19. If an indurated (hardened), erythematous area is observed, measure and record results in millimeters with metric ruler	❏	❏	_____
20. Return to assess patient's response to medication	❏	❏	_____
21. Document assessment in nurse's notes	❏	❏	_____
22. At designated time, compare control with agent; document results in chart	❏	❏	_____

Student Name_____ Date_____ Instructor's name_____

Giving a Subcutaneous Injection

	S	U	Comments
1. Follow the six rights	❏	❏	_____
2. Perform the three label checks	❏	❏	_____
3. Follow standard precautions	❏	❏	_____
4. Perform hand hygiene	❏	❏	_____
5. Check for allergies	❏	❏	_____
6. Prepare medication according to standard procedure for injectables	❏	❏	_____
7. Identify room, bed, patient, and patient's birthdate; explain procedure	❏	❏	_____
8. Don gloves	❏	❏	_____
9. Recheck for allergies	❏	❏	_____
10. Select and expose site (check which site was used previously and rotate site); the abdomen is the usual preferred site when administering heparin or Lovenox	❏	❏	_____
11. Clean site with alcohol swab from center outward using circular motion; let dry	❏	❏	_____
12. **Method A (thin patient or child):** Spread skin of selected site taut and hold firmly; insert needle at 45-degree angle and aspirate; inject medication slowly; do not aspirate if heparin or Lovenox is being administered	❏	❏	_____
Method B (average-size or obese patient): Grasp and press together skin of selected site so that it forms roll between fingers; insert needle at a 90-degree angle and aspirate; do not aspirate if heparin or Lovenox is being given; inject medication slowly	❏	❏	_____
13. Withdraw needle quickly and apply an antiseptic swab or a 2 x 2 gauze sponge; do not massage the site if heparin or Lovenox is administered because this will increase local bleeding and ecchymosis will occur	❏	❏	_____

	S	U	Comments
14. Do not recap needle (if safety glide needle used, advance protective glide); dispose directly into sharps container	❏	❏	_____
15. Remove gloves and perform hand hygiene	❏	❏	_____
16. Chart site used and amount and type of medication; subcutaneous; record initials, date, and time	❏	❏	_____
17. Return to assess patient's response to medication	❏	❏	_____
18. Document assessment in nurse's notes	❏	❏	_____

Student Name_____ Date_____ Instructor's name_____

APPLYING A TOURNIQUET

	S	U	Comments
1. Use a strong, wide, flat piece of material if possible (for example, towel, necktie, wide belt)	❏	❏	_____
2. Place pressure on the nearest pressure point to control bleeding while applying the tourniquet	❏	❏	_____
3. Apply a pad (piece of cloth, handkerchief, dressing) over the artery to be compressed to prevent impairment of skin integrity	❏	❏	_____
4. Place the tourniquet between the wound and the heart: allow some uninjured skin between the wound and the tourniquet; wrap the material around the limb twice, and tie a half-knot on the upper surface of the limb	❏	❏	_____
5. Place a stick or rod (approximately 6 inches long) over the knot, and secure it in place	❏	❏	_____
6. Twist the stick enough times to stop the bleeding	❏	❏	_____
7. Secure the stick firmly with the free ends of the tourniquet; do not cover the tourniquet	❏	❏	_____
8. Write "T" or "TK" (meaning tourniquet) on the victim's forehead and the time it was applied; attach a note to the victim's clothing describing the time and location of the tourniquet	❏	❏	_____
9. Treat for shock, and transport to the nearest medical facility	❏	❏	_____
10. Never loosen a tourniquet once it has been applied; always seek medical attention once tourniquet has been applied	❏	❏	_____